Violence in Health Care

Understanding, Preventing and Surviving Violence: A Practical Guide for Health Professionals

Edited by

JONATHAN SHEPHERD

Professor of Oral and Maxillofacial Surgery,
Director: Violence Research Group
University of Wales College of Medicine

Honorary Consultant Oral and Maxillofacial Surgeon
University Hospital of Wales, Cardiff

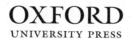

OXFORD
UNIVERSITY PRESS

OXFORD
UNIVERSITY PRESS

Great Clarendon Street, Oxford OX2 6DP

Oxford University Press is a department of the University of Oxford.
It furthers the University's objective of excellence in research, scholarship,
and education by publishing worldwide in

Oxford New York

Auckland Bangkok Buenos Aires Cape Town Chennai
Dar es Salaam Delhi Hong Kong Istanbul Karachi Kolkata
Kuala Lumpur Madrid Melbourne Mexico City Mumbai Nairobi
São Paulo Shanghai Singapore Taipei Tokyo Toronto

and an associated company in Berlin

Oxford is a registered trade mark of Oxford University Press
in the UK and in certain other countries

Published in the United States
by Oxford University Press Inc., New York

© Oxford University Press 2001 J. Shepherd

The moral rights of the author have been asserted

Database right Oxford University Press (maker)

First published 2001
Reprinted 2002

A catalogue record for this title is available from the British Library

Library of Congress Cataloging in Publication Data

Violence in health care: understanding, preventing, and surviving violence:
a practical guide for health professionals / edited by Jonathan Shepherd—2nd ed.
Originally published with subtitle: a practical guide to coping with violence and caring for victims.
Includes bibliographical references and index.
1. Medical personnel—Violence against. 2. Violence in hospitals. 3. Victims of crimes—Services for.
4. Family violence. 5. Violence—Prevention. I. Shepherd, Jonathan.
R727.2.V56 2001   362.1'1'0684—dc21   2001021703
ISBN 0 19 263143 8 (Pbk)

1 3 5 7 9 10 8 6 4 2

Typeset by J&L Composition Ltd, Filey, N. Yorkhire
Printed in Great Britain on acid-free paper by
Biddles Ltd, Guildford and King's Lynn

Preface to second edition

There have been many developments in the understanding and management of violence since the first edition of this book was published in 1994. The problem of violence however has not gone away and there is no room for complacency or tolerance of violence in the workplace. It is clear that every branch of health care has its own particular problems in terms of the experience and prevention of physical and verbal abuse of health-care staff and patients. Violence prevention in health-care facilities is now not just the concern of the health-care team but of architects, managers, psychologists, and governments. In the UK, for example, in 1999 the Government completed a wide-ranging, cross-departmental exercise to combat violence in the National Health Service, which resulted — among other things — in the concept of 'Zero Tolerance Zones'. Part of this exercise, and of other initiatives in most industrialized countries, has been greater commitment to law enforcement as part of the answer.

Similarly, after two decades in which overall rates of community violence in the UK have risen and rates of conviction of violent offenders have fallen, the emphasis is once again on law enforcement and criminal deterrence. Coupled with this is the realization that health services, and particularly accident and emergency departments and primary care, have an important role to play in reporting and helping patients to report violence known to them. It should not be possible for a violent offender to put someone in hospital without fear of investigation. This more collaborative approach also helps victims, many of whom are susceptible to repeat injury, and helps to ensure that they are assessed for their wide-ranging mental health needs.

This second edition reflects these important changes while keeping to the core purposes of the first edition. All the chapters have been comprehensively revised. There are new chapters on the care of victims, domestic violence, and limiting violence through good design. This last additional chapter includes some excellent illustrations of tranquil, airy health-care facilities.

I am very grateful to the numerous reviewers of the first edition, not only for the kind comments that helped to make it such a success, but also for their helpful, if sometimes blunt, suggestions on where improvements might be made. These have all been acted upon.

Jonathan Shepherd
Cardiff 2001

Foreword

Dame Helen Reeves, OBE
Chief Executive, Victim Support

I am delighted once again to be invited to write the forward for this important book. When the first edition was published in 1994, there was scant information available about the essential role that health care workers play in dealing with the aftermath of criminal violence. Since then, the subject has received significantly more attention. In particular, research has been focused on the risks of violence to health care workers who are called upon to work with some of the more distressed and unstable members of the community. In addition, a great deal of research and guidance has been published on the needs of victims of domestic or racial violence and sexual abuse, looking specifically at how these needs relate to the medical professions.

Many practical problems still persist. For example, the percentage of unreported crime has remained constant. The British Crime Survey, which was introduced during the 1980s and continues to gather information on a two-yearly basis, reveals that less than half of all crime is reported to the police, and this includes many serious crimes of violence. The victims in many cases have been too fearful to seek help from the police, because of their anxiety that the involvement of the criminal justice process might increase their vulnerability to repeated attacks and harassment. At Victim Support we have taken a series of measures to try to make our services more accessible to these individuals, for example by the launch of a national telephone Victim Supportline in 1998.

It remains true that many victims of crime, whether or not they report the offence or hear about Victim Support, are more likely to contact health care workers for medical advice and assistance. Health care workers are likely to meet those individuals whom nobody else sees. Obviously they need to be prepared to provide a good response. This will include some knowledge about the possible effects of the crime on the individual, an explanation of any proposed treatment and also some information about the other sources of help available. This book will provide much of the information that is required.

To provide an effective response it is important that we recognize the value of cooperation between different agencies; acknowledging that we do not have to work in isolation. Many GPs and Accident and Emergency departments already enjoy close links with their local Victim Support services. In 1995, we published a booklet *Treating victims of crime: guidelines for health professionals*, which looked at how health professionals could contribute to making victims' experiences less distressing.

This booklet was distributed to all GPs and medical teams in Accident and Emergency departments. In writing the booklet we were assisted by Professor Jonathan Shepherd, who has continued to further the interests of victims of violence through his prominent position in both the medical profession and in Victim Support.

I believe that this is a very important book, providing as it does a wealth of information on the whole array of issues that health care workers may face when they become involved with the problems caused by crime. I hope it will prove a much used resource helping individuals to become aware of the issues and to develop strategies to tackle these issues. Health care professionals have a key role to play in dealing with the consequences of crime and I believe this book will enhance the vital working relationships that are forming between health care professions and those of us who work with victims of crime.

Contents

List of contributors

Dr Jonathan Bisson
Consultant Liason Psychiatrist
University Hospital of Wales

Dr Henrietta Bullard
Consultant Forensic Psychiatrist
Oxfordshire Mental Healthcare NHS
Trust

Dr Stefan Cembrowicz
General Practioner
Montpelier Health Centre, Bristol

Ms Debbie Crisp
Department of Social and Political
Science
Royal Holloway College
University of London

Dr Alan Emond
Consultant Community Paediatrician
United Bristol Healthcare NHS Trust

Professor David Farrington
Institute of Criminology
University of Cambridge

Ms Susan Francis
Medical Architecture Research Unit
South Bank University, London

Dr Gillian Mezey
Department of Forensic Psychiatry
St George's Hospital, London

Professor David Miers
Law School
University of Cardiff

Dr Duncan Raistrick
Leeds Addiction Unit,
Leeds Community and Mental Health
NHS Trust

Ms Sue Ritter
Health Services Research Department
Institute of Psychiatry
University of London

Professor Jonathan Shepherd
Professor of Oral and Maxillofacial
Surgery
University Hospital of Wales
University of Wales College of Medicine
Cardiff

Professor Betsy Stanko
Department of Social and Political
Science
Royal Holloway College
University of London

Mr Steve Wright
Health Services Research Department
Institute of Psychiatry
University of London

Chapter 1

The causes and prevention of violence

David Farrington

Introduction

The most basic definition of violence is behaviour that is intended to cause, and that actually causes, physical or psychological injury. The most important violent offences defined by the criminal law are homicide, assault, robbery, and rape.

This chapter is in three sections. This first section reviews basic knowledge about violence: changes over time, measurement and prevalence, continuity from childhood to adulthood, specialization or versatility, and demographic correlates (age, gender, and race). The second section reviews risk factors for violence and presents a theory of violence, while the third section reviews effective prevention programmes.

The main emphasis is on results obtained in Great Britain and the United States and on stranger or street violence rather than domestic or within-family violence. Most research focuses on male offenders and on the most common offences of assault and robbery. Within a single chapter, it is impossible to review everything that is known about violence; for more extensive information, see Reiss and Roth (1993), Loeber and Farrington (1998), and Tonry and Moore (1998).

Changes over time

In recent years, criminal violence has been increasing in England and Wales. According to police records (Home Office 1998), homicide has increased from 559 crimes in 1987 to 739 in 1997 (from 1.1 to 1.4 per 100 000 population). Serious assault (wounding) has increased from 98 021 to 239 326 crimes over the same time period (from 2.0 to 4.6 per 1000 population). Robbery has increased from 20 282 to 63 072 crimes (from 0.4 to 1.2 per 1000 population). Rape of a female has increased from 1068 to 6281 crimes (from 4 to 24 per 100 000 females).

The national victimization survey (the British Crime Survey) also indicates that violence is increasing in England and Wales, but less dramatically. Serious assaults increased from 507 000 in 1981 to 811 000 in 1995, but then decreased to 660 000 in 1997; this was an overall increase from 13 per 1000 population in 1981 to 16 per 1000 in 1997. (These figures were corrected for changes in the questions about domestic violence; see Langan and Farrington 1998, p.58.) The British Crime Survey also found that robberies increased from 163 000 in 1981 to 313 000 in 1995 before decreasing to 309 000 in 1997; an overall increase from 4.2 to 7.4 per 1000 population.

In contrast to England and Wales, rates of violence in the United States have generally decreased over the same time period (Langan and Farrington 1998). According to the US National Crime Victimization Survey, serious (aggravated) assault decreased from 12.0 per 1000 population in 1981 to 8.8 in 1996, and robbery decreased from 7.4 per 1000 population in 1981 to 5.2 in 1996. According to the Uniform Crime Reports (police-recorded crimes), homicide decreased from 9.8 per 100 000 population in 1981 to 7.4 in 1996, while the incidence of rape was the same in both years (71 per 100 000 females).

Measurement and prevalence

The most common ways of identifying violent offenders are by using police or court records or self-reports of offending. For example, Elliott (1994) in the US National Youth Survey enquired about aggravated assault (attacking someone with the idea of seriously hurting or killing that person), being involved in a gang fight, and robbery (using force or strongarm methods to get money or things from people). Prevalences were surprisingly high. In the first wave of the survey (age 11–17 in 1976), 31% of African-American boys and 22% of Caucasian boys admitted a felony assault in the previous year (aggravated assault, gang fight, or sexual assault). At the same time, 13% of African-American boys and 6% of Caucasian boys admitted robbery (of teachers, students, or others) in the previous year.

The comparison between self-reports and official records gives some indication of the probability of a violent offender being caught and convicted. In the Cambridge Study in Delinquent Development, which is a longitudinal survey of about 400 London boys from age 8 to age 40, 45% of boys admitted starting a physical fight or using a weapon in a fight between ages 15 and 18, but only 3% were convicted of assault between these ages (Farrington 1989). Hence, only 7% of self-reported violent offenders between ages 15 and 18 were convicted. Self-reported violence had predictive validity: 10% of those who admitted assault up to age 18 were subsequently convicted of assault, compared with 5% of the remainder.

Continuity

In general, there is continuity from juvenile to adult violence and from childhood aggression to youth violence. In Columbus, Ohio, 59% of violent juveniles were arrested as adults in the next 5–9 years, and 42% of these adult offenders were charged with at least one Index (serious) violent offence (Hamparian et al. 1985). More of those arrested for Index violence as juveniles were re-arrested as adults than of those arrested for minor violence (simple assault or molesting) as juveniles. In the Cambridge Study, one-third of the boys convicted of violence between ages 10 and 20 were reconvicted of violence between ages 21 and 40, compared with only 8% of those not convicted of youth violence (Farrington, 2001).

Generally, violent males have an early age of onset of offending of all types (Farrington 1991). Both in official records and self-reports, an early age of onset of violent offending predicts a relatively large number of violent offences (Elliott 1994; Hamparian et al. 1978). Moffitt (1993) suggested that the 'life-course-persistent' offenders who started early (around age 10) and had long criminal careers were fundamentally different from the 'adolescence-limited' offenders who started later (around age 14) and had short criminal careers lasting no longer than 5–6 years.

Childhood aggression predicts youth violence. In the Orebro (Sweden) follow-up of about 1000 youths (Stattin and Magnusson 1989), two-thirds of boys who were officially recorded for violence up to age 26 had high aggressiveness scores at ages 10 and 13 (rated by teachers), compared with 30% of all boys. Similarly, in the Jyvaskyla (Finland) follow-up of nearly 400 youths (Pulkkinen 1987), peer ratings of aggression at ages 8 and 14 significantly predicted officially recorded violence up to age 20.

One possible explanation of the continuity over time is that there are persisting individual differences in an underlying potential to commit aggressive or violent behaviour. In any cohort, the people who are relatively more aggressive at one age also tend to be relatively more aggressive at later ages, even though absolute levels of aggressive behaviour and behavioural manifestations of violence are different at different ages.

Specialization or versatility

Generally, violent offenders tend to be versatile rather than specialized. They tend to commit many different types of crimes and also show other problems such as truancy, substance use, persistent lying, and sexual promiscuity. However, there is a small degree of specialization in violence superimposed on this versatility (Brennan *et al.* 1989). There is also versatility in violent offending. For example, males who assault their female partners are significantly likely to have convictions for other types of violent offences (Farrington 1994).

As an indication of their versatility, violent people typically commit more nonviolent offences than violent offences. In the Cambridge Study, the convicted violent delinquents up to age 21 had nearly three times as many convictions for non-violent offences as for violent offences (Farrington 1978). In the Oregon Youth Study, which is a longitudinal survey of over 200 boys from age 10, the boys arrested for violence had an average of 6.6 arrests of all kinds (Capaldi and Patterson 1996).

Age and violence

Offending tends to peak in the teenage years in many different countries. In 1997, the peak age for convictions and cautions for indictable offences in England and Wales was 18 for males and females (Home Office 1998, p.120). Tarling (1993) also found that the peak age for serious assault, robbery, and rape was at 17–18. In 1997, there were 7.8 recorded violent offenders per 1000 males aged 14–17 and 8.3 per 1000 males aged 18–20; there were 2.2 recorded violent offenders per 1000 females aged 14–17 and 1.1 per 1000 females aged 18–20.

Similar results are obtained in self-report surveys. For example, in the English national self-report survey of Graham and Bowling (1995), the peak age for violence was 16 for males and females. For males, the percentage admitting violence decreased from 12% at age 14–17 to 9% at age 18–21 and 4% at age 22–25; for females, the figures were 7%, 4%, and less than 1%, respectively.

Many theories have been proposed to explain why offending (especially by males) peaks in the teenage years. For example, offending (and especially violence) has been linked to testosterone levels in males, which increase during adolescence and early adulthood and decrease thereafter (Archer 1991). Other explanations focus on changes with age in physical capabilities and opportunities for crime, linked to changes in 'routine activities' (Cohen and Felson 1979), such as going to pubs in the evenings with other males. The most popular explanation emphasizes the importance of social influences (Farrington 1986). From birth, children are under the influence of their parents, who generally discourage offending. However, during their teenage years, juveniles gradually break away from the control of their parents and become influenced by their peers, who may encourage offending in many cases. After age 20, offending declines again as peer influences give way to a new set of family influences hostile to offending, originating in spouses and female partners.

Gender and violence

In general, males commit offences more frequently and more seriously than females. In 1997 in England and Wales, 421 000 males were found guilty or cautioned for indictable offences, compared with 88 000 females, yielding a gender (male : female) ratio of 4.8 : 1 (Home Office 1998, p. 108). For violence, the ratio was higher (5.8 : 1); for robbery, it was higher still (9.3 : 1). The lowest gender ratios were for fraud and forgery (2.6 : 1) and theft and handling (2.8 : 1). Cumulatively, 34% of males and 9% of females born in 1953 were convicted of non-traffic offences before age 40 (Home Office Statistical Bulletin 1995).

Official gender ratios for crime in England and Wales are among the lowest in the world. Harvey *et al.* (1992) found that, for both 1980 and 1985, the gender ratio for convictions in England and Wales of 4.9 : 1 was the lowest out of 19 countries in a United Nations survey. The highest gender ratios for convictions were for Indonesia and Japan.

Self-report surveys yield lower gender ratios. In their English national survey, Graham and Bowling (1995) found that 28% of males and 12% of females (aged 14–25) admitting offending in the previous year; 9% of males and 4% of females admitted violence in the previous year. The cumulative prevalence of violence up to the time of the survey was 28% for males and 10% for females. Various explanations have been put forward to explain the discrepancy between police records and self-reports, including the fact that self-reported offences are generally less serious and the possibility that the police and the courts discriminate in favour of females (especially those who are pregnant or who have small children).

Numerous explanations of gender differences in crime and violence have been proposed. Maccoby and Jacklin (1974) pointed out that gender differences in aggressiveness are found very early in life, before any differential reinforcement of aggression in boys and girls. Furthermore, they argued that males were more aggressive than females in all human societies for which evidence was available, that similar gender differences in aggressiveness were found in sub-human primates as in humans, and that aggression was related to levels of sex hormones such as testosterone (which are much higher in males). In seems obvious that, because on average males are bigger and stronger than females, males will be better able to commit offences that require physical strength.

Not all offences are linked to aggression or physical strength, of course. Another possible explanation is that boys and girls are socialized differently by their parents. Generally, girls are supervised more closely, and girls stay at home more. Hence, if they behave in a socially disapproved fashion, their parents are more likely to notice this and react to it. Adults are generally more tolerant of incipient delinquency in boys than in girls, and they may encourage boys to be tough and take risks. On the theory that the strength of the conscience depends on the reinforcement of appropriate behaviour and the punishment of socially disapproved acts, it follows that girls will develop a stronger conscience and will be less likely to commit delinquent acts than boys.

The gender ratio can also be explained by reference to sex roles, social habits, and opportunities. Boys are more likely than girls to spend time hanging around on the street at night, especially in groups, and therefore are more likely to commit violent acts, which may often arise in this social situation. Girls are more likely than boys to spend time shopping, and so it is not surprising that shoplifting is the most common female offence. Boys have more interest in cars and weapons, and more knowledge about how to use them, and so are more likely to commit car thefts and robberies. Later on in life, women have more opportunity to commit minor frauds because they are more likely to be collecting welfare benefits.

Race and violence

Most research on race and crime in Great Britain has compared blacks (persons with an ethnic origin in Africa or the Caribbean), Asians (persons with an ethnic origin in India, Pakistan, or Bangladesh), and whites. Blacks are more likely to be arrested than Asians, and whites are least likely to be arrested. In 1998–99 in England and Wales, 117 blacks per 1000 population were arrested for indictable offences, compared with 44 Asians and 27 whites (Home Office 1999, p.22). The black: white ratio was 2.7 : 1, while the Asian : white ratio was 1.6 : 1.

The black : white disproportionality was particularly high for violent offences, and especially for robbery. For example, in London, the rate of arrests for robbery in 1998–99 was 8.07 per 1000 blacks, 1.41 per 1000 Asians, and 0.47 per 1000 whites. The rate of arrests for violence was 17.42 per 1000 blacks, 6.48 per 1000 Asians, and 3.95 per 1000 whites. For homicide in 1996–99, the annual rate of 'principal suspects' was 5.5 per 100 000 blacks, 2.8 per 100 000 Asians, and 1.0 per 100 000 whites. Black offenders usually killed black victims, just as Asian offenders usually killed Asian victims, and white offenders usually killed white victims. Killings of black victims were disproportionally committed using guns (37% of black victims, compared with 11% of Asian victims and 5% of white victims; Home Office 1999, p. 18).

Racial disproportionalities in offending are much lower in self-reports than in official records. In their English national survey, Graham and Bowling (1995, p. 15) found that 25% of blacks, 19% of whites, 18% of Pakistanis, 13% of Indians, and 7% of Bangladeshis admitted violence. Two main classes of reasons have been put forward to explain the discrepancy between official record and self-report findings (Rutter *et al.* 1998): that ethnic minorities under-report their offences; or that there is police and court bias against ethnic minorities.

Victim reports of offender characteristics are another source of evidence. Based on the 1987 and 1991 British Crime Surveys, Fitzgerald and Hale (1996, p. 16) reported that 87% of white victims had at least one white offender, 8% had a black offender, and 2% had an Asian offender. For black victims, the figures were 50% (white offender), 44% (black offender), and 1% (Asian offender). For Asian victims, the figures were 68% (white offender), 23% (black offender), and 16% (Asian offender). They also reported that the population was 94.5% white, 1.8% black, and 2.9% Asian. Based on these figures (and neglecting the fact that they refer to 'at least' one offender), the black : white ratio for offenders can be estimated to be 5.6 : 1, compared with 0.9 : 1 for the Asian : white ratio.

Based on existing evidence, reviewers such as Smith (1997) and Rutter *et al.* (1998) have concluded that black people (but not Asian people) in Great Britain are disproportionally likely to commit offences, especially violent offences. Many possible explanations of this disproportionality have been put forward. Most suggest that race itself is not an important factor, and that race differences in offending are attributable to race differences in important risk factors such as poverty, bad neighbourhoods, single-parent families, teenage mothers, poor parental supervision, harsh physical punishment, low intelligence, low school attainment, and so on. There is little British research on this topic, but in the Pittsburgh Youth Study of 1500 boys, Farrington and Loeber (in press) found that most of the black : white differences in violence could be explained by reference to differences in these risk factors.

Risk factors for violence

Violent offences, like other crimes, arise from interactions between offenders and victims in situations. Some violent acts are probably committed by people with relatively stable and enduring violent tendencies, while others are committed by more 'normal' people who find themselves in situations that are conducive to violence. This chapter summarizes knowledge about the development of violent persons (i.e. persons with a relatively high probability of committing violent acts in any situation) and the occurrence of violent acts. Risk factors for violence are defined as factors that predict a high probability of violence. In order to determine whether a risk factor (e.g. school failure, poor parental supervision, delinquent peers) is a predictor or possible cause of violence, the risk factor needs to be measured before the violence. Hence, longitudinal follow-up studies are needed, and especially longitudinal studies of large community samples of several hundred persons containing information from several data sources (to maximize validity).

In the interests of throwing light on possible causes of violence and prevention methods, the emphasis in this chapter is on risk factors that can change over time. Thus, genetic factors that are fixed at birth, such as the XYY chromosome abnormality, are not discussed, but biological factors that can change, such as the resting heart rate, are included. The main focus is on individual-level studies as opposed to aggregate-level ones (e.g. of rates of violence in different areas), and on violent offenders rather than victims of violence. However, it should be noted that victims of violence overlap significantly with violent offenders (Rivara *et al.* 1995).

Biological risk factors

According to Raine (1993), one of the most replicable findings in the literature is that antisocial and violent people tend to have low resting heart rates. This can be easily demonstrated by taking pulse rates. The main theory underlying this finding is that a low heart rate indicates low autonomic arousal and/or fearlessness. Low autonomic arousal, like boredom, leads to sensation-seeking and risk-taking in an attempt to increase stimulation and arousal levels. Conversely, high heart rates, especially in infants and young children, are associated with anxiety, behavioural inhibition, and a fearful temperament (Kagan 1989), which tend to inhibit violence.

In the British National Survey of Health and Development, which is a prospective longitudinal survey of over 5300 children born in England, Scotland, or Wales in 1946, heart rate was measured at age 11 (Wadsworth 1976). A low heart rate predicted convictions for violence and sexual offences up to age 21; 81% of violent offenders and 67% of sexual offenders had below-average heart rates. There was also an interaction between heart rate and family background. A low heart rate was especially characteristic of boys who had experienced a broken home before age 5, but among these boys it was not related to violence or sexual offences. A low heart rate was significantly related to violence and sexual offences among boys who came from unbroken homes.

In the Cambridge Study, resting heart rate was measured at age 18 and was significantly related to convictions for violence and to self-reported violence at age 18, independently of all other variables (Farrington 1997b). More than twice as many of the boys with low heart rates (65 beats per minute or less) were convicted of violence as of the remainder.

Perinatal (pregnancy and delivery) complications have been studied, because of the hypothesis that they might lead to neurological damage, which in turn might lead to violence. In a Danish perinatal study, Kandel and Mednick (1991) followed up over 200 children born in Copenhagen during 1959–61. They found that delivery complications predicted arrests for violence up to age 22; 80% of violent offenders scored in the high range of delivery complications, compared with 30% of property offenders and 47% of non-offenders. However, pregnancy complications did not significantly predict violence.

Interestingly, delivery complications especially predicted violence when a parent had a history of psychiatric illness; in this case, 32% of males with high delivery complications were arrested for violence, compared with only 5% of those with low delivery complications (Brennan et al. 1993). Unfortunately, these results were not replicated by Denno (1990) in the Philadelphia Biosocial Project, which is a follow-up of nearly 1000 African-American births in Philadelphia during 1959–62. It may be that pregnancy and delivery complications predict violence only or mainly when they occur in combination with other family adversities. Interactions between biological and psychosocial factors are quite common.

Psychological/personality factors

Among the most important personality dimensions that predict violence are hyperactivity, impulsiveness, poor behavioural control, and attention problems. Conversely, nervousness and anxiety are negatively related to violence. In the Dunedin (New Zealand) follow-up of over 1000 children, ratings of poor behavioural control (e.g. impulsiveness, lack of persistence) at age 3–5 significantly predicted boys convicted of violence up to age 18, compared to those with no convictions or with non-violent convictions (Henry et al. 1996). In the same study, the personality dimensions of constraint (e.g. cautiousness, avoiding excitement) and negative emotionality (e.g. nervousness, alienation) at age 18 were significantly correlated with convictions for violence (Caspi et al. 1994).

Many other studies show linkages between these personality dimensions and violence. In the Copenhagen perinatal project, hyperactivity (restlessness and poor concentration) at age 11–13 significantly predicted arrests for violence up to age 22, especially among boys experiencing delivery complications (Brennan et al. 1993). More than half of those with both hyperactivity and high delivery complications were arrested for violence, compared to less than 10% of the remainder. Similarly, in the Orebro longitudinal study in Sweden, hyperactivity at age 13 predicted police-recorded violence up to age 26. The highest rate of violence was among males with both motor restlessness and concentration difficulties (15%), compared to 3% of the remainder (Klinteberg et al. 1993).

Similar results were obtained in the Cambridge and Pittsburgh studies (Farrington 1998). High daring or risk-taking at age 8–10 predicted both convictions for violence and self-reported violence in the Cambridge Study. Poor concentration and attention difficulties predicted convictions for violence in the Cambridge Study and reported violence (by boys, mothers, and teachers) in Pittsburgh. High anxiety/nervousness was negatively related to violence in both studies, and low guilt significantly predicted court referrals for violence in the Pittsburgh study.

The other main group of psychological factors that predict violence comprise low intelligence and low school attainment. In the Philadelphia Biosocial Project (Denno 1990), low verbal and performance IQ at ages 4 and 7, and low scores on the California Achievement Test at age 13–14 (vocabulary, comprehension, maths, language, spelling), all predicted arrests for violence up to age 22. In Project Metropolitan in Copenhagen, which is a follow-up study of over 12 000 boys born in 1953, low IQ at age 12 significantly predicted police-recorded violence between ages 15 and 22. The link between low IQ and violence was strongest among lower class boys (Hogh and Wolf 1983).

Similar results were obtained in the Cambridge and Pittsburgh studies (Farrington 1998). Low non-verbal IQ at age 8–10 predicted both official and self-reported violence in the Cambridge Study, and low school achievement at age 10 predicted official violence in both studies. The extensive meta-analysis by Lipsey and Derzon (1998) also showed that low IQ, low school attainment, and psychological factors such as hyperactivity, attention deficit, impulsivity, and risk-taking, were important predictors of later serious and violent offending.

Impulsiveness, attention problems, low intelligence, and low attainment could all be linked to deficits in the executive functions of the brain, located in the frontal lobes. These executive functions include sustaining attention and concentration, abstract reasoning and concept formation, goal formulation, anticipation and planning, programming and initiation of purposive sequences of motor behaviour, effective self-monitoring and self-awareness of behaviour, and inhibition of inappropriate or impulsive behaviours (Moffitt and Henry 1991). Interestingly, in the Montreal longitudinal-experimental study, which is a follow-up of over 1100 children from age 6, a measure of executive functions based on cognitive–neuropsychological tests at age 14 was the strongest neuropsychological discriminator of violent and non-violent boys (Seguin *et al.* 1995). This relationship held independently of a measure of family adversity (based on parental age at first birth, parental education level, broken family, and low socio-economic status).

Family factors

Numerous family factors predict violence. In her follow-up of 250 treated Boston boys in the Cambridge–Somerville Study, McCord (1979) found that the strongest predictors at age 10 of later convictions for violence (up to age 45) were poor parental supervision, parental aggression (including harsh, punitive discipline), and parental conflict. An absent father was almost significant as a predictor, but the mother's lack of affection was not significant. McCord (1977) also demonstrated that fathers convicted for violence tended to have sons convicted for violence. In the Cambridge Study, the strongest childhood predictor of adult convictions for violence was having a convicted parent (Farrington, 2001). In her later analyses, McCord (1996) showed that violent offenders were less likely than non-violent offenders to have experienced parental affection and good discipline and supervision, but equally likely to have experienced parental conflict.

Similar results have been obtained in other studies. In the Chicago Youth Development Study, which is a longitudinal follow-up of nearly 400 inner-city boys initially studied at age 11–13, poor parental monitoring and low family cohesion predicted self-reported violent offending (Gorman-Smith *et al.* 1996). Also, poor parental monitoring and low attachment to parents predicted self-reported violence in the Rochester Youth Development Study, which is a longitudinal study of nearly 1000 children originally studied at age 13–14 (Thornberry *et al.* 1995). Broken families between birth and age 10 predicted convictions for violence up to age 21 in the British National Survey (Wadsworth 1978), and single parent status at age 13 predicted convictions for violence up to age 18 in the Dunedin study (Henry *et al.* 1996). Parental conflict and a broken family predicted official violence in the Cambridge and Pittsburgh studies, and coming from a single-parent female-headed household predicted official and reported violence in Pittsburgh (Farrington 1998).

Harsh physical punishment by parents, and child physical abuse, typically predict violent offending by sons (Malinosky-Rummell and Hansen 1993). Harsh parental discipline predicted official and self-reported violence in the Cambridge Study (Farrington 1998). In a follow-up study of nearly 900 children in New York State, Eron *et al.* (1991) reported that parental punishment at age 8 predicted not only arrests for violence up to age 30, but also the severity of the man's punishment of his child at age 30 and also his history of spouse assault. In a longitudinal study of over 900 abused children and nearly 700 controls, Widom (1989) discovered that recorded child physical abuse and neglect predicted later arrests for violence, independently of other predictors such as gender, ethnicity, and age. In the Rochester Youth Development Study, Smith and Thornberry (1995) showed that recorded childhood maltreatment under age 12 predicted self-reported violence between ages 14 and 18, independently of gender, ethnicity, socio-economic status, and family structure.

Large family size (number of children) predicted youth violence in both the Cambridge and Pittsburgh studies (Farrington 1998). In the Oregon Youth Study, large family size at age 10 predicted self-reported violence at age 13–17 (Capaldi and Patterson 1996). Young mothers (mothers who had their first child at an early age, typically as a teenager) also tend to have violent sons, as Morash and Rucker (1989) demonstrated in the Cambridge Study for the prediction of self-reported violence at age 16. Interestingly, the relationship between a young mother and a convicted son in this study disappeared after controlling for other variables, notably large family size, a convicted parent, and a broken family (Nagin *et al.* 1997). A young mother also predicted official and reported violence in the Pittsburgh Youth Study (Farrington 1998).

Peer, socio-economic, and neighbourhood factors

Having delinquent friends is an important predictor of youth violence; peer delinquency predicted self-reported violence in the Rochester Youth Development Study (Thornberry *et al.* 1995). What is less clear is how far the link between delinquent friends and delinquency is a consequence of co-offending, which is particularly common under age 21 (Reiss and Farrington 1991). Elliott and Menard (1996) concluded both that delinquency caused delinquent peer-bonding and that delinquent peer-bonding caused delinquency. However, there seems to be no information specifically about the link between peer violence and youth violence.

In general, coming from a low socio-economic status (SES) family predicts youth violence. For example, in the US National Youth Survey, the prevalences of self-reported felony assault and robbery were about twice as high for lower class youth as for middle class ones (Elliott *et al.* 1989). Similar results have been obtained for official violence in Project Metropolitan in Stockholm (Wikström 1985), in Project Metropolitan in Copenhagen (Hogh and Wolf 1983), and in the Dunedin Study in New Zealand (Henry *et al.* 1996). Interestingly, all three of these studies compared the SES of the family at the boy's birth, based on the father's occupation, with the boy's later violent crimes. The strongest predictor of official violence in both the Cambridge and Pittsburgh studies was family dependence on welfare benefits (Farrington 1998).

Generally, boys living in urban areas are more violent than those living in rural ones. In the US National Youth Survey, the prevalence of self-reported felony assault and robbery was considerably higher among urban youth (Elliott *et al.* 1989). Within urban areas, boys living in high-crime neighbourhoods are more violent than those living in low-crime neighbourhoods. In the Rochester Youth Development Study, living in a high-crime neighbourhood significantly predicted self-reported violence (Thornberry *et al.* 1995). Similarly, in the Pittsburgh Youth Study, living in a bad neighbourhood (either as rated by the mother or based on census measures of poverty, unemployment, and female-headed households) significantly predicted official and reported violence (Farrington 1998).

Situational factors

It might be argued that all the risk factors reviewed so far in this section — biological, psychological/personality, family, peer, socio-economic, and neighbourhood — essentially influence the development of a long-term individual potential for violence. In other words, they contribute to between-individual differences: why some people are more likely than others, given the same situational opportunity, to commit violence. Another set of influences — situational factors — explain how the potential for violence becomes the actuality in any given situation. Essentially, they explain short-term within-individual differences: why a person is more likely to commit violence in some situations than in others. Situational factors may be specific to particular types of crimes: robberies as opposed to rapes, or even street robberies as opposed to bank robberies. One of the most influential situational theories of offending is routine activities theory (Cohen and Felson 1979). This suggests that, for a predatory crime to occur, the minimum requirement is the convergence in time and place of a motivated offender and a suitable target, in the absence of a capable guardian.

Much work on describing situations leading to violence has been carried out in Great Britain under the heading of crime analysis (Ekblom 1988). This begins with a detailed analysis of patterns and circumstances of crimes and then proceeds to devising, implementing, and evaluating crime-reduction strategies. For example, Barker *et al.* (1993) analysed the nature of street robbery in London. Most of these crimes occurred in predominantly ethnic minority areas, and most offenders were 16–19-year-old African Caribbean males. The victims were mostly white females, alone, and on foot. Most offences occurred at night, near the victim's home. The main motive for robbery was to get money, and the main factor in choosing victims was whether they had a wealthy appearance.

In their Montreal longitudinal study of delinquents, LeBlanc and Frechette (1989) provided detailed information about motives and methods used in different offences at different ages. For example, for violence at age 17, the main motivation was utilitarian or rational. For all crimes, however, the primary motivation changed from hedonistic (searching for excitement, with co-offenders) in the teenage years, to utilitarian (with planning, psychological intimidation, and use of instruments such as weapons) in the twenties (Le Blanc 1996). In the US National Survey of Youth, which was a cross-sectional survey of nearly 1400 American youth aged 11–18, assaults were usually committed for retaliation or revenge or because of provocation or anger (Agnew 1990).

In the Cambridge Study, motives for physical fights depended on whether the boy fought alone or with others (Farrington 1993a). In individual fights, the boy was usually provoked, became angry, and hit out to hurt his opponent and to discharge his own internal feelings of tension. In group fights, the boy often said that he became involved to help a friend or because he was attacked, and rarely said that he was angry. The group fights were more serious, occurring in bars or streets, and they were more likely to involve weapons, produce injuries, and lead to police intervention. Fights often occurred when minor incidents escalated, because both sides wanted to demonstrate their toughness and masculinity, and were unwilling to react in a conciliatory way.

Many of the boys in the Cambridge Study fought after drinking alcohol and it is clear that alcohol intoxication is an immediate situational factor that precipitates violence. In Sweden, Wikström (1985) found that about three-quarters of violent offenders and about half of the victims of violence were intoxicated at the time. Conventional wisdom suggests that alcohol consumption has a disinhibiting effect on behaviour that encourages both offending and victimization. However, the biological links between alcohol and violence are complex (Miczek *et al.* 1994).

Behaviours leading up to violence have been studied. Wolfgang (1958) classified actions leading to homicide in Philadelphia based on police records. Most commonly, homicides arose from trivial altercations (insults or jostling), domestic quarrels, jealousy, or altercations over money. Similarly, violent offences in London usually arose from family disputes or quarrels between neighbours or persons working together (McClintock 1963). In Sweden, most violent crimes were preceded by arguments, either arising out of the situation or based on existing social relationships (Wikström 1985). However, in all these studies, a minority of violent acts were basically unprovoked attacks or robberies. Pallone and Hennessy (1993) referred to 'tinderbox criminal violence', defined as violence occurring between similar types of people, known to each other, ostensibly to settle long-lasting or emerging disputes.

Much is known about the situations in which violence occurs (Sampson and Lauritsen 1994). For example, in Sweden, violence preceded by situational arguments typically occurred in streets or restaurants, while violence preceded by relationship arguments typically occurred in homes (Wikström 1985). In England, stranger assaults typically occurred in streets, bars, or discotheques, non-stranger assaults typically occurred at home or work, and robberies typically occurred in the street or on public transport (Hough and Sheehy 1986). Violence in public places could be investigated using systematic observation, for example, recording incidents from closed-circuit television cameras mounted on buildings. More research on situational influences on violent acts needs to be incorporated in prospective longitudinal studies, in order to link up the developmental and situational perspectives.

A theory of violence

In order to develop theories of violence, it is important to establish how risk factors have independent, additive, interactive, or sequential effects. Generally, the probability of violence increases with the number of risk factors. For example, in the Cambridge Study, a 'vulnerability' score was developed on the basis of five risk factors measured at age 8–10: low family income, large family size, a convicted parent, low IQ, and poor parental child-rearing behaviour. The percentage of boys convicted for violence between ages 10 and 20 increased from 3% of those with none of these risk factors to 31% of those with four or five (Farrington 1997a). This type of research gives some indication of how accurately violence might be predicted.

Theories can help to explain how and why biological factors such as a low heart rate, psychological/personality factors such as impulsivity or a low IQ, family factors such as poor parental supervision, peer factors, socio-economic factors, and neighbourhood factors influence the development of an individual potential for violence. For example, living in a bad neighbourhood and suffering socio-economic deprivation may in some way cause poor parenting, which in some way causes impulsivity and school failure, which in some way causes a high potential for violence. Theories can also help in specifying more general concepts that underlie violence potential, such as low self-control or weak bonding to society. Theories can also help in specifying how a potentially violent person interacts with situational factors to produce violent acts.

A theory of violence, shown diagrammatically in Fig. 1.1, is intended to be consistent with existing theories and with knowledge about risk factors (Farrington 1998). The theory suggests that long-term influences (biological, psychological/ personality, family, peer, school, community, etc.) lead to the development of long-term, fairly stable, slowly changing differences between individuals in the potential for violence. Superimposed on these long-term between-individual differences in violence potential are short-term within-individual variations in violence potential. The short-term

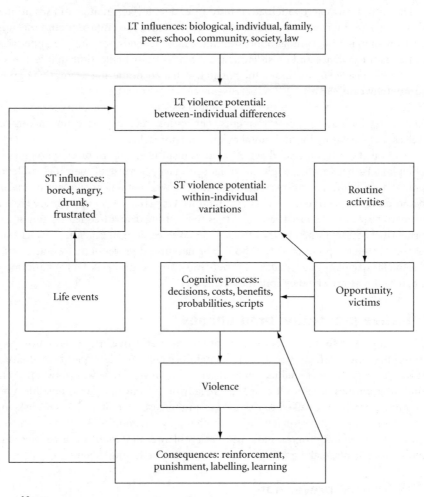

Notes:
ST = Short-term; LT = Long-term

Fig. 1.1 Diagrammatic theory of violence.

variations depend on short-term motivating influences such as being bored, angry, drunk, or frustrated, and on situational opportunities, including the availability of potential victims.

Faced with an opportunity for violence, whether a person actually is violent depends on cognitive (thinking) processes, including considering the subjectively perceived costs and benefits of violence and their associated subjective probabilities or risks, and taking account of stored behavioural repertoires. It is also assumed that the consequences of violence (rewards, punishment, labelling, etc.) can have feedback effects in a learning process on long term violence potential and on the decision-making process (e.g. by influencing subjective perceptions of costs, benefits, and probabilities).

This approach is an explicit attempt to integrate developmental and situational theories. The interaction between the individual and the environment is seen in decision-making in criminal opportunities, which depends both on the underlying potential for violence and on situational factors (costs, benefits, probabilities). Also, the double-headed arrow shows the possibility that encountering a tempting opportunity may cause a short-term increase in violence potential, just as a short-term increase in potential may motivate a person to seek out an opportunity for violence. The theory includes cognitive elements (perception, memory, decision-making) as well as the social learning and causal risk factor approaches.

As in most criminological theories, there is insufficient attention to typologies of offenders. Perhaps some people are violent primarily because of their high violence potential (e.g. 'life-course-persistent' offenders), while others are violent primarily because they happen to be in violent situations. Or perhaps some people are violent primarily because of short-term influences (e.g. getting drunk frequently) and others primarily because of the way they think and make decisions in potentially violent situations. From the point of view of both explanation and prevention, it would be useful to classify people according to their most influential risk factors and most important reasons why they commit violent acts.

Effective prevention programmes

This section briefly summarizes some of the most effective crime-reduction programmes, whose effectiveness has been demonstrated in high-quality evaluation research. Programmes to reduce crime in general are reviewed because most intervention programmes have not focused specifically on violence. As far as possible, programme elements are linked to risk factors and to cost–benefit analyses (Welsh and Farrington 2000). Unfortunately, there is often only a tenuous link between risk factors and prevention programmes. Another problem is that many programmes have multiple elements, making it difficult to isolate their 'active ingredients'.

Risk-focused prevention

The basic idea of risk-focused prevention is very simple: identify the key risk factors for offending and implement prevention methods designed to counteract them. There is often a related attempt to identify key protective factors against offending and to implement prevention methods designed to enhance them. Typically, longitudinal surveys provide knowledge about risk and protective factors, and experiments are used to evaluate the impact of prevention and intervention programmes. Thus, risk-focused prevention links explanation and prevention, links fundamental and applied research, and links scholars, policy makers, and practitioners. The book *Serious and violent juvenile offenders: risk factors and successful interventions* (Loeber and Farrington 1998) contains a detailed exposition of this approach as applied to serious and violent juvenile offenders.

Risk-focused prevention was imported into criminology from medicine and public health by pioneers such as Hawkins and Catalano (1992). This approach has been used successfully for many years to tackle illnesses such as cancer and heart disease. For example, the identified risk factors for heart disease include smoking, a fatty diet, and lack of exercise. These can be tackled by encouraging people to stop smoking, to have a more healthy low-fat diet, and to take more exercise. Typically, the effectiveness of risk-focused prevention in the medical field is evaluated using the 'gold standard' of randomized controlled trials, and there has been increasing emphasis in medicine on cost–benefit analyses of interventions. Not surprisingly, therefore, there has been a similar emphasis in criminology on high-quality evaluations and on cost–benefit analyses.

Risk factors tend to be similar for many different outcomes, including violent and non-violent offending, mental health problems, alcohol and drug problems, school failure, and unemployment. Therefore, a prevention programme that succeeds in reducing a risk factor for violent offending will, in all probability, have wide-ranging benefits in reducing other types of social problems as well.

Individual and family programmes

Four types of programmes are particularly successful: parent education (in the context of home visiting), parent management training, child skills training, and pre-school intellectual-enrichment programmes (Farrington and Welsh 1999). Generally, these programmes are targeted on the risk factors of: poor parental child-rearing, supervision, or discipline (parent education or parent management training); high impulsivity, low empathy and self-centredness (child skills training); and low intelligence and attainment (pre-school programmes).

In the most famous intensive home-visiting programme, Olds *et al.* (1986) in Elmira (New York) randomly allocated 400 mothers either to receive home visits from nurses during pregnancy, or to receive visits both during pregnancy and during the first two years of life, or to a control group who received no visits. Each visit lasted about one and a quarter hours, and the mothers were visited on average every two weeks. The home visitors gave advice about pre-natal and post-natal care of the child, about infant development, and about the importance of proper nutrition and the avoidance of smoking and drinking during pregnancy.

The results of this experiment showed that the post-natal home visits caused a decrease in recorded child physical abuse and neglect during the first two years of life, especially by poor unmarried teenage mothers; 4% of visited versus 19% of non-visited mothers of this type were guilty of child abuse or neglect. This last result is important because children who are physically abused or neglected tend to become violent offenders later in life (Widom 1989). In a 15-year follow-up, the main focus was on lower class unmarried mothers. Among these mothers, those who received pre-natal and post-natal home visits had fewer arrests than those who received pre-natal visits or no visits (Olds *et al.* 1997). Also, children of these mothers who received pre-natal and/or post-natal home visits had less than half as many arrests as children of mothers who received no visits (Olds *et al.* 1998).

Several economic analyses show that the benefits of this programme outweighed its costs for the lower class unmarried mothers. The most important are by Karoly *et al.* (1998) and Aos *et al.* (1999). However, both measured only a limited range of benefits. Karoly *et al.* measured only benefits to the government or taxpayer (welfare, education, employment, and criminal justice), not benefits to crime victims, consequent upon reduced crimes. Aos *et al.* measured only benefits to crime victims (tangible, not intangible) and in criminal justice savings, excluding other types of benefits (e.g. welfare, education, and employment). Nevertheless, both reported a benefit : cost ratio greater than 1 for this programme : 4.1 according to Karoly *et al.* and 1.5 according to Aos *et al.* The benefit : cost ratio was less than 1 for the low risk part of the sample.

The most famous pre-school intellectual enrichment programme is the Perry project carried out in Ypsilanti (Michigan) by Schweinhart and Weikart (1980). This was essentially a 'Head Start' programme targeted on disadvantaged African-American children, who were allocated (approximately at random) to experimental and control groups. The experimental children attended a daily pre-school programme, backed up by weekly home visits, usually lasting two years (covering ages 3–4). The aim of the 'plan-do-review' programme was to provide intellectual stimulation, to increase thinking and reasoning abilities, and to increase later school achievement.

This programme had long-term benefits. Berrueta-Clement *et al.* (1984) showed that, at age 19, the experimental group was more likely to be employed, more likely to have graduated from high school, more likely to have received college or vocational training, and less likely to have been arrested. By age 27, the experimental group had accumulated only half as many arrests on average as the controls (Schweinhart *et al.* 1993). Also, they had significantly higher earnings and were more likely to be homeowners. More of the experimental women were married, and fewer of their children were born out of wedlock.

Several economic analyses show that the benefits of this programme outweighed its costs. The benefit : cost ratio was 2.1 according to Karoly *et al.* (1998) and 1.5 according to Aos *et al.* (1999). For reasons explained above, both of these figures are underestimates. The Perry project's own calculation (Barnett 1993) was more comprehensive, including crime and non-crime benefits, intangible costs to victims, and even including projected benefits beyond age 27. This generated the famous benefit : cost ratio of 7.2. Most of the benefits (65%) were derived from savings to crime victims.

The Montreal longitudinal-experimental study was based on child skills training and parent management training. Tremblay *et al.* (1995) identified 366 disruptive (aggressive/hyperactive) boys at age 6, and randomly allocated 319 of these to experimental or control conditions. Between ages 7 and 9, the experimental group received training designed to foster social skills and self-control. Coaching, peer modelling, role playing, and reinforcement contingencies were used in small group sessions on such topics as 'how to help', 'what to do when you are angry' and 'how to react to teasing'. Also, their parents were trained using the parent management training techniques developed by Patterson (1982), which focus on promoting the use of consistent and contingent rewards and penalties.

This prevention programme was quite successful. By age 12, the experimental boys committed less burglary and theft, were less likely to get drunk, and were less likely to be involved in fights than the controls (according to self-reports). Also, the experimental boys had higher school achievement. At every age from 10 to 15, the experimental boys had lower self-reported delinquency scores than the control boys. Interestingly, the differences in antisocial behaviour between experimental and control boys increased as the follow-up progressed. Unfortunately, no cost–benefit analysis of this programme has yet been carried out.

Even where a programme is effective, its costs may outweigh its benefits if the programme is expensive. For example, in the Syracuse (New York) Family Development Research Programme of Lally et al. (1988), the researchers began with a sample of pregnant women (mostly poor African-American single mothers) and gave them weekly help with child-rearing, health, nutrition, and other problems. In addition, their children received free full-time day care, designed to develop their intellectual abilities, up to age 5. This was not a randomized experiment, but a matched control group was chosen when the children were aged 3.

Ten years later, 119 treated and control children were followed up to about age 15. Significantly fewer of the treated children (2% as opposed to 17%) had been referred to the juvenile court for delinquency offences, and the treated girls showed better school attendance and school performance. However, the benefit : cost ratio of this programme was only 0.3 according to Aos et al. (1999). This was largely because of the cost of the programme ($45 000 per child in 1998 dollars, compared with $14 000 for Perry and $7000 for Elmira); providing free full-time day care up to age 5 was very expensive. Against this, it must be repeated that the Aos et al. benefit : cost ratios are underestimates.

Peer, school, and community programmes

Peer, school, and community risk factors are less well-established than individual and family risk factors. For example, while it is clear that having delinquent peers, attending a high-delinquency-rate school, and living in a high-crime-rate area all predict a person's offending, the precise causal processes are not well understood.

There are no outstanding examples of effective intervention programmes for offending based on peer risk factors. The most hopeful programmes involve using high-status conventional peers to teach children ways of resisting peer pressure; this has been effective in reducing drug use (Tobler et al. 1999). Also, in a randomized experiment in St. Louis, Feldman et al. (1983) showed that placing antisocial adolescents in activity groups dominated by prosocial adolescents led to a reduction in their antisocial behaviour (compared with antisocial adolescents placed in antisocial groups). This suggests that the influence of prosocial peers can be harnessed to reduce offending.

The most important intervention programme, whose success seems to be based mainly on reducing peer risk factors, is the Children at Risk programme (Harrell *et al.* 1997), which targeted high-risk youths (average age 12.4) in poor neighbourhoods of five cities across the United States. Eligible youths were identified in schools and randomly assigned to experimental or control groups. The programme was a comprehensive community-based prevention strategy targeting risk factors for delinquency, including case management and family counselling, family skills training, tutoring, mentoring, after-school activities, and community policing. The programme was different in each neighbourhood.

The initial results of the programme were disappointing, but a one-year follow-up showed that (according to self-reports) experimental youths were less likely to have committed violent crimes and used or sold drugs (Harrell *et al.* 1999). The process evaluation showed that the greatest change was in peer risk factors. Experimental youths associated less often with delinquent peers, felt less peer pressure to engage in delinquency, and had more positive peer support. In contrast, there were few changes in individual, family, or community risk factors, possibly linked to the low participation of parents in parent training and of youths in mentoring and tutoring (Harrell *et al.* 1997, p.87). In other words, there were problems of implementation of the programme linked to the serious and multiple needs and problems of the families. No cost–benefit analysis of this programme has yet been carried out, but its relatively low cost ($9000 per youth) and its targeting of high-risk youths suggests that its benefits would probably outweigh its costs.

One of the most important school-based prevention experiments was carried out in Seattle by Hawkins *et al.* (1991). This combined parent management training, teacher training, and child skills training. About 500 first-grade children (aged 6) in 21 classes in eight schools were randomly assigned to be in experimental or control classes. The children in the experimental classes received special treatment at home and school, which was designed to increase their attachment to their parents and their bonding to the school. Also, they were trained in interpersonal cognitive problem-solving. Their parents were trained to notice and reinforce socially desirable behaviour in a programme called 'Catch them being good'. Their teachers were trained in classroom management, for example, to provide clear instructions and expectations to children, to reward children for participation in desired behaviour, and to teach children prosocial (socially desirable) methods of solving problems.

This programme had long-term benefits. O'Donnell *et al.* (1995) focused on children in low-income families and reported that, in the sixth grade (aged 12), experimental boys were less likely to have initiated delinquency, while experimental girls were less likely to have initiated drug use. In the latest follow-up, Hawkins *et al.* (1999) found that, at age 18, the full intervention group (receiving the intervention from grades 1–6) admitted less violence, less alcohol abuse, and fewer sexual partners than the late intervention group (grades 5–6 only) or the controls. The benefit : cost ratio of this programme according to Aos *et al.* (1999) was 1.8.

School bullying, of course, is a risk factor for offending (Farrington 1993b). Several school-based programmes have been effective in reducing bullying. The most famous of these was implemented by Olweus (1994) in Norway. It aimed to increase awareness and knowledge of teachers, parents, and children about bullying and to dispel myths about it. A 30-page booklet was distributed to all schools in Norway describing what was known about bullying and recommending what steps schools and teachers could take to reduce it. Also, a 25-min video about bullying was made available to schools. Simultaneously, the schools distributed to all parents a four-page folder containing information and advice about bullying. In addition, anonymous self-report questionnaires about bullying were completed by all children.

The programme was evaluated in Bergen. Each of the 42 participating schools received feedback information from the questionnaire about the prevalence of bullies and victims, in a specially arranged school conference day. Also, teachers were encouraged to develop explicit rules about bullying (e.g. do not bully, tell someone when bullying happens, bullying will not be tolerated, try to help victims, try to include children who are being left out) and to discuss bullying in class, using the video and role-playing exercises. Also, teachers were encouraged to improve monitoring and supervision of children, especially in the playground. The programme was successful in reducing the prevalence of bullying by half.

A similar programme was implemented in 23 Sheffield schools by Smith and Sharp (1994). The core programme involved establishing a 'whole-school' anti-bullying policy, raising awareness of bullying and clearly defining roles and responsibilities of teachers and students, so that everyone knew what bullying was and what they should do about it. In addition, there were optional interventions tailored to particular schools: curriculum work (e.g. reading books, watching videos), direct work with students (e.g. assertiveness training for those who were bullied), and playground work (e.g. training lunch-time supervisors). This programme was successful in reducing bullying in primary schools, but had relatively small effects in secondary schools. The effects of these anti-bullying programmes on violent offending need to be investigated.

Programmes targeting community risk factors have not been notably effective (Hope 1995). However, community-based programmes have been effective. For example, Jones and Offord (1989) implemented a skills training programme in an experimental public housing complex in Ottawa and compared it with a control complex. The programme centred on non-school skills, both athletic (e.g. swimming and hockey) and non-athletic (e.g. guitar and ballet). The aim of developing skills was to increase self-esteem, to encourage children to use time constructively, and to provide desirable role models. Participation rates were high: about three-quarters of age-eligible children in the experimental complex took at least one course in the first year. The programme was successful: delinquency rates decreased significantly in the experimental complex compared to the control complex. The benefit : cost ratio (focusing on taxpayer savings, excluding costs to crime victims) was 2.5.

One of the most important community-based treatment programmes is multisystemic therapy (MST), which is a multiple component programme (Henggeler et al. 1998). The particular type of treatment is chosen according to the particular needs of the youth; therefore, the nature of the treatment is different for each person. The treatment may include individual, family, peer, school, and community interventions, including parent training and child skills training.

Typically, MST has been used with juvenile offenders. For example, in Missouri, Borduin *et al.* (1995) randomly assigned 176 juvenile offenders (mean age 14.8) either to MST or to individual therapy focusing on personal, family, and academic issues. Four years later, only 29% of the MST offenders had been re-arrested, compared with 74% of the individual-therapy group. According to Aos *et al.* (1999), the benefit : cost ratio for MST is very high (13.5), largely because of the potential crime and criminal justice savings from targeting chronic juvenile offenders.

Situational and policing programmes

Several situational crime prevention programmes are effective and have benefits out-weighing their costs (Welsh and Farrington 1999). Two studies show that improved street lighting can lead to reductions in crime. In the first, in Dudley, crimes commit-ted before and after the improved lighting were measured using victimization surveys in experimental (relit) and control areas (Painter and Farrington 1997). Comparing the year before with the year after, crimes decreased significantly more in the experi-mental area than in the control area. Personal crimes (robberies, assaults, threats, and pestering) decreased by 41%. Based only on the financial savings from reduced crimes, the benefit : cost ratio was 6.2 when the full capital cost of the improved light-ing was taken into account and 74 when it was written off over its expected life of 20 years (Painter and Farrington 1999a, in press).

In the second study, in Stoke-on-Trent, crimes committed before and after the improved lighting were measured in experimental (relit), adjacent, and non-adjacent control areas (Painter and Farrington 1999b). Comparing the year before with the year after, crimes decreased significantly in the experimental and adjacent areas (which were not clearly delimited) but not in the control area. Personal crimes decreased by 68% in the experimental area. It was suggested that there might have been a diffusion of benefits to the adjacent area. Based only on the financial savings from reduced crimes in the experimental area, the benefit : cost ratio was 2.4 when the full capital cost of the improved lighting was taken into account and 24 when it was written off over its expected life of 20 years (Painter and Farrington 1999a, in press).

From the viewpoint of crime prevention, the most important policing projects are those targeting 'hot-spots', or places where large numbers of crimes occur. Other important policing projects are based on the general-deterrent effects of new laws and policing policies (e.g. the impact of the British breathalyser on drunk driving: see Ross *et al.* 1970, and Homel 1988), or on the individual-deterrent effects of police arrests and their consequences (e.g. the impact of arresting men committing domestic violence: see Sherman 1992).

In one of the most important 'hot spot' studies, Sherman and Weisburd (1995) car-ried out a randomized experiment in Minneapolis; over 100 high-crime places were randomly assigned either to receive increased police patrolling (a target of 3 h per day) or not, on the assumption that increased police presence would deter offending. Calls for police service for crime were monitored in the year before and the year of the experiment. Crime and disorder was also measured in the second year using systematic observation in all places. The experiment showed that the increased patrolling led to decreased crime in the experimental places.

Conclusions

The major long-term risk factors for youth violence are biological (low resting heart rate), psychological/personality (high impulsiveness and low intelligence, possibly linked to the executive functions of the brain), family (poor supervision, harsh discipline, child physical abuse, a violent parent, large family size, a young mother, a broken family), peer delinquency, low socio-economic status, urban residence, and living in a high-crime neighbourhood. Important short-term situational factors include the motives of potential offenders (e.g. anger, a desire to hurt), alcohol consumption, and actions leading to violent events (e.g. the escalation of a trivial altercation). More research is needed specifically searching for protective factors against youth violence, for example, by investigating why aggressive children do not become violent adults. Protective factors could have important policy implications.

In order to investigate developmental and risk factors for youth violence, longitudinal studies are needed. Such studies should include multiple cohorts, in order to draw conclusions about different age groups from birth to the mid-twenties. They should include both males and females and the major racial/ethnic groups. They should measure a wide range of risk and especially protective factors. They should be based on large, high-risk samples, especially in inner-city areas, incorporating screening methods to maximize the yield of violent offenders, while simultaneously making it possible to draw conclusions about the total population. They should include long-term follow-ups to permit conclusions about developmental pathways. They should make a special effort to study careers of violence and to link developmental and situational data.

High-quality evaluation research shows that many programmes are effective in reducing offending, and that in many cases the financial benefits of these programmes outweigh their financial costs. The best programmes include general parent education, parent management training, pre-school intellectual enrichment programmes, child skills training, teacher training, peer influence resistance training, anti-bullying programmes, improving street lighting, and increased police patrolling of crime 'hot spots'. Since most of these evaluation projects were carried out in the United States, it is obvious that more high-quality evaluation research is urgently needed in Great Britain. Also, better methods of summarizing existing knowledge are needed, based on the Campbell collaboration (Farrington and Petrosino, 2000). The time is ripe to invest in risk-focused prevention, not only to prevent crime and violence, but also to improve mental and physical health and life success in areas such as education, employment, relationships, housing, and child-rearing.

References

Agnew, R. (1990). The origins of delinquent events: an examination of offender accounts. *Journal of Research in Crime and Delinquency*, **27**, 267–94.

Aos, S., Phipps, P., Barnoski, R., and Lieb, R. (1999). *The comparative costs and benefits of programs to reduce crime* (version 3.0). Washington State Institute for Public Policy, Olympia, Washington.

Archer, J. (1991). The influence of testosterone on human aggression. *British Journal of Psychology*, **82**, 1–28.

Barker, M., Geraghty, J., Webb, B., and Kay, T. (1993). *The prevention of street robbery*. Home Office Police Department, London.

Barnett, W.S. (1993). Cost–benefit analysis. In *Significant benefits: the High/Scope Perry preschool study through age 27* (ed. L.J. Schweinhart, H.V. Barnes, and D.P. Weikart), pp.142–73. High/Scope Press, Ypsilanti, Michigan.

Berrueta-Clement, J.R., Schweinhart, L.J., Barnett, W.S., Epstein, A.S., and Weikart, D.P. (1984). *Changed lives: the effects of the Perry preschool program on youths through age 19*. High/Scope Press, Ypsilanti, Michigan.

Borduin, C.M., Mann, B.J., Cone, L.T., Henggeler, S.W., Fucci, B.R., Blaske, D.M., and Williams, R.A. (1995). Multisystemic treatment of serious juvenile offenders: long-term prevention of criminality and violence. *Journal of Consulting and Clinical Psychology*, **63**, 569–87.

Brennan, P.A., Mednick, S.A., and John, R. (1989). Specialization in violence: evidence of a criminal subgroup. *Criminology*, **27**, 437–53.

Brennan, P.A., Mednick, B.R., and Mednick, S.A. (1993). Parental psychopathology, congenital factors, and violence. In *Mental disorder and crime* (ed. S. Hodgins), pp.244–61. Sage, Newbury Park, California.

Capaldi, D.M., and Patterson, G.R. (1996). Can violent offenders be distinguished from frequent offenders? Prediction from childhood to adolescence. *Journal of Research in Crime and Delinquency*, **33**, 206–31.

Caspi, A., Moffitt, T.E., Silva, P.A., Stouthamer-Loeber, M., Krueger, R.F., and Schmutte, P.S. (1994). Are some people crime-prone? Replications of the personality–crime relationship across countries, genders, races, and methods. *Criminology*, **32**, 163–95.

Cohen, L.E., and Felson, M. (1979). Social change and crime rate trends: a routine activity approach. *American Sociological Review*, **44**, 588–608.

Denno, D.W. (1990). *Biology and violence: from birth to adulthood*. Cambridge University Press, Cambridge.

Ekblom, P. (1988). *Getting the best out of crime analysis*. Home Office, London.

Elliott, D.S. (1994). Serious violent offenders: onset, development course,, and termination. *Criminology*, **32**, 1–21.

Elliott, D.S., and Menard, S. (1996). Delinquent friends and delinquent behaviour: temporal and developmental patterns. In *Delinequency and crime: current theories* (ed. J.D. Hawkins), pp.28–67. Cambridge University Press, Cambridge.

Elliott, D.S., Huizinga, D., and Menard, S. (1989). *Multiple problem youth: delinquency, substance use, and mental health problems*. Springer–Verlag, New York.

Eron, L.D., Huesmann, L.R., and Zelli, A. (1991). The role of parental variables in the learning of aggression. In *The development and treatment of childhood aggression* (ed. D.J. Pepler and K.J. Rubin), pp. 169–88. Lawrence Erlbaum, Hillsdale, NJ.

Farrington, D.P. (1978). The family backgrounds of aggressive youths. In *Aggression and antisocial behaviour in childhood and adolescence* (ed. L. Hersov, M. Berger, and D. Shaffer), pp. 73–93. Oxford: Pergamon.

Farrington, D.P. (1986). Age and crime. In *Crime and justice*, Vol. 7 (ed. M. Tonry and N. Morris), pp.189–250. University of Chicago Press, Chicago.

Farrington, D.P. (1989). Self-reported and official offending from adolescence to adulthood. In *Cross-national research in self-reported crime and delinquency* (ed. M. Klein), pp.399–425. Kluwer, Dordrecht, Netherlands.

Farrington, D.P. (1991). Childhood aggression and adult violence: early precursors and later life outcomes. In *The development and treatment of childhood aggression* (ed. D.J. Pepler and K.H. Rubin), pp.5–29. Lawrence Erlbaum, Hillsdale, NJ.

Farrington, D.P. (1993a). Motivations for conduct disorder and delinquency. *Development and Psychopathology*, **5**, 225–41.

Farrington, D.P. (1993b). Understanding and preventing bullying. In *Crime and justice*, Vol. 17 (ed. M. Tonry and N. Morris), pp.381–458. University of Chicago Press, Chicago.

Farrington, D.P. (1994). Childhood, adolescent and adult features of violent males. In *Aggressive behavior: current perspectives* (ed. L.R. Huesmann), pp.215–40. Pleum Press, New York.

Farrington, D.P. (1997a). Early prediction of violent and non-violent youthful offending. *European Journal on Criminal Policy and Research*, **5**(2), 51–66.

Farrington, D.P. (1997b). The relationship between low resting heart rate and violence. In *Biosocial bases of violence* (ed. A. Raine, P.A. Brennan, D.P. Farrington, and S.A. Mednick), pp.89–105. Plenum, New York.

Farrington, D.P. (1998). Predictors, causes and correlates of male youth violence. In *Youth violence* (ed. M. Tonry and M.H. Moore), pp.421–75. University of Chicago Press, Chicago.

Farrington, D.P. (2001). Predicting adult official and self-reported violence. In *Clinical assessment of dangerousness: empirical contributions* (ed. G-F. Pinard and L. Pagani), pp.66–88. Cambridge University Press, Cambridge.

Farrington, D.P., and Loeber, R. How can the relationship between race and violence be explained? In *Violent crimes: the nexus of ethnicity, race and class* (ed. D.F. Hawkins). Cambridge University Press, Cambridge. (In press)

Farrington, D.P., and Petrosino, A. (2000). Systematic reviews of criminological interventions: the Campbell collaboration crime and justice group. *International Annals of Criminology*, **38**, 49–66.

Farrington, D.P., and Welsh, B.C. (1999). Delinquency prevention using family-based interventions. *Children and Society*, **13**, 287–303.

Feldman, R.A., Caplinger, T.E., and Wodarski, J.S. (1983). *The St. Louis conundrum*. Prentice-Hall, Englewood Cliffs, NJ.

Fitzgerald, M., and Hale, C. (1996). *Ethnic minorities: victimization and racial harassment*. Home Office, London.

Gorman-Smith, D., Tolan, P.H., Zelli, A., and Huesmann, L.R. (1996). The relation of family functioning to violence among inner-city minority youths. *Journal of Family Psychology*, **10**, 115–29.

Graham, J., and Bowling, B. (1995). *Young people and crime*. Home Office, London.

Hamparian, D.M., Schuster, R., Dinitz, S., and Conrad, J.P. (1978). *The violent few: a study of dangerous juvenile offenders*. D.C. Heath, Lexington, Massachusetts.

Hamparian, D.M., Davis, J.M., Jacobson J.M., and McGraw, R.E. (1985). *The young criminal years of the violent few*. Office of Juvenile Justice and Delinquency Prevention, Washington DC.

Harrell, A.V., Cavanagh, S.E., Harmon, M.A., Koper, C.S., and Sridharan, S. (1997). *Impact of the children at risk program: comprehensive final report*, Vol. 2. The Urban Institute, Washington, DC.

Harrell, A.V., Cavanagh, S.E., and Sridharan, S. (1999). *Evaluation of the children at risk program: results one year after the program*. National Institute of Justice, Washington, DC.

Harvey, L., Burnham, R.W., Kendall, K., and Pease, K. (1992). Gender differences in criminal justice: an international comparison. *British Journal of Criminology*, **32**, 208–17.

Hawkins, J.D., and Catalano, R.F. (1992). *Communities that care.* Jossey–Bass, San Francisco.

Hawkins, J.D., von Cleve, E., and Catalano, R.F. (1991). Reducing early childhood aggression: results of a primary prevention program. *Journal of the American Academy of Child and Adolescent Psychiatry*, **30**, 208–17.

Hawkins, J.D., Catalano, R.F., Kosterman, R., Abbott, R., and Hill, K.G. (1999). Preventing adolescent health risk behaviors by strengthening protection during childhood. *Archives of Pediatrics and Adolescent Medicine*, **153**, 226–34.

Henggeler, S.W., Schoenwald, S.K., Borduin, C.M., Rowland, M.D., and Cunningham, P.B. (1998). *Multisystemic treatment of antisocial behavior in children and adolescents.* Guilford, New York.

Henry, B., Caspi, A., Moffitt, T.E., and Silva, P.A. (1996). Temperamental and familial predictors of violent and non-violent criminal convictions: age 3 to age 18. *Developmental Psychology*, **32**, 614–23.

Hogh, E., and Wolf, P. (1983). Violent crime in a birth cohort: Copenhagen 1953–1977. In *Prospective studies of crime and delinquency* (ed. K.T. van Dusen and S.A. Mednick), pp. 249–67. Kluwer–Nijhoff, Boston.

Home Office (1998). *Criminal statistics, England and Wales, 1997.* The Stationery Office, London.

Home Office (1999). *Statistics on race and the criminal justice system, 1999.* Home Office, London.

Home Office Statistical Bulletin (1995). *Criminal careers of those born between 1953 and 1973.* Home Office, London.

Homel, R. (1988). *Policing and punishing the drinking driver: a study of general and specific deferrence.* Springer–Verlag, New York.

Hope, T. (1995). Community crime prevention. In *Building a safer society: strategic approaches to crime prevention* (ed. M. Tonry and D.P. Farrington), pp.21–89. University of Chicago Press, Chicago.

Hough, M., and Sheehy, K. (1986). Incidents of violence: findings from the British Crime Survey. *Home Office Research Bulletin*, **20**, 22–6.

Jones, M.B., and Offord, D.R. (1989). Reduction of antisocial behavior in poor children by non-school skill-development. *Journal of Child Psychology and Psychiatry*, **30**, 737–50.

Kagan, J. (1989). Temperamental contributions to social behavior. *American Psychologist*, **44**, 668–74.

Kandel, E., and Mednick, S.A. (1991). Perinatal complications predict violent offending. *Criminology*, **29**, 519–29.

Karoly, L.A., Greenwood, P.W., Everingham, S.S., Hoube, J., Kilburn, M.R., Rydell, C. *et al.* (1998). *Investing in our children: what we know and don't know about the costs and benefits of early childhood interventions.* RAND Corporation, Santa Monica, California.

Klinteberg, B.A., Andersson, T., Magnusson, D., and Stattin, H. (1993). Hyperactive behaviour in childhood as related to subsequent alcohol problems and violent offending: a longitudinal study of male subjects. *Personality and Individual Differences*, **15**, 381–8.

Lally, J.R., Mangione, P.L., and Honig, A.S. (1988). The Syracuse University Family Development Research Program: long-range impact of an early intervention with low-income children and their families. In *Parent education as early childhood intervention: emerging directions in theory, research and practice.* (ed. D.R. Powell). Norwood, N.J.: Ablex.

Langan, P.A., and Farrington, D.P. (1998). *Crime and justice in the United States and in England and Wales, 1981–96.* US Bureau of Justice Statistics, Washington, DC.

LeBlanc, M. (1996). Changing patterns in the perpetration of offences over time: trajectories from early adolescence to the early 30s. *Studies on Crime and Crime Prevention,* **5**, 151–65.

LeBlanc, M., and Frechette, M. (1989). *Male criminal activity from childhood through youth.* Springer–Verlag, New York.

Lipsey, M.W., and Derzon, J.H. (1998). Predictors of violent or serious delinquency in adolescence and early adulthood: a synthesis of longitudinal research. In *Serious and violent juvenile offenders: risk factors and successful interventions* (ed. R. Loeber and D.P. Farrington), pp.86–105. Sage, Thousand Oaks, California.

Loeber, R., and Farrington, D.P. (edn.) (1998). *Serious and violent juvenile offenders: risk factors and successful interventions.* Sage, Thousand Oaks, California.

Maccoby, E.E., and Jacklin, C.N. (1974). *The psychology of sex differences.* Stanford University Press, Stanford, California.

Malinosky-Rummell, R., and Hansen, D.J. (1993). Long-term consequences of childhood physical abuse. *Psychological Bulletin,* **114**, 68–79.

McClintock, F.H. (1963). *Crimes of violence.* Macmillan, London.

McCord, J. (1977). A comparative study of two generations of native Americans. In *Theory in criminology: contemporary views* (ed. R.F. Meier), pp.83–92. Sage, Beverly Hills, California.

McCord, J. (1979). Some child-rearing antecedents of criminal behaviour in adult men. *Journal of Personality and Social Psychology,* **37**, 1477–86.

McCord, J. (1996). Family as crucible for violence: comment on Gorman-Smith *et al.* (1996). *Journal of Family Psychology,* **10**, 147–52.

Miczek, K.A., DeBold, J.F., Haney, M., Tidey, J., Vivian, J., and Weeris, E.M. (1994). Alcohol, drugs of abuse, aggression and violence. In *Understanding and preventing violence,* Vol. 3: *Social influences.* (ed. A.J. Reiss and J.A. Roth), pp.377–570. National Academy Press, Washington, DC.

Moffitt, T.E. (1993). Adolescence-limited and life-course-persistent antisocial behavior: a developmental taxonomy. *Psychological Review,* **100**, 674–701.

Moffitt, T.E., and Henry, B. (1991). Neuropsychological studies of juvenile delinquency and juvenile violence. In *Neuropsychology of aggression* (ed. J.S. Milner), pp. 131–46. Kluwer, Boston.

Morash, M., and Rucker, L. (1989). An exploratory study of the connection of mother's age at childbearing to her children's delinquency in four data sets. *Crime and Delinquency,* **35**, 45–93.

Nagin, D.S., Pogarsky, G., and Farrington, D.P. (1997). Adolescent mothers and the criminal behaviour of their children. *Law and Society Review,* **31**, 137–62.

O'Donnell, J., Hawkins, J.D., Catalano, R.F., Abbott, R.D., and Day, L.E. (1995). Preventing school failure, drug use, and delinquency among low-income children: long-term intervention in elementary schools. *American Journal of Orthopsychiatry,* **65**, 87–100.

Olds, D.L., Henderson, C.R., Chamberlin, R., and Tatelbaum, R. (1986). Preventing child abuse and neglect: a randomized trial of nurse home visitation. *Pediatrics,* **78**, 65–78.

Olds, D.L., Eckenrode, J., Henderson, C.R., Kitzman, H., Powers, J., Cole, R. *et al.* (1997). Long-term effects of home visitation on maternal life course and child abuse and neglect: Fifteen-year follow-up of a randomized trial. *Journal of the American Medical Association,* **278**, 637–43.

Olds, D.L., Henderson, C.R., Cole, R., Eckenrode, J., Kitzman, H., Luckey, D. *et al.* (1998). Long-term effects of nurse home visitation on children's criminal and antisocial behavior: Fifteen-year follow-up of a randomized controlled trial. *Journal of the American Medical Association*, **280**, 1238–44.

Olweus, D. (1994). Bullying at school: basic facts and effects of a school based intervention program. *Journal of Child Psychology and Psychiatry*, **35**, 1171–90.

Painter, K.A., and Farrington, D.P. (1997). The crime reducing effect of improved street lighting: the Dudley project. In *Situational crime prevention: successful case studies* (2nd edn) (ed. R.V. Clark), pp.209–26. Harrow and Heston, Guilderland, NY.

Painter, K.A., and Farrington, D.P. (1999a). Improved street lighting: crime reducing effects and cost-benefit analyses. *Security Journal*, **12**(4), 17–32.

Painter, K.A., and Farrington, D.P. (1999b). Street lighting and crime: diffusion of benefits in the Stoke-on-Trent project. In *Surveillance of public space: CCTV, street lighting and crime prevention* (ed. K.A. Painter and N. Tilley), pp.77–122. Criminal Justice Press, Monsey, NY.

Painter, K.A., and Farrington, D.P. The financial benefits of improved street lighting, based on crime reduction. *Lighting Research and Technology*. (In press.)

Pallone, N.J., and Hennessy, J.H. (1993). Tinderbox criminal violence: neurogenic impulsivity, risk-taking, and the phenomenology of rational choice. In *Advances in criminological theory*, Vol. 5: *Routine activity and rational choice* (ed. R.V. Clarke and M. Felson), pp.127–157. New Brunswick, NJ: Transaction.

Patterson, G.R. (1982). *Coercive family process.* Castalia, Eugene, Oregon.

Pulkkinen, L. (1987). Offensive and defensive aggression in humans: a longitudinal perspective. *Aggressive Behavior*, **13**, 197–212.

Raine, A. (1993). *The psychopathology of crime: criminal behavior as a clinical disorder.* Academic Press, San Diego, California.

Reiss, A.J., and Farrington, D.P. (1991). Advancing knowledge about co-offending: results from a prospective longitudinal survey of London males. *Journal of Criminal Law and Criminology*, **82**, 360–95.

Reiss, A.J., and Roth, J.A. (ed.) (1993). *Understanding and preventing violence* (Four volumes). National Academy Press, Washington, DC.

Rivara, F.P., Shepherd, J.P., Farrington, D.P., Richmond, P.W., and Cannon, P. (1995). Victim as offender in youth violence. *Annals of Emergency Medicine*, **26**, 609–14.

Ross, H.L., Campbell, D.T., and Glass, G.V. (1970). Determining the social effects of a legal reform: the british 'Breathalyzer' crackdown of 1967. *American Behavioral Scientist*, **13**, 493–509.

Rutter, M., Giller, H., and Hagell, A. (1998). *Antisocial behaviour by young people.* Cambridge University Press, Cambridge.

Sampson, R.J., and Lauritsen, J.L. (1994). Violent victimization and offending: individual, situational and community-level risk factors. In *Understanding and preventing violence*, Vol. 3: *Social influences* (ed. A.J. Reiss and J.A. Roth), pp. 1–114. National Academy Press, Washington, DC.

Schweinhart, L.J., and Weikart, D.P. (1980). *Young children grow up: the effects of the Perry preschool program on youths through age 15.* High/Scope Press, Ypsilanti, Michigan.

Schweinhart, L.J., Barnes, H.V., and Weikart, D.P. (1993). *Significant benefits: the High/Scope Perry preschool study through age 27.* High/Scope Press, Ypsilanti, Michigan.

Seguin, J., Pihl, R.O., Harden, P.W., Tremblay, R.F., and Boulerice, B. (1995). Cognitive and neuropsychological characteristics of physically aggressive boys. *Journal of Abnormal Psychology*, **104**, 614–24.

Sherman, L.W. (1992). *Policing domestic violence: experiments and dilemmas.* Free Press, New York.

Sherman, L.W., and Weisburd, D. (1995). General deterrent effects of police patrol in crime 'hot spots': a randomized controlled trial. *Justice Quarterly,* **12,** 625–48.

Smith, D.J. (1997). Ethnic origins, crime and criminal justice. In *The Oxford handbook of criminology* (2nd edn.) (ed. M. Maguire, R. Morgan, and R. Reiner), pp.703–59. Clarendon Press, Oxford.

Smith, P.K., and Sharp, S. (1994). *School bullying.* Routledge, London.

Smith, C., and Thornberry, T.P. (1995). The relationship between childhood maltreatment and adolescent involvement in delinquency. *Criminology,* **33,** 451–81.

Stattin, H., and Magnusson, D. (1989). The role of early aggressive behaviour in the frequency, seriousness, and types of later crime. *Journal of Consulting and Clinical Psychology,* **57,** 710–8.

Tarling, R. (1993). *Analysing offending: data, models and interpretations.* Her Majesty's Stationery Office, London.

Thornberry, T.P., Huizinga, D., and Loeber, R. (1995). The prevention of serious delinquency and violence: Implications from the program of research on the causes and correlates of delinquency. In *Sourcebook on serious, violent, and chronic juvenile offenders* (ed. J.C. Howell, B. Krisberg, J.D. Hawkins, and J.J. Wilson), pp.213–37. Sage, Thousand Oaks, California.

Tobler, N.S., Lessard, T., Marshall, D., Ochshorn, P., and Roona, M. (1999). Effectiveness of school-based drug prevention programs for marijuana use. *School Psychology International,* **20,** 105–37.

Tonry, M., and Moore, M.H. (ed.) (1998). *Youth violence.* University of Chicago Press, Chicago.

Tremblay, R.E., Pagani-Kurtz, L., Masse, L.C., Vitaro, F., and Pihl, R.O. (1995). A bimodal preventive intervention for disruptive kindergarten boys: its impact through mid-adolescence. *Journal of Consulting and Clinical Psychology,* **63,** 560–8.

Wadsworth, M.E.J. (1976). Delinquency, pulse rates, and early emotional deprivation. *British Journal of Criminology,* **16,** 245–56.

Wadsworth, M.E.J. (1978). Delinquency prediction and its uses: the experience of a 21-year follow-up study. *International Journal of Mental Health,* **7,** 43–62.

Welsh, B.C., and Farrington, D.P. (1999). Value for money? A review of the costs and benefits of situational crime prevention. *British Journal of Criminology,* **39,** 345–68.

Welsh, B.C., and Farrington, D.P. (2000). Monetary costs and benefits of crime prevention programs. In *Crime and justice,* Vol. 27 (ed. M. Tonry), pp.305–61. University of Chicago Press, Chicago.

Widom, C.S. (1989). The cycle of violence. *Science,* **244,** 160–6.

Wikström, P-O. H. (1985). *Everyday violence in contemporary Sweden.* National Council for Crime Prevention, Stockholm.

Wolfgang, M.E. (1958). *Patterns in criminal homicide.* University of Pennsylvania Press, Philadelphia.

Chapter 2

Alcohol, other drugs, and violence

Duncan Raistrick

Introduction

Drinking and taking other drugs are not only activities that most people in the UK engage in but they are also activities that, for many people, are interwoven with their leisure-time pursuits. The General Household Survey (Office for National Statistics 1998) reports on trends in alcohol consumption: in 1996, 15% of men and 33% of women were categorized as non-drinkers or very light drinkers; 27% of men and 14% of women were categorized as drinking over the recommended safe limits of 21 units and 14 units per week, respectively. Over the last 10 years the proportion of men drinking over safe limits has remained more or less constant, while the number of women has slowly increased. Information on illicit drug use is much more difficult to collect and there have been no regular population surveys of the kind undertaken for alcohol. Social Trends 29 (Office for National Statistics 1999) collated data from a number of surveys: in 1996, 57% of men and 43% of women aged 20–24 years said that they had not used drugs 'ever', while 24% and 12% had used drugs in the 'last month'. Aside from people seeking help specifically for their substance-use, a significant number of these drinkers and drug-users come into contact with social and health care services for all manner of reasons, which may or may not have roots in substance use.

The consequences of drinking and taking drugs have an enormous impact upon the health service. Broadly speaking accidents, trauma, and aggressive behaviour can be thought of as problems of intoxication, whereas physical illness is more likely to be associated with regular drinking or injecting drugs. In a study of Accident and Emergency attenders who had a blood alcohol >80 mg%, 50% had been involved in an assault incident, 8.1% in a road traffic accident, 6.3% in accidents in the home, and 3.7% in accidents at work (Walsh and MacLeod 1983). A high proportion of road traffic fatalities occur in people who have a blood alcohol level in excess of the legal driving limit of 80 mg%: 23% of car drivers, 37% of pedestrians, and 16% of cyclists in one study. In another study of prescribed and illicit drug-use in road user fatalities, 22% of drivers, 30% of passengers, and 16% of pedestrians tested positive. Alcohol intoxication is also implicated in suicide and self-harm. In one survey (Chick 1994), alcohol was found to contribute to 28% of overdoses, 20% of head injuries, 18% of road traffic accidents, and 11% of gastro-intestinal hemorrhages in the general hospital.

Suffice to say that people who misuse alcohol or other drugs will, for a variety of reasons, be commonplace in both primary and secondary health care settings. Different health service departments will experience different problems in building a working relationship with people who misuse alcohol and other drugs, but common sense and common experience create the expectation that aggressive or violent behaviour and substance use sometimes go together. It is important to make sense of any violent incident *post hoc*. It may be helpful to attribute the cause of violence to interactions between the drug, the individual, and the setting, each of which is discussed below.

The drug

The pharmacopoeia of psychoactive drugs, licit and illicit, is so extensive that any attempt at a typology will quickly reveal shortcomings. Nonetheless, it will be useful for practical purposes to bring together those substances that have similar effects and, in the main, similar withdrawal states. Four groups have been selected:

1 stimulant drugs;
2 depressant drugs;
3 opiate drugs; and
4 perception-altering drugs.

These groups are not mutually exclusive: for example, alcohol, a depressant, and LSD, a perception-altering drug, both have an initial stimulant effect; while morphine, an opiate, has powerful depressant properties. Nonetheless, there is an established utility to this classification. See Stahl (1996) for a more detailed account of pharmacology. There are some general characteristics of drugs to be aware of before considering the effects of specific drug groups.

Intoxication, tolerance, and withdrawal

Some drugs are thought of in the public's mind as more likely to cause violent episodes than others, however, common beliefs are often distorted by frequency of exposure to a substance, so that its connection with violence may prove, on close examination, a spurious one. For example, Accident and Emergency staff will see more cases of alcohol-related violence than, say, drug-clinic staff who may experience more problems related to amphetamine use. What then are the pharmacological effects of a drug that are likely to contribute to a violent episode?

An alteration of mental state that impairs judgement, releases inhibitions, causes confusion, increases confidence, increases activity, induces paranoia, distorts percep- tions, or increases irritability might be expected to be one of the ingredients of a violent episode. There are many drugs that can cause such shifts in mental state, either as an effect of intoxication or as a result of withdrawal from the drug. Intoxication refers to the pharmacological effect of taking a particular psychoactive substance, and should be distinguished from being 'drunk' or 'stoned', which refer to the behaviour associated with taking a particular drug. Behaviour has much to do with circum- stances and expectations: studies have repeatedly found experienced observers unable to predict intoxication, meaning plasma levels of a drug, from behaviour. The effect of a drug is more pronounced during the phase of increasing plasma levels when com- pared with that of a similar but decreasing plasma concentration.

As individuals use a drug on a regular basis over a period of time they become accustomed to its effect and require a higher dose of the drug in order to achieve the same effect as on initial use. This phenomenon is referred to as tolerance, which is largely accounted for by a reduced sensitivity of the central nervous system. Learning to handle being intoxicated may contribute significantly to the overall tolerance and, for some drugs, an increase in their rate of metabolism plays a part. Tolerance does not develop evenly for all the effects of a substance. For example, tolerance to the sedative effect of alcohol is not matched by tolerance to its amnesic effect, and toleiance to the euphoriant effects of opiates is not matched by tolerance to their analgesic properties. In some situations tolerance may appear to decrease. For example, cannabis-smokers often improve their smoking technique so as to enhance, at least for a time, the drug effect, and drinkers may report a decline in tolerance, usually attributed to liver damage, in the later stages of their drinking careers.

Withdrawal symptoms may occur in individuals who develop tolerance to a drug. In developing tolerance, a kind of resistance or opposition to the effects of a drug is built up by changes in biochemical activity within the central nervous system: balance is restored, so that the individual feels and functions more or less as normal only when intoxicated with the drug or with a drug from a similar pharmacological group. If this drug is suddenly stopped, then the biochemical shifts that were opposing and neutralizing the drug effect are released and manifest as withdrawal symptoms. Typically withdrawal symptoms are opposite in direction to the drug effect (see Nutt 1999).

Method of use

The intensity of a desired drug effect and the propensity for the emergence of undesired effects, possibly with potential for aggression and violence, owes much to the particular preparation that is taken and how it is taken. In terms of both speed of onset and dose of drug delivered, there is a hierarchy of methods of use that holds good for most substances. The least efficient is the oral route, which is both slow in terms of onset and costly in terms of liver metabolism of the drug ingested; subcutaneous and intramuscular injection are probably on a par with snorting; intravenous injection and inhalation are the most effective routes. It is not just the route but also the preparation that is important: for example, cocaine smoked in the form known as 'crack' will produce plasma levels five times those of a large dose of snorted crystalline cocaine. Alcohol, which is normally taken as a drink, is most rapidly absorbed at a strength of 10–30%, which coincides with the strength of drinks such as gin and tonic, sherry, and beer with a whisky chaser. In short, the route of administration and of preparation of a substance may be chosen, usually as a result of experience, to maximize the drug effect. The more profound the disturbance of mental state, the more likely are aggression and violence.

The severity of withdrawal symptoms depends upon the rate of fall of plasma levels of a substance, which in turn depends upon the dose taken and the speed with which the substance is metabolized. A convenient measure is the half-life of a substance, which is defined as the time taken to reduce the plasma level by 50%. The practical implication is that, all other things being equal, a drug with a short half-life, such as morphine, will require a booster dose every 6–8 h in order to avoid withdrawal symptoms, whereas a different opioid drug, such as methadone, with a very long half-life, will require only a once-daily dose. It follows that the drug with the shorter half-life will have the greater potential for aggression and violence, in terms of both procurement needs and more rapid shifts to unpleasant mental states.

Plasticity

The effect of a drug may be modified, and indeed wholly altered, because of the circumstances in which it is taken. For example, being at a football match or clubbing may, of itself, be more potent than a drug in heightening the level of arousal and excitement; equally, to be arrested by the police or to find oneself alone in an unfamiliar place may be a sobering experience. This capacity of a drug for its effects to be moulded is known as plasticity. Drugs that are said to be low in plasticity, such as heroin and amphetamine, have very predictable effects irrespective of the circumstances of their use, whereas high-plasticity drugs, such as solvents and LSD, are dependent upon setting to define the drug experience. The most popular recreational drugs, alcohol and cannabis, fall between these two extremes. It is perhaps not surprising that highly plastic drugs fail to find favour for general recreational purposes. The practical implications will be apparent after considering drug-specific effects.

Dependence

Dependence is a psychological phenomenon that evades precise definition. It is to do with the extent to which thinking about substance-use and behaviour related to substance-use come to dominate a person's life. Dependence is best understood within the framework of social learning theory; it is not therefore seen as an all-or-none phenomenon, but rather as existing across a spectrum from low to high. The high-dependence individual is characterized by a preoccupation with a need to use a drug or drugs in order to modulate every emotion, every physical experience, every life-event. The perceived need for a drug will be more important than anything else happening at that time. The high-dependence individual will be a regular, probably daily user, and will often have a fairly stereotyped pattern of use; intake may well be high and there may be episodes of intoxication, but not necessarily so.

Dependence *per se* probably makes only a modest direct contribution to the association between violence and substance misuse; the indirect implications are much greater. The cost, both financial and in time, of maintaining a high level of dependence on any substance is likely to be significant, and liable to end in conflict with a partner, workmates, or suppliers of drink or other drugs. Equally, a failure to maintain a substance-use pattern can provoke craving and interpersonal conflicts. So dependence will contribute to the likelihood of aggression and violence by indirect means, and to a lesser degree by associated episodes of intoxication.

Stimulant drugs

The most powerful compounds in this group are cocaine and amphetamine; less potent compounds include caffeine, nicotine, and a variety of sympathomimetics,

such as pseudoephedrine, used in such proprietary preparations as nasal deconges-
tants. Typically the effect of taking cocaine or amphetamine is a feeling of confidence
and general well-being; thoughts are sharper and come more quickly, speech is quick-
ened, and there is a general overactivity. Intoxicated people are usually witty and
infectious fun to be with; however, if crossed or interrupted they may become irritable and aggressive. Stimulants remove the need for sleep, reduce the appetite, and
heighten sexual drive.

As the dose of stimulant increases to toxic levels, so the picture changes to one of
extreme agitation, persecutory ideas, visual hallucinations, confusion, and physical
abnormalities, which include hypertension, seizures, and eventually coma. The early
stages can be controlled using minor tranquillizers and beta-blockers within a supportive environment. Both intoxication and overdose with stimulant drugs may be
mistaken for a hypomanic illness.

Intoxication and overdose with stimulant drugs both have a potential for violence.
Overactive people are more likely to come into contact with other people and conflict
is likely as they try to take other people along with their latest good ideas, which may
include sexual propositions. Add to this picture feelings of great physical strength and
suspicious or frankly deluded thinking, and violence becomes more inevitable.
Interestingly, regular users of stimulants are familiar with the experience of paranoid
thoughts, and often retain sufficient insight to remove themselves from the company
of others until their thoughts return to normal, which usually happens without
recourse to specific treatment over 3–10 days.

The withdrawal, or come down, from cocaine and amphetamine is characterized by
a depression of mood, which may be so profound as to require short-term hospitalization. Exhaustion is matched by an excess of sleep, but disturbed by troublesome
and morbid nightmares. In short, any aggression at this stage is likely to be turned
inwards.

Ecstasy is often included as a stimulant drug but can be seen as belonging to a separate group, if preferred. Ecstasy and similar drugs combine amphetamine and LSD
effects. Tolerance to the perception-altering properties happens quite quickly but the
emotional bonding, which is seen to be the hallmark feature of the drug, persists. It
may well be that commonly reported effects of ecstasy have as much to do with the
setting in which it is taken, usually clubbing, as with pharmacology.

Biographical snapshot

Around the turn of the century, medical practitioners were more likely than members
of any profession to be addicted to cocaine. Sigmund Freud was perhaps the most
famous of these physicians. After about 1892, biographers write of a change in Freud's
personality characterized by marked swings of mood, an outpouring of work, indis-
criminately placing sex at the centre of his analytical theories, and an intolerance,
even a hatred, for old friends and colleagues, most notably Joseph Breuer. Freud's
potential for violence was in fact contained, not least because he enjoyed the reputation of a genius rather than of a psychotic. Interestingly, Freud failed to connect the
'murderous and sadistic lusts' of his own dreams with cocaine use, preferring an analytical interpretation. So the picture with cocaine is of a drug with little respect for

setting or character; stimulants induce a sense of arousal and power coupled with paranoia (Thornton 1983).

Depressant drugs

Numerically this is the largest group of psychoactive substances, and includes alcohol, minor tranquillizers, barbiturates, hypnotics, and other sedatives. It is probably useful to include cannabis within this group, since it is normally smoked, in the UK at least, as a relaxant. If preferred cannabis can, however, be set in a group of its own. It is usually held that drugs with a relatively non-specific mode of action, such as alcohol and barbiturates, impair higher cortical control centres in the brain, thereby disinhibiting the expression of emotions, thoughts, and behaviours normally not seen. The intoxicated person becomes more talkative, and may feel highly confident or even omnipotent, but in reality is less able to process information and is operating with impaired judgement. Setting aside any latent aggression or antisocial personality characteristics, there is scope here for any normal, well-adjusted person to misinterpret interactions or events, thereby increasing the potential for a violent outcome. The benzodiazepine transquillizers, such as diazepam (Valium) and lorazepam (Ativan) have a specific effect on neurotransmitters, and the mode of action of cannabis is unknown; for practical purposes, however, the consequences of intoxication are very similar to those found with other depressants.

In contrast to the stimulant drugs, the dangers of violence diminish as the dose of depressant increases, the capacity for co-ordinated movement is lost, and ultimately coma supervenes. There is a benzodiazepine antagonist available but otherwise no specific treatment for depressant overdose. Care should be taken to protect against inhalation of vomit, especially when alcohol has been consumed, and hospitalization may be necessary when a cocktail of depressants has been taken or when consciousness is difficult to maintain. Cannabis is again an anomaly here, in that overdose is characterized by a state of anxiety and fear, which may progress into paranoid and confused state akin to that described for stimulants, but without the overactivity; talking down is usually sufficient.

There are three distinct phases of depressant withdrawal. First, and by far the most common, is the tremulous state, which is characterized by shakiness of hands, tremulousness of the face and whole body, tachycardia, anxiety, and dysphoria; in more severe cases there may be fleeting hallucinations and illusory distortions of the immediate environment. In short, the potential for violence stems from a state of over-arousal. These symptoms emerge within 6–8 h of stopping drinking. A similar tremulousness and irritability may be seen after heavy cannabis smoking.

For alcohol, benzodiazepines, and barbiturates a second phase of withdrawal may be manifest as seizures; for alcohol these usually occur 24–36 h after stopping drinking. A third and still later phase, usually 72 h after stopping drinking, is delirium: the delirium is often characterized by very frightening visual hallucinations, often brightly coloured images of menacing animals such as rats, snakes or spiders, and is often associated with paranoid ideas. There is a marked increase in the likelihood of violence, which will be directed against the hallucinations or delusions.

Biographical snapshot

In Western countries, alcohol is the most widely used legal recreational drug, and is often used by lovers and friends in social settings. Caitlin Thomas, in her biography of Dylan Thomas, describes him as a passive man, indeed a pacifist, and yet their drinking sessions together were frequently scenes of argument, though it seems not physical violence. Writing of one row she says, 'I can't remember how it started but . . . everywhere was covered in green toothpaste . . . neither of us could remember what happened . . . probably something to do with women' She describes herself as ashamed of a visit to America because of 'all that drinking and fighting [verbal]', and yet excuses her husband on the grounds of his being a poet! In fact, the picture is one of family and marital neglect related to drinking, interspersed with frequent arguments while intoxicated (Thomas 1987).

Opiates

Opiates include all those substances that have a morphine-like effect. Most commonly misused are diamorphine (heroin), morphine, methadone (Physeptone), dihydrocodeine (DF118), codeine, and buprenorphine (Temgesic). The opiates work through specific receptors within the brain and receptors associated with the intestines. The most striking effect is a state of euphoria, or feeling of being on 'cloud nine', but in a dreamy sort of way and one that is detached from the immediate surroundings. An overdose of opiates increases this state but will cause respiratory depression and possibly death from respiratory failure. The effects of opiates can be reversed with naloxone (Narcan). Violence is an unusual companion of the opiate effect.

Withdrawal from opiates may be quite trivial, rather like a cold: a runny nose and eyes, and hot and cold sweats, but progressing in more severe withdrawal to muscle cramps, and sometimes to spasm, vomiting, and diarrhoea, with some degree of agitation. Because opiates work at specific receptors, the effect of giving more opiate is completely and quickly to reverse the withdrawal state. It is in the pursuit of more opiates to avoid or relieve withdrawal that there is risk of violence. One of the arguments for long-term prescribing of methadone is that, because methadone is very long acting, repeated withdrawals, the associated cravings for more opiates, and the potential for violence are reduced.

Biographical snapshot

It is generally the case that naturally occurring substances are moderate in their effects, and it is purified forms that take on the mantle of dangerousness. So it is with opiates. Nonetheless, Thomas De Quincey in *Confessions of an English opium eater* captures very vividly the essence of opiate use (opium being the 'milk' of the opium poppy). Contrasting opium with alcohol, he writes 'the man who is inebriated is in a condition which calls up into supremacy the merely human, too often the brutal, part of his nature, but the opium eater feels that the diviner part of his nature is paramount; that is the moral attentions are in a state of cloudless serenity'. Later on he declares 'opium had long ceased . . . spells of pleasure; it was solely by the tortures connected with the attempt to abjure it, that it kept its hold', giving an insight that the opiate effect, rather than withdrawal, is central to opiate addiction. (De Quincey 1971).

Perception-altering drugs

Perception-altering drugs are something of a mixed bag, which contains solvents, butane gas, and other volatile substances, LSD, and magic mushrooms. In contrast to the previous drug categories described, where the drug effect is essentially an extension of normal experience, the perception-altering drugs have the capacity to cause experiences outside the usual perceptual experience of reality or, in other words, transient psychotic states. Volatile substances in particular endow the user with the capacity to experience illusory images, which may amuse, but which may bring fear, aggression, or morbid thoughts. Volatile substances commonly act as depressants, and so a picture similar to alcohol intoxication may be superimposed on the illusory state; at higher doses there may also be hallucinations. LSD is an extremely potent drug that induces colourful and vibrant visual hallucinations. It is also a highly plastic drug, and so the content of the hallucinations may vary from being fun to being threatening and fear provoking; the potential for violence varies accordingly. The psychosis of intoxication is best dealt with by reassurance from a trusted person who will encourage concentration to be focused on real verbal and visual stimuli; hypnotics may be useful, and major tranquillizers should be used if the psychosis persists beyond a few days. Some volatile substances have a withdrawal state similar to the tremulousness of depressants. There is no equivalent for LSD, even though experienced users become tolerant to doses 10–20 times those sufficient for naive users.

Biographical snapshot

Because LSD is such a highly plastic drug, its potential for causing violence is largely determined by the circumstances of its use, and so the link between LSD and violence may be difficult to prove. The multiple murders committed by Charles Manson and his followers have, however, been linked to LSD. It may well be that Manson's underlying delusional symptoms were born out of a schizophrenic illness but enriched by his daily use of 'acid'. LSD may have had an additional and even more important role in altering the mental state of his followers, so that they became more receptive and committed to an ideology embracing the need for ritual killing. In short, the picture is of a drug with so-called 'mind-expanding' properties, often appealing to those interested in 'alternative' life-styles, but with an effect conditioned by the setting in which it is taken.

The individual

Personality

The previous section has argued that the pharmacological effects of different drugs and the withdrawal symptoms associated with some substance-use are, of themselves, likely to increase the risk of violence. Equally, some individuals will be more susceptible to the pharmacological processes than others. Students are often taken as the subjects for research in the addiction field, since they tend to use rather more alcohol and other drugs than the general population. As a group, students are privileged in terms of educational achievement and future prospects, and so it might be expected that there would be low levels of violence among this group. The opposite has been found: in one study, 20% of males and 6% of females admitted to damaging property after drinking, and 4% of males and 5% of females admitted to involvement in an assault. Some 20% of males and 10% of females had been assaulted by another college member who had been drinking. Assaults and vandalism have been associated with heavier drinking patterns; but there is no way of knowing whether alcohol was a causal agent or whether those people who drank heavily were also more aggressive. However, with such large numbers of students reporting involvement in assaults or vandalism it is reasonable to believe that, given the combination of the right circumstances and intoxication, *any* individual has the potential for violence (West *et al.* 1990).

Drinking or drug-use probably potentiates antisocial behaviour, and vice versa, though some would go so far as to say that without adverse personality character-istics, drinkers or drug-users are no more likely than anyone else to be violent. While it may be possible to support this view by studying the co-variance of the disorders antisocial personality and substance misuse, the thesis depends upon acceptance of antisocial personality as a discrete condition. In reality definitions of antisocial personality tend to be circular, and the characteristic is best understood as existing as a continuum. Equally, the extent of substance-use or severity of dependence are understood as existing as a continuum. The two continua are not entirely independent of each other, and interactions can be expected at all points. A variant of the antisocial personality is the impulsive personality, meaning people who act without thinking and without awareness of the consequences; again the definition is somewhat circular. Impulsivity is not seen as a condition or disorder, but as a character trait that is distributed throughout the population. More impul-sive individuals are more likely to be involved in a range of so-called impulsive behaviour, such as excessive drinking, drug-use, gambling, bulimia, aggression, and self-harm (Abram 1989).

A society that lives with and expects violence will be one where violence is generally more likely, but also one where it is more likely as a first-resort solution to problems. Nonetheless, some kinds of violence have been associated with physiological factors. Taking homicide as the extreme of violence, where homicide is substance-related the offenders are more likely to have abnormal brain function. One study found that half the alcohol abusers who had caused another's death had a degree of dementia, and/or withdrawal seizures, and/or alcoholic delirium. Equally, the users of other drugs were likely to have a brain lesion or a history of psychotic episodes.

Victims

In the study of homicides referred to above, both the offender and victim were intoxi-cated, except in a very small minority of cases. Where alcohol was misused, the victim and offender were more intimate both in terms of their relationship and the method of killing: repeated stabbing, kicking, beating, and strangling were most common. Killings associated with illicit drug-use are more likely to take place in public and are more likely to be motivated by illicit drug trading than by passion. This probably reflects the fact that alcohol is the drug most commonly taken for social and recreational purposes (Lindqvist 1991).

The availability within a population of different substances and different weapons will determine the general level of their use, and this proposition also holds within subsections of the populations. A North American study, for example, found that some 10% of pregnant women were physically and sexually abused; the chances of being subject to violence increased up to 40%, however, if the women drank heavily or took illicit drugs. One follow-up study of the victims of battery has found that, of those killed by their batterers, the men killed were much more likely to be intoxicated on a daily basis and have a greater intake of both street and prescription drugs.

About 70% of assault victims attending Accident and Emergency departments in Britain have taken alcohol in the 6 h prior to assault: broadly speaking, the victims have higher consumption levels and spend proportionately more of their income on alcohol than would be expected from the general population. In younger age groups, however, drinking alone does not distinguish victims. Consistent with this, there is a relationship between high binge consumption and severe injury in assault. Violence is often instigated by the eventual victim.

A rather different problem arises where individuals believe they have been assaulted, usually sexually, while under the influence of drugs: complaints of sexual assault, when assault could have happened, are well known in association with benzodiazepine sedation or anaesthesia. Equally, benzodiazepines, alcohol, and other drugs have been given, usually to women, to facilitate rape and to fog the women's recollections of the sexual assault. The concept of so-called 'date rape' once again brings substance misuse and violence out of the closet. It is not good enough to pretend that these behaviours are the monopoly of deviant or mentally disturbed people, rather there is a need to change social attitudes and values more generally.

The setting

The number of intoxicated people that are seen in different health care settings varies quite markedly. Accident and Emergency departments, general practice surgeries, out-patient clinics, and people's homes are all places where people who misuse alcohol or other drugs are likely to be intoxicated. It may be tempting for health-care professionals to try and minimize their contact with people who are intoxicated but to do so risks missing concurrent physical or mental illness, and also risks communicating rejection of the drinker or drug-taker, which may be a trigger for confrontation and violence. People who are intoxicated are more likely to be accompanied by friends or relatives who are also intoxicated and who are equally likely to misunderstand and misinterpret communications.

For the most part, health-care professionals see the consequences of aggression or violence that occurred elsewhere rather than experiencing it first-hand. Most violence associated with substance-misuse is thought to occur in the domestic setting, and therefore has implications for the transmission of both behaviours to new generations. This mechanism does not explain all the associations between crime, violence in particular, and substance-misuse; much debate has revolved around the question 'does drug-misuse lead to crime or does crime lead to drug-misuse?'. There seems to be agreement that intoxication, rather than regular use, is behind much substance-related violence. At a very crude level of analysis it can be said that the criminal career, not necessarily violence, antedates the substance-misuse career about as often as the opposite is true. There is a strong association between progression of the substance-misuse career from licit to soft drugs, soft to hard drugs, and hard drugs to injecting drugs, and criminal activity of all kinds. Violence, including gang fights, assault, and armed robbery, has been reported as happening, on average, from 5 days a year for licit users to 36 days a year for injectors, though variations are quite marked within each group: violence may be related not only to the severity of drug-taking but also friends' drug-taking and to the extent of previous criminal history. The overview is of a teenage group where delinquent behaviour, including violence, vandalism, and experimentation with alcohol, solvents, cannabis, and to a lesser extent hard drugs, co-vary; each element nudges the other on a stage further (Hammersley *et al.* 1990).

Why do some adolescents grow out of this phase and others not? A lack of conventional social support and associating with friends that have criminal or drug-using backgrounds have also been shown to be important factors in the process of pushing an individual towards a lifestyle that embraces both crime and substance-misuse, the one feeding the other. Not all illegal drug-use involves violence, and not all legal use is peaceful. The difference is that the repertoire of violent behaviour grows with the progression from soft, legal to hard, illegal substance-use. Unfortunately these findings open up few easy opportunities for intervention, suggesting a need for fairly intensive individualized programmes.

The family has been identified as a source of learning that violence is an acceptable and normal part of a relationship: studies have found 50–90% of violent incidents in the home occur while at least one family member is intoxicated, and about two-thirds of the cases involve alcohol, while one-third involve other drugs. What constitutes violence in the home has generally been defined in subjective terms of what is unacceptable to the recipient, rather than in terms of categorizing the behaviour. So, unacceptable aggression may be anything from pushing or slapping through to forced sex or assaults with weapons.

Support for a link between child abuse, physical or sexual, and substance-misuse being transmitted in families is claimed from studies of young offenders. Among these young people there are high prevalence rates for misuse of illicit drugs and a consistent positive association with a range of childhood abuse, accounting directly for as much as 30% of illicit drug use.

Disturbances of child development are difficult to rectify later in life, and especially so where there is dependence on alcohol or other drugs. It follows that it may be useful for carers to develop skills of remedial work with children in families where violence and substance-misuse coexist. It has been argued that intoxication serves to excuse violent behaviour with the aim of maintaining family integrity: this is another example of the user, retrospectively, making sense of an unwanted behaviour; but, in common with defence mechanisms, understanding is insufficient to inform action. So what protective interventions are available to the carer? Two general principles are useful: first, the less the disruption to family life the greater the chance of survival;

and, second, the less the violence and substance-misuse, the greater the chance of survival.

The first principle can be supported in different ways depending on how much family cohesion remains. At one extreme the task may simply involve securing stricter adherence to family routines such as meal times, taking the children to school, quality time with parents, and regular bedtimes; at the other extreme remedial work may have more to do with practical, self-preservation ploys for the children, such as having a key to get in and out of the house, knowing who and how to telephone for help, and having a safe place to go. The second principle may be difficult to support. The violent behaviour and substance-misuse behaviour should be tackled separately, possibly involving specialist help. The more unwanted behaviour there is in a household, then the more coping strategies have to be used by partners and, to some extent, children; clearly a point may be reached where these coping strategies are failing or become exhausted altogether. So, alongside efforts to treat the unwanted behaviours directly, it may also be useful to teach partners coping skills: the general principle will be selectivity, and judiciously choosing to attack or ignore substance-misuse behaviours, while encouraging agreeable interpersonal contacts. This is best done by working individually with partners and listing their responses to episodes of intoxication: having done this it is usually easy for partners to see which of their coping behaviours are likely to exacerbate substance misuse and possibly aggression, and which will achieve the opposite and desired effect (Orford *et al.* 1998).

Understanding and dealing with violence

The well-established association between violence and substance-misuse is seen to be crude when account is taken of violence as an end-point that can be reached by many routes. Take, for example, a serious assault causing actual bodily harm, and consider the possible reasons. First, an assault may be an act of enforcement. A drug dealer or liquor trader has a business to protect, and any weakness in collecting payment or defending a particular patch could quickly lead to the collapse of the business; this kind of violence may well occur as part of organized crime, and spill over into gang wars. A similar kind of problem may arise from disputes about the quality and quantity of the usually illicit drugs being dealt. 'Enforcement' violence is clearly a police matter.

Second, an assault may be to do with the effects of intoxication. In this case violence may be a way of communication for the inarticulate, an expression of anger for the introverted, or a consequence of misunderstanding for the person who has impaired judgement. People tend to get intoxicated with people they know and, in so far as this happens, then 'communication' violence will be directed at a friend, partner, or relative; in another sense the violence will be undirected and lack real purpose. It may be possible to deal with simple intoxication without involving the police and much depends upon the willingness of the individual to move to a safe place, which may be home, a hospital, or designated 'drying out' centre.

A third reason for an assault is mental illness as a result of intoxication or withdrawal. Mental illness in this context does not include personality problems, but rather refers to a state, albeit temporary, where there is a loss of contact with reality. In these states it becomes apparent that an individual's behaviour is actually a response to frightening hallucinations or delusional ideas that contain some element of threat. Drug-induced psychotic states are to be distinguished from functional psychosis by the presence of confusional and affective elements in the mental state. Individuals thought to be in danger can be detained under the Mental Health Act, even though the mental illness is substance-related. Many such psychotic states are ephemeral, lasting only a few hours or days. Nonetheless, any case of delirium (meaning confusion, disorientation, or hallucinations, which are usually visual and secondary delusions), or any case of paranoid psychosis (meaning well-formed delusions or disorganized thought), where some threat is perceived, should be treated in a hospital setting, or at least under the direction of a clinician experienced in the field of mental illness and substance-use.

Checking out substance-misuse

Whatever the cause of violence, the behavioural management, from the viewpoint of health professionals, is initially the same: the objective will be to ensure the safety of staff, patients, and others present. The precise action will depend upon circumstances, and the general principles are discussed elsewhere in this book. It may or may not be obvious at the outset that a violent situation, potential or actual, is substance-related, and so it is useful for health care professionals to have a checklist in mind. Naturally the checklist will need the application of common sense to modify the approach in different settings.

Is the aggression substance-related?

In the majority of cases, it is self-evident that substance-use at least contributes to a situation. The individual will often be known, both sober and intoxicated, and there will often be a history from friends or relatives. In the absence of obvious signs it is still most likely that abnormal behaviour, particularly in young people, is substance-related; if appropriate, check pockets or handbags for drugs, enquire in a matter-of-fact, non-judgemental tone about possible use, and look for external signs such as injection marks, abnormal pupillary reactions, or indicator stains or marks on clothing. If possible a urine sample for toxicology screening and a blood sample for an alcohol level will be useful investigations. Depending on the sensitivity of the assay, substances are likely to be detected in urine for 3–4 half-lives after ingestion. For example, cocaine will very rarely be detected, except as its metabolite; whereas cannabis may be detected for more than one week after a single smoke.

Is the aggression caused by simple intoxication?

It may only be possible to make a preliminary judgement. The ideal solution is to place the person somewhere that they can 'sleep it off', 'come down', 'sober up': in other words, environmental manipulation without prescribing medication is usually adequate. A 'carrot and stick' approach is worth practising: first apply the 'stick' in the form of overwhelming odds, discreetly available in the background; then apply the 'carrot' in the form of a personal approach that will be sympathetic and concerned to resolve immediate problems. The intoxicated person may misunderstand conversation, leading to further aggression, and is likely to be amnesic for some parts of the discussion. It follows that the carer should give very clear and simple statements about what is going on and not expect a therapeutic session at this point. The immediate task is to isolate the source of violence in a safe place where further assessment can be made. Any appointments, perhaps with a local addiction service, should be given in writing, with the sentiment that the carer is anxious that the person or client should seek help.

Is the aggression caused by an abnormal mental state?

It is probable that containment of any aggression caused by psychosis will be symptom- rather than diagnosis-based. However, medication should, if possible, be withheld until after a psychiatric assessment. The important exception to this rule is Wernicke's encephalopathy, which is caused by thiamin deficiency commonly associated with chronic alcoholism, and which should be dealt with as an emergency, with the administration of intravenous thiamin. Drug-induced psychoses are frequently associated with confusion and disorientation: the essential action here is for a staff member to remain in constant contact as far as possible, to keep external stimuli to a minimum, and to give regular reality orientation. The environment should be well-lit, but with plain furnishings. The same principles apply where an individual is experiencing abnormal perceptions, particularly visual hallucinations, as part of delirium or intoxication with perception-altering drugs. Paranoid states either emerge from intoxication with drugs such as stimulants or cannabis, or present as secondary symptoms as part of delirium, and in either event they require non-specific treatment; chronic paranoid states, particularly when occurring in clear consciousness, should be treated as a functional psychosis.

Are there other problems to check out?

Having decided that someone is intoxicated, there is always a danger of becoming blind to the possibility of coexisting illness such as diabetes, chest infection, heart failure, head injury, or meningitis—all these are over-represented among people who misuse alcohol and other drugs. These conditions may themselves lead to aggression. In short, beware of intoxication masking other conditions, which may require urgent attention. Equally, be aware of the possibility of future complications: check out the likelihood of a single drug or a polydrug overdose, a history of seizures, delirium, or any other medication or condition that would indicate hospital admission.

The attempt here has been to highlight some issues specific to substance-use and violence. Always these specific points are to be taken alongside general approaches to containing violence, and always to be applied with generous amounts of common sense, drawing upon any relevant disciplines and established knowledge concerned with treating the problems of addiction.

Summary

Tackling alcohol together (Raistrick *et al.* 1999) sets out the evidence base for a UK Alcohol Policy: the recommended policy mix includes specific measures to minimize 'drunkenness' and maximize community and domestic safety. Similarly, for illicit drugs, in the report *Drug Misuse and the Environment* (ACMD 1998) there is a new emphasis on community action safety. The relationship between substance-misuse and violence is, however, complex: the more illicit and more deviant addictive behaviours are associated with more violence, but each potentiates the other.

Violence most commonly accompanies intoxication, but may also be associated with withdrawal symptoms and, usually in indirect ways, with high levels of dependence. The four major categories of psychoactive substances, namely stimulant drugs, depressant drugs, opiates, and perception-altering drugs can all cause, in some way or another, changes of mental state that increase the possibility of violence. Given the right mix of circumstances and drug effect, most individuals have a potential for aggression or violence. Subgroups of the population with histories of physiological disturbance in brain function or organic brain syndromes are more prone to extremes of violence under the influence of psychoactive drugs.

The appropriate management of aggression depends upon an accurate assessment of its meaning. Health-care workers need to be clear about which situations demand a response from the police and which demand medical interventions. Health-care workers need to adapt general principles of management violence to suit their particular work setting and professions.

References

Abram, K.M. (1989). The effect of co-occurring disorders on criminal careers: interaction of antisocial personality, alcoholism, and drug disorders. *International Journal of Law and Psychiatry*, **12**, 133–48.

Advisory Council on the Misuse Drugs (1998). *Drug misuse and the environment.* The Stationery Office, London.

Chick, J. (1994). Alcohol problems in the general hospital. In *Alcohol and alcohol problems, British Medical Bulletin* 50 G. Edwards, and T. J. Peters (ed) pp. 200–10. Churchill Livingstone, London.

De Quincey, T. (1971). *Confessions of an English opium eater.* Penguim Harmondsworth.

Hammersley, R., Forsyth, A., and Lavelle, T. (1990) The criminality of new drug users in Glasgow. *British Journal of Addiction*, **85**, 1538–94.

Lindqvist, P. (1991). Homicides committed by abusers of alcohol and illicit drugs. *British Journal of Addiction*, **86**, 321–6.

Nutt, D. (1999). Alcohol and the brain. Pharmacological insights for psychiatrists. *The British Journal of Psychiatry*, **175**, 114–9.

Office for National Statistics (1999). *Social Trends 29*, The Stationary Office, London.

Office for National Statistics (1998). *Living in Britain: results from the 1996 General Household Survey: a survey carried by Social Survey Division.* The Stationery Office, London.

Orford, J., Natera, G., Davies, J., Nava, A., Mora, J., Rigby, K. *et al.* (1998). Tolerate, engage or withdraw: a study of the structure of families coping with alcohol and drug problems in South West England and Mexico City. *Addiction*, **93**, 1799–1813.

Raistrick, D., Hodgson, R., and Ritson, B. (1999). *Tackling alcohol together, The evidence base for a UK alcohol policy.* Free Association Books, London.

Stahl, S.M. (1996). *Essential psychopharmacology.* Cambridge University Press, Cambridge.

Thomas, C. (1987). *Caitlin, a warring absence*, Pan Books, London.

Thornton, E.M. (1983). *Freud and cocaine, the Freudian fallacy*. Blond and Briggs, London.

Walsh, M.E. and Macleod, D.A.D. (1983). Breath alcohol analysis in the accident and emergency department. *Injury: the British Journal of Accident Surgery*, **15**, 62–6.

West, R., Drummond, C., and Eames, K. (1990). Alcohol consumption, problem drinking and antisocial behaviour in a sample of college students. *British Journal of Addiction*, **85**, 479–86.

Chapter 3

Mental disorder and violence

Henrietta Bullard

Mental disorder and violent crime

The relationship between mental disorder and violence is complex and the assessment of risk is difficult and imprecise. Although there is an association between mental disorder and violence, the risk of violence in those with mental disorder is dependent on a number of variables including the type of disorder, the nature and severity of the illness, the influence of co-morbidity with drug and alcohol misuse, the history of any previous violence, and the effectiveness of treatment and management. Clinicians are poor at predicting future violence and are accurate in no more than one out of three cases (Gunn 1993). This high rate of false-positive assessments must result in the restriction of the liberty of individuals who do not pose a risk. Actuarial methods of assessing risk are based on unchanging empirical data and do not help the clinician to predict the probability of a violent outcome without considering dynamic variables, such as the patient's willingness to be supervised, his compliance with medication, co-morbid substance-misuse and his response to treatment (Buchanon 1999).

Epidemiological studies have shown that substance-misuse is a major risk factor in violent offending (Coid 1996; Swanson, 1994). This is true for people with mental illness and for those without. For persons with mental illness alone, the risk of violent offending is three times that found in those who do not have a mental illness. For persons who are mentally ill and have a substance-misuse disorder, the risk rises to three times that found in people with mental illness alone. Of people with mental illness, 40% are co-morbid for substance-misuse (Johns 1997).

Serious violence, and particularly homicides, perpetrated by the mentally disordered have had a profound effect on clinical practice and on government policy (Department of Health 1994). Since 1994, inquiries to investigate the circumstances surrounding homicides committed by mentally disordered offenders have been mandatory (Appleby *et al.* 1999). These inquiries have shown that most mentally abnormal offenders who kill are already known to the psychiatric services (Ritchie *et al.* 1994). Successive inquiries have been critical of the care offered to these patients and in many cases have concluded that inadequate risk assessments, poor knowledge of previous violence, failure to record violent incidents, and a tendency to minimize the seriousness of violent behaviour have contributed to the fatal outcomes. An analysis of 40 homicide inquiries between 1988 and 1997 concluded that more homicides could be prevented by improved mental health care than by attempts at better risk assessment and management (Taylor *et al.* 1999). There are about 40 homicides attributed to mentally disordered offenders each year, out of a total of 600 homicides recorded by the police. There are a further 300 killings resulting from dangerous driving. Although the actual risk of homicide by the mentally disordered is small and has shown no increase over the years, the government has emphasized its commitment to the protection of the public by enacting new legislation on stalking, introducing registers for sex offenders, making homicide inquiries mandatory, introducing the Supervision Register and, most recently, announcing plans to incarcerate (and treat) those deemed to suffer from severe personality disorders (dangerous people with severe personality disorder, DSPD), whether or not they have committed a crime. A review of the Mental Health Act 1983 is underway and includes proposals for a Community Treatment Order. As a result, there is a risk that resources will be increasingly targeted on patients known to be violent or on those assessed as posing a high risk of violence. The public opprobrium, which attaches to doctors and psychiatric services resulting from a critical inquiry report, will inevitably substantially lower the threshold for deciding levels of perceived risk.

Mental disorders

Mental disorder is defined in the Mental Health Act 1983 as meaning 'mental illness, arrested or incomplete development of mind (mental impairment), psychopathic disorder and any other disorder or disability of mind'. Mental illness is not defined in the Mental Health Act or in the ICD-10 Classification of Mental and Behavioural Disorders, but by convention is used to include the psychotic, neurotic, and organic brain disorders.

Schizophrenia

Schizophrenia is a common and often damaging mental illness. The majority of patients in psychiatric hospitals, and now increasing numbers in the community, have schizophrenia. It affects nearly 1% of the population and its effects on the lives of sufferers and their relatives are profound. There is a slight preponderance of males, and the illness characteristically presents in late adolescence and early adult life. The onset of the illness may be abrupt or insidious. There is often a prodromal period when the young person becomes less sociable and fails to achieve his or her potential at school. They may 'drop out' and behave in an uncharacteristic manner: neglecting their appearance, and sometimes abusing illegal drugs. Some patients become interested in psychology, philosophy, and the paranormal. This period of the illness is followed by increasingly bizarre behaviour, associated with hallucinations, abnormal beliefs (delusions), and difficulty with language. Many patients experience paranoid delusions, which they hold with unshakeable conviction. These delusions cause great distress, and some patients feel persecuted and victimized all their lives. They may complain that their minds or bodies have been 'taken over', and that none of their thoughts are their own. One patient killed himself in prison after many years of believing that the Home Office was electronically spying on his brain. He wore a metal foil hat to prevent penetration of the 'rays'. This patient was not susceptible to rational argument and had no insight into his illness. He was nevertheless suffering as a result of his delusions, and during a period of low mood killed himself. It is sometimes not appreciated that the life-time risk of suicide in schizophrenia is 10%. Suicide may be the result of intolerable and protracted paranoid delusions or, tragically, can occur when patients develop insight into their illness and recognize the hopelessness of their situation.

One of the most serious consequences of schizophrenia is the gradual deterioration in the personality. Once lively and energetic young people with a zest for life become strange and withdrawn. They may have difficulty in caring for themselves and neglect their personal hygiene. As the illness progresses, the more florid symptoms usually subside and patients are left with a 'defect state'. This describes a state in which there is loss of drive and initiative, and patients may not even be able to get up in the morning without prompting. Our large psychiatric hospitals, now closed, were home for thousands of schizophrenic patients who were thought to need asylum. The concept of asylum and institutional care is now an unfashionable one, and the current trend is for care in the community.

Effective medication is available for patients with schizophrenia. Antipsychotic drugs, for example, the 'typical antipsychotics' such as chlorpromazine, haloperidol, and the depot preparations, do help most patients. Newer drugs, termed 'novel atypical antipsychotics', which include risperidone and olanzapine, have fewer side-effects. Claims that the newer drugs are superior still need evaluation with well-designed clinical trials. Both typical and atypical neuroleptic drugs are used to suppress or alleviate florid symptoms, including delusions and hallucinations, which are commonly found in schizophrenia. Patients who do respond to treatment regain insight, and are often willing to continue medication when they leave hospital. This is known to be important, and patients who relapse are often found to have discontinued medication before becoming ill (Swanson *et al.* 1998). A proportion of patients remain psychotic and resistant to modern drugs. These patients cannot hope to live normal lives in the community.

Most patients with schizophrenia never show physical violence and never commit offences (Coid 1996). Patients with schizophrenia tend to be withdrawn and non-assertive. However, a minority of patients do become verbally and physically aggressive, and it is important that for this minority the circumstances leading to violent episodes are understood and properly monitored. Many of the patients who commit serious offences of violence and require treatment in one of the three special hospitals (Broadmoor, Rampton, and Ashworth) have a history of previous psychiatric treatment associated with threats of violence or actual violence. The prediction of violence is fraught with difficulties, but doctors and other professionals must be alert to the possibility of dangerous behaviour. The risk will be higher where patients have a history of assaults, have used weapons or have expressed an intention to harm or kill, have a named victim or victims, and where there is evidence of relapse of a psychotic illness (Noble and Rodger 1989). Recent research points to the importance of 'threat/control override' symptoms in predicting violence (Beck-Sander and Clark 1998; Link 1998). This confirms the clinical view that patients with paranoid schizophrenia act violently when they feel threatened, to the point where they feel justified in overriding legal and moral objections. Families are often at most risk and, because of the hopelessness associated with mental illness (schizophrenia in particular), the mentally ill are often cared for by elderly parents. The presence of a mentally ill son or daughter in the family home is stressful and, if patients harbour paranoid delusions about their families and are not receiving any psychiatric treatment, they may, in response to their illnesses, erupt into violence. There is evidence that where family violence and schizophrenia are associated, the mother is most at risk.

Epidemiological studies suggest that a diagnosis of a DSM III Axis I diagnosis (schizophrenia and affective disorders) increases the prevalence of violence four times compared with controls, and where psychotic disorders and substance misuse coexist, the prevalence is 10 times that of controls (Johns 1997). Psychotic symptomatology, particularly delusions associated with thought control, thought insertion, and persecution, increase the risk of violence (Taylor *et al.* 1993). Studies in prisons have shown a high prevalence of mental disorder amongst both sentenced and remand prisoners. Mental disorders over-represented in prisons include personality disorders and psychoses, often complicated by Drug misuse. Drug misuse has reached epidemic proportions in prisons and the mentally ill are particularly susceptible and vulnerable to bullying by drug dealers.

Manic–depressive psychosis

The manic and the depressed patient both suffer from a disorder of mood, and both conditions may coexist in the same patient at different times. Manic–depressive psychosis is the name given to an illness characterized by pathological fluctuations in mood. The manic patient is irritable, overactive, and disinhibited. They feel wonderful and may describe grandiose delusions, perhaps believing themselves to be a famous brain surgeon or related to royalty. They talk incessantly and ideas come tumbling out: some make sense, some do not. Although manic patients pose a risk to themselves by spending their money recklessly, making unconsidered sexual liaisons, and by restless overactivity, they rarely inflict serious violence. Such patients are difficult to manage in the community and urgently need hospital admission. Because of their exuberance in public places they are often picked up by the police. The police need to exercise skill and judgement when handling a manic patient, who will probably not want to co-operate. The police are often subjected to assaults, usually punches and kicks, by manic patients, who may cause a considerable disturbance in a police station. A police cell is not an appropriate place for someone who is mentally ill, but it usually has to do until the patient can be detained under the Mental Health Act and transferred to hospital.

The depressed patient suffers from a pathologically low mood, as a consequence of which they are unable to make rational judgements. Their whole outlook on life is coloured by their depressive disorder, which will also influence their behaviour. Suicidal ideas are common, and 15% of depressed patients succeed in committing suicide. There is a high risk of suicide in women who kill their children and in men who kill their wives. While depression is associated with homicide, this is always in the context of the family, while homicides committed by patients suffering from schizophrenia are more random. Depressed patients rarely, if ever, kill strangers.

Neurotic disorders

The neurotic disorders include anxiety states, obsessive compulsive disorders, post-traumatic stress disorder (PTSD), and somatiform disorders. Neuroses are life-long disabling conditions, but they do not involve the patient in loss of contact with reality. Neurotic patients know there is no substance to their anxiety, but continue to suffer as if there were. There is a condition called a 'dissociative state', which is commonly seen in neurotic patients who are under stress. These patients react to stress by psychological denial. They no longer feel in contact with themselves or their problems, and during these periods of altered consciousness may behave bizarrely. It is very rare for patients to be violent while in a dissociative state, although less serious acquisitive offending may occur.

Post-traumatic stress disorder often follows exposure to major trauma and can be the precipitant for serious violence. Childhood physical and sexual abuse (see below) appear to be the precursors of both post-traumatic stress disorder and self-harm and violence. In women victims of childhood sexual abuse, self-harm is rather more common than violence to others. Self-harm and violence do occur together and the risk of either event occurring has to be assessed for each individual. The battered woman syndrome is thought to be a variant of PTSD (Roth and Coles 1995). Women who have been subjected to prolonged physical or psychological abuse experience PTSD symptoms. When women have killed the perpetrator, usually a partner, the courts have come to accept that they do suffer from PTSD, which 'substantially impaired their responsibility'. In these cases a charge of murder is reduced to manslaughter on the grounds of diminished responsibility.

Personality disorders

People are not all the same, but most people conform to the basic rules of a civilized society. We do not kill unless seriously provoked or in self-defence; we do not rape or cause physical harm to others. If we do harm to or injure another person we feel guilt and remorse. There are some people who know the rules but do not or cannot comply with them. Aggressive psychopaths who are persistently assaultative probably have little or no control over aggressive impulses. They themselves may have been the victims of violence, and their reactions and behaviour have been modelled on those of their parents. They can be very dangerous, and particularly when under the influence of alcohol. They may however show genuine remorse; and not all psychopathic personalities have the cold, emotionless inner world that is usually ascribed to them.

There is a group of personality disordered patients who account for much of the violence both in hospital and in the community. They are often diagnosed as having emotionally unstable personality disorders characterized by impulsivity, disturbance of mood, sensitivity to rejection, and low self-esteem. They react to stress by impulsive acts of violence or self-harm. Patients who suffer from emotionally unstable personality disorders often give a history of childhood physical and sexual abuse, sometime persisting over many years. There is a gender difference in the expression of symptoms in these patients and male patients tend to be more assaultative and destructive, while female patients demonstrate more self-harm. However, the potential for violence in female patients should not be underestimated, and in special hospitals not only is the percentage of female patients higher than in any other psychiatric setting but the severity, persistence, and frequency of violent incidents on female wards is higher than that on male wards.

Emotionally unstable personality disorder is the most common diagnosis in men who kill their wives or partners and in women who kill their children. Such people find intimate relationships difficult and constantly strive to ward off feelings of loss, rejection, and abandonment. Men who kill their wives are usually both dependent and depressed. There may have been a deterioration in the relationship, possibly due to the partner's need for more freedom and autonomy. He may interpret her interest outside the home as a criticism and rejection of himself. These feelings may then turn to rejection and anger. An insecure, emotionally unstable man may decompensate in his ability to cope with the stress of real or imagined loss and, in a mood of depression mixed with anger and resentment, he loses control and kills his wife.

Delusional or pathological jealousy is the term used to describe a syndrome where the patient becomes convinced his wife or girlfriend (usually wife) is unfaithful. He goes to extreme lengths to 'catch her out', and may examine her knickers for semen stains and go through her handbag for clues of infidelity. The underlying disorder may be secondary to an alcohol psychosis or, more commonly, to a schizophrenic psychosis. The outlook for recovery is poor. Pathological jealousy differs from normal jealousy not only in degree but also in quality.

The sexual psychopath, who is fortunately very rare, may only demonstrate his potential for violence in a sexual context. Abnormal sadistic sexual fantasies are private and hidden until they are acted out in a sexual assault. The sadistic sexual psychopath needs violence, in either fantasy or reality, to fulfil his sexual needs. The number of previous sexual offences is the best predictor of future offending. Subsequent sexual offences often have an identical *modus operandi* to previous offences.

Mental impairment

Mental impairment is defined in the Mental Health Act as a 'state of arrested or incomplete development of mind which includes significant impairment of intelligence and social functioning and is associated with abnormally aggressive or seriously irresponsible conduct'. Mental retardation is the term used in the ICD-10 Classification of Mental and Behavioural disorders and in clinical practice the term used is learning disability. The learning disabled have difficulties in learning and acquiring sufficient skills to confront a complex world. The severely impaired lack capacity to make decisions about their lives and require long-term residential care. A small minority demonstrate unpredictable and violent behaviour and need to be compulsorily detained in hospital. Their aggression is usually non-directional and unpredictable. Nursing staff need to have accepted procedures for controlling and restraining severely mentally impaired patients during aggressive outbursts. The minimum of force must be used, and every effort needs to be made to calm and relax the patient.

Mild degrees of learning disability may be associated with minor sexual offending, and occasionally with more serious offences, including arson and sexual violence. The physical and sexual abuse of children may occur in families where both partners are intellectually impaired. Social deprivation, including poor social functioning, poor housing, inadequate state-supported child-care, illiteracy, unemployment, and excessive alcohol consumption may all contribute to violence in the family. Families where both partners are intellectually impaired need regular social supervision. There is a higher prevalence of psychotic disorders, mood disorders, and emotionally unstable personality disorders in persons with learning disability. These patients often present with aggressive and challenging behaviour, which may lead to offending and imprisonment. In prison they are under stress and at risk of exploitation. Self-harm, suicide, and violence (mostly directed towards property) are common. It is important that patients with multiple handicaps are correctly diagnosed and managed.

Organic brain syndromes

The organic dementias are a rare cause of dangerous behaviour. They include senile and pre-senile organic psychosis, alcohol psychosis, alcohol dementia (Korsakov's psychosis), drug psychoses, and transient organic psychotic condition. These disorders are characterized by confusion, disorientation, memory loss, poor concentration, lack of judgement, and sometimes hallucinations. Most people with severe memory loss require institutional care. For example, a man with an alcohol dementia could play the piano and converse reasonably convincingly, but could not remember who he was, where he was, or what he had said a few minutes earlier. Unpredictably, when in hospital, he killed the man in the next bed. He had no memory of the incident, and was found unfit to plead at his trial. He had never been violent before, but when assessing his potential for future violence caution needed to be exercised, and it was concluded that, as his condition was untreatable and his mental state unchanged, he represented a risk to other patients. He is detained in Broadmoor Hospital under the Criminal Procedure (Insanity and Unfitness to Plead) Act 1991.

The brain-damaged patient is usually a young male with a frontal lobe syndrome following a road-traffic accident. He has intellectual impairment and memory loss, and often demonstrates disinhibited behaviour. He is usually mobile, and may make inappropriate sexual advances to women, which include touching, indecent exposure, and improper suggestions. Violence is uncommon but, when it does occur, is usually minor. Patients with organic brain disorders are often childish, and have a lowered tolerance of frustration.

Epilepsy is not associated with an increased tendency to violent behaviour. The concept of the 'epileptic personality' has been discredited. It used to be thought that persons suffering from epilepsy were more likely to be irritable and aggressive. Violent incidents do, rarely, occur in epileptic fugue states, when patients are in an altered state of consciousness. They may be able to perform motor activities like driving a car, but, afterwards, have no recollection of what they have done during that period.

Treatment and management of the mentally disordered and violent patient

General approach

Psychiatric treatment incorporates the skills of doctors, nurses, psychologists, occupational therapists, and, perhaps most important, the family and the patient. There is no cure for schizophrenia or for disorders of personality and we have no understanding of causation. Schizophrenia cannot be prevented, but the effects of the illness can be modified. Depressive illness can be treated successfully with antidepressant drugs, and the duration of the illness can be dramatically reduced. However, in most cases it is not possible to predict whether the illness will recur. Thus, psychiatric treatment can broadly be seen as encompassing everything that happens to a patient between diagnosis and recovery and post-recovery.

The diagnosis is of crucial importance, and the doctor must take a thorough history of the illness, the presenting symptoms, the personal and family background, any previous medical and psychiatric treatment (including drug and alcohol use), and any violence or offending behaviour. While eliciting the history, she or he will be observing the appearance, the behaviour, and the demeanour of the patient. Even if the patient says nothing, or is too restless to be interviewed, a provisional diagnosis should be attempted, and arrangements should be made for further assessment and treatment. This is usually referred to as 'management'. The final diagnosis may not be arrived at immediately, but as full an assessment as possible should be made. What is wrong with the patient? How long has something been wrong? Why is he or she behaving like this? Who can provide more information about the patient's background and history? Is the patient under the influence of alcohol or drugs? Has the patient a history of psychiatric illness? Has the patient a record of violence, and in what context? Could this be an organic as opposed to a functional psychosis? This may seem a tall order when confronted in casualty or in the police station by an excited patient, but much of this information will be obtained at a glance. Or the patient may be accompanied by a relative or the police, who will tell you what they know.

However disturbed or threatening a patient may seem, there is usually a part of that person in touch with reality. There is a condition known as catatonic schizophrenia, where the patient is completely withdrawn, mute, and inaccessible; but this is not common. It is important to approach patients the right way, and to explain who one is and that one wants to help. Sometimes small gestures are more important than words: perhaps offering the patient a seat or something to drink. It is often appropriate to empathize with what one thinks the patient may be experiencing. If patients look suspicious and are guarded in their answers, this may be a cue to enquire whether they feel someone is trying to harm them or is talking about them in a pejorative or malevolent way. It is usually not a good idea to try and persuade patients that they are wrong in their beliefs; this inevitably leads to confrontation, which can result in further distress, and sometimes violence.

Social workers have difficult decisions to make about the safety of children, and may themselves be at risk from assaults. Social and other professional workers have been threatened, assaulted, and in some cases killed by people for whom they have had a statutory responsibility. Social workers and others who have contact with aggressive clients should not stay alone in the same room as someone who has threatened violence or shown signs of losing control. It is best to terminate the interview, or to request help from a colleague where this is possible. It is also important to recognize that isolated and inadequate people do become dependent on social workers, nurses, doctors, etc., and occasionally react with violence when the relationship is terminated. Patients and clients have damaged the property of professionals, threatened violence, taken hostages, and caused great fear. It is difficult to assess how dangerous it is for doctors, social workers, nurses, the police, and others to visit disturbed people in their homes. The risk can be minimized by taking sensible precautions (see Chapter 2). It is unwise for any professional with a statutory responsibility for taking children into care, for removing people to hospital, or for detaining under the Mental Health Act, to pursue these objectives while unaccompanied. The disturbed patient, or even someone who is simply angry, will be more reassured by someone who is confident, feels safe, and knows what he or she is doing. It is possible to be compassionate and understanding, and at the same time to exercise one's professional duties and responsibilities.

Management of physical violence

The management of the acutely disturbed patient may require physical restraint. Methods of control and restraint have been developed that enable nurses who have been trained in the technique and other professionals to restrain a violent or aggressive patient without causing injury to the patient or to the nursing staff. Once restrained, it is usually necessary to sedate the patient and seclude them until they can safely be reintegrated into the ward. Seclusion is used only when absolutely necessary, and never as a punishment. Patients in conditions of seclusion need constant observation, and accurate records must be kept. Dangerous objects that could be used as weapons should be removed, and precautions taken to ensure that the patients cannot harm themselves. When patients are not responsible or in control of their behaviour, a few hours in seclusion, adequate medication, and good nursing care can help them much more than allowing them their freedom, which may result in dangerous behaviour and injuries to other patients and staff.

Disturbed patients in the casualty departments of hospitals and in police stations present special problems. Patients may be brought in by the police or wander in unaccompanied. They may be aggressive or noisy or both. They are probably incapable of giving an account of themselves, and may resent any questioning. They may be injured or smell of alcohol, and professional staff have to make a provisional diagnosis and decide what to do. If the patient is thought to be suffering from a psychiatric disorder, the police surgeon in a police station, or the duty psychiatrist in a general hospital, should be asked for advice. Preparations may need to be made for the patient's detention under the Mental Health Act, and this will involve contacting an Approved Social Worker and two doctors, one of whom must be approved under Section 12 of the Mental Health Act. Where possible, the patient's general practitioner should provide one of the opinions. The general practitioner or police surgeon will request advice from the duty psychiatrist. Immediate treatment can be given under common law but has to be given with caution. There have been deaths in custody and in hospital that have followed the administration of medication, usually by injection. Clinicians need training in the use and dangers of rapid tranquilization, and should be familiar with the drugs used and be able to assess the risks of cardio-pulmonary complications. An organic cause of the patient's behaviour must be excluded before the administration of medication. Patients may have taken an overdose of alcohol or narcotic drugs and be dehydrated or physically ill. A less common cause of disturbed and violent behaviour is a cerebral tumour.

In the police station there may be concern about restraining and secluding a psychiatric patient. This is understandable, as a police cell is not an appropriate 'place of safety'. Under Section 136 of the Mental Health Act the police may remove a person thought to be suffering from a mental disorder and considered in need of care or control to a place of safety. Unfortunately, the 'place of safety' is all too often a police station. Most psychiatric hospitals have no reception facilities, and disturbed psychiatric patients are either taken to general hospital casualty departments or to police stations. This is not the fault of the police, who would much prefer to take the mentally disordered to psychiatric hospitals. The person may be detained in the place of safety for up to 72 h. The purpose of Section 136 is to enable the person to be examined by a doctor and interviewed by an Approved Social Worker. In some cases an application may be made for compulsory admission of the patient to hospital for assessment or for assessment followed by treatment.

Psychiatric provision

The psychiatric services are commissioned by the health authorities and primary care groups, and managed by mental health and community trusts. Health authorities and primary care groups have a statutory duty to fund provision for both in-patient and community services. Social services are responsible for the provision of residential and day care for all patients who need this level of support. Case Management is the term used to describe the delivery and monitoring of care through the Care Programme Approach (Department of Health 1995). This is an integrated multidisciplinary model of care, which is designed to help professionals share information, monitor progress, assess unmet needs, and make an assessment of risk. A prediction is made of the risk of harm to the patient or others, and factors thought to increase the risk of untoward events are identified. The importance of suitable accommodation, compliance with medication, daytime occupation, and evidence of adequate self-care cannot be overstressed.

Local psychiatric services provide a comprehensive service for patients who need psychiatric care in hospital and in the community. A minority of patients need nursing in conditions of physical security. Whether patients need security depends on whether they are likely to abscond from an open ward, whether they have demonstrated any serious violence recently or in the past, and whether they are thought to represent a risk in terms of violent behaviour or personal harm. Physical security can be perimeter security, ward security, or room security, or a mixture of all these. A locked door may be all that is required to detain patients physically so that they can benefit from medical and nursing care. The general rule is that patients should be nursed in the least restrictive environment compatible with the patient's safety and the safety of others. In the past the 'locked ward' had a bad reputation, which in many cases was justified. These wards were overcrowded and understaffed, and there was little creative therapy to occupy the patients. Where physical security is thought to be necessary, patients can be nursed in low, medium, or high security.

Low secure units

Patients who are acutely psychotic sometimes need to be nursed in conditions of low security. Low security usually means a locked door to prevent patients from leaving, combined with a high ratio of nursing staff to patients. Wards are small and, ideally, the number of patients should not exceed ten. The physical environment is important as disturbed patients, and the nurses caring for them, need space, airiness, natural light, and access to fresh air. A seclusion room is required for patients who are assaultative or who are judged to be at risk of imminent violence. Seclusion should only be used when other methods to calm the patient have failed. It should never be used as a punishment. Nursing staff should be trained in control and restraint techniques, and in the care of patients who are secluded. It is particularly important to keep good records of violent incidents and follow all procedures and policies that relate to seclusion These records should be regularly examined by senior medical and nursing staff, and be available to the Mental Health Act Commission for scrutiny.

Medium secure units

Medium secure units were developed in response to growing concern about the plight of the mentally disordered in prison. In 1992, the Department of Health instructed health authorities to include mentally disordered offenders in their strategic and purchasing plans (Department of Health 1992). In the same year, the Government published the final report, by the Home Office and Department of Health, of a joint review of services for mentally disordered offenders and others requiring similar services (Department of Health, Home Office 1992). The final report recommended that high-quality care should be provided near to a patient's home and, where possible, in the community, but otherwise in the least restrictive conditions justified. The committee recommended that mentally disordered offenders should be cared for by general psychiatry and learning disability services. The committee made 276 recommendations and these had far-reaching implications for services for the mentally disordered. At the same time, the principles of Case Management and the Care Programme Approach were being implemented and high-profile homicide enquiries focused the Government's policy-making on the protection of the public (Department of Health 1995).

Medium secure units have, as the name suggests, a medium level of security. The physical security consists of a perimeter fence of 3–4 m in height and locked internal security. The ratio of staff to patients is high and the physical environment is spacious and should allow for good observation. Patients are admitted to medium security from courts and the prisons, and most patients are detained under Part III of the Mental Health Act 1983. The majority of patients in medium security are male, the ratio being about six to one. The main diagnostic category is mental illness, although most medium secure units admit patients suffering from psychopathic disorder.

In recent years the numbers of medium secure beds nationally has risen and much of the provision has been provided by the private sector. There is a need for medium secure provision for adolescents, the learning disabled, and the severely brain damaged. There is also an urgent need for services for patients who require long-term care in conditions of medium security.

Special hospitals

Special hospitals are constituted by Section 4 of the National Health Service Act 1977 by which the Secretary of State for Social Services is required to provide special hospitals 'for patients subject to detention' who 'require treatment under conditions of special security on account of their dangerous, violent and criminal propensities'. The special hospitals were managed by the Department of Health and Social Security until they were reorganized in 1989 and a new Special Hospitals Services Authority was constituted. This authority managed the three special hospitals, Broadmoor, Rampton and Ashworth, but each hospital had its own local management. The SHSA was disbanded in 1998 and its responsibilities subsumed by the High Security Commissioning Board. In 1999, following complaints about the activities of patients on the personality disorder unit at Ashworth Hospital, the Fallon Report published its findings in 1999. The report criticized the management of the hospital, both that at a local level and the Special Hospitals Service Authority. One of the recommendations of the Fallon Report was that the special hospitals should be integrated within the general psychiatric services and they are now managed by local NHS Trusts.

The level of security in special hospitals is high and there is perimeter and internal security. At Broadmoor Hospital, 75% of the patients are classified as suffering from mental illness and 25% are classified as suffering from psychopathic disorder. At Rampton Hospital there is provision for patients suffering from mental impairment and severe mental impairment. There is a preponderance of males in special hospitals, in a ratio of four to one. All the patients in special hospitals are detained, and at Broadmoor Hospital 60% of patients are subject to special restrictions and can only be discharged by a tribunal or by the Secretary of State.

The treatments available in special hospitals are as good, if not better, than those found in regional secure units and psychiatric hospitals. The perimeter security allows patients more freedom to move from their wards to the workshops and the occupations department. Although security is higher in special hospitals, the atmosphere is less oppressive for the patients than the ward security of medium secure units. Patients usually move to medium secure units before they are discharged to the community.

Legal aspects of management

The mental health act 1983

While most patients are admitted informally, the Mental Health Act makes provision for the compulsory detention of patients suffering from any of the four forms of mental disorder as defined in the Act. Admission to hospital can be for assessment or for treatment, and there is provision for the detention of patients who are already in hospital. Admissions for assessment are for 72 h and, where two doctors make a recommendation under Section 2, for 28 days. Admission for treatment (Section 3) allows a patient to be admitted to a hospital and detained for a period of 6 months. The grounds for admission under the Mental Health Act are that the patient is suffering from one of the four forms of mental disorder of a nature or degree that makes it appropriate for them to receive treatment in hospital, and it is necessary for the health or safety of the patient or for the protection of other persons that they should receive such treatment. In the case of psychopathic disorder or mental impairment, the doctors have to confirm that treatment is likely to alleviate or prevent a deterioration of the patient's condition.

Part III of the Mental Health Act 1983 is concerned with the mentally disordered offender. There is provision in Section 48 for the transfer to hospital of the mentally ill and severely mentally impaired who have been remanded in custody. Section 47 allows the transfer to hospital of a mentally disordered offender who is serving a sentence of imprisonment. Section 35 empowers the court to remand an accused to hospital for a report, and Section 36 allows the Crown Court to remand an accused to hospital for treatment. Hospital orders (Section 37, Mental Health Act 1983) can be made in the Magistrates Court and the Crown Court. The Magistrates Court can, in certain circumstances, make a hospital order without recording a conviction. In most cases, a hospital order is made in the Magistrates Court following conviction on lesser charges and in the Crown Court following conviction on more serious charges. The hospital order is the most frequently used section for the detention of mentally disordered offenders. If the safety of the public is thought to be at risk, the court can apply a restriction order under Section 41. The restriction order makes the patient liable to be detained in hospital unless absolutely discharged by a Mental Health Review Tribunal or by the Secretary of State. Restriction orders can be for a limited period or without limit of time. There are also provisions under the Mental Health Act for the transfer by the Home Office of remand and sentenced prisoners to hospital for treatment. There has been some concern expressed about the transfer of sentenced prisoners to hospital towards the end of their sentence. Once transferred to hospital, the person concerned then finds themself subject to what can be indeterminate detention.

Patients' rights

A patient detained under the Mental Health Act has a right to apply to a Mental Health Review Tribunal for discharge, except where the order for detention is for 72 h. Mental Health Review Tribunals were established in 1960 following the introduction of the Mental Health Act 1959. The Tribunal is appointed by the Lord Chancellor, and consists of a legal, a medical, and a lay member. Medical members are usually psychiatrists, and the Tribunal is chaired by the legal member. In the case of a restricted patient, the legal member is drawn from a panel of specially appointed lawyers, who are usually circuit judges or recorders. Patients are entitled to legal advice, and solicitors may obtain the services of an independent psychiatrist to prepare a report. The

Tribunal also obtains a medical report from the patient's responsible medical officer, who usually represents the detaining authority at the hearing. The medical member of the Tribunal examines the patient before the hearing, and both he and the independent psychiatrist have access to the patient's medical records. At the hearing, the Tribunal has powers to discharge unrestricted patients and to discharge restricted patients conditionally or absolutely. Patients who have been transferred from prison and who are subject to a restriction order cannot be discharged by a Tribunal. The Tribunal can make recommendations to the Secretary of State concerning its view as to whether the patient should be returned to prison or should remain in hospital for further treatment.

Patients have no right to refuse medication during the first three months following detention, but after that it is unlawful to give patients medication without their informed consent. If it is felt to be in the interests of the patient to continue with medication, a second opinion can be obtained from a doctor appointed by the Mental Health Act Commission. Electro-convulsive therapy cannot be given to a patient without either their consent or a second opinion.

Mental health act commission

Between 1959 and 1983 there was no statutory independent body designated to visit psychiatric hospitals and to protect the interests of patients. During this period there were a succession of scandals and allegations of ill-treatment, cruelty, and neglect. The Mental Health Act Commission was established in 1983 as a Special Health Authority, and is responsible to the Secretary of State for Health. It is an independent body with a chairperson and 91 part-time members. The functions of the Commission are laid down in Section 121 of the Mental Health Act 1983.

The role of the home office and the protection of the public

The Home Office is responsible for ordering the transfers of remand and sentenced prisoners to hospital and for the supervision of conditionally discharged restricted patients. This latter function is administered by the Mental Health Unit at the Home Office, and officials remain in close contact with both the patient's responsible medical officer and the social worker who is managing the patient in the community. Regular reports are submitted to the Home Office, who have the power to recall a patient to hospital at any time. The Home Office usually only exercises its power to recall if there is a serious risk to the safety of the public. Once recalled to hospital, a patient has the right to apply to a Mental Health Review Tribunal.

The Home Office may also commission the advice of the Advisory Board on restricted patients. This is an independent non-statutory body whose members are appointed by the Home Secretary. The Advisory Board was set up in 1973 following a report chaired by Sir Carl Aarvold, which reviewed the procedures for the discharge and supervision of psychiatric patients subject to restriction. The Aarvold Committee considered that there were patients in special hospitals who, because of the nature of their offending, did require special care in assessing their suitability for conditional discharge. The selection of cases is made by officials in the Home Office, who seek the agreement of the Minister concerned that the case should be referred to the Advisory Board.

Diversion of mentally disordered offenders from custody

In 1990 the Home Office issued Circular 66/90 entitled 'Provision for Mentally Disordered Offenders' to encourage a policy of diversion of mentally disordered offenders from custody (Home Office 1990). Circular 66/90 was circulated to health authorities, social services, the probation service, and Magistrates and Crown Courts. Circular 66/90 recognized that diversion from custody could occur at a number of different stages in the criminal justice process, and made recommendations about a multidisciplinary approach to the problem. Court liaison services have been set up in various parts of the country to study the size of the problem and to initiate procedures aimed at diverting the mentally disordered from the criminal justice system to hospital.

Predicting and preventing violence

Risk assessment and risk management

Dangerousness can be defined as violence involving injury or lasting psychological harm. It is easier to predict that someone will repeat a violent act if they have shown a tendency to behave in a similar way on previous occasions. If someone habitually becomes aggressive when drunk, it is reasonably safe to assume that while they continue to drink to excess, they will present a danger. On the other hand, if someone has committed a single offence involving violence and has otherwise been a stable person, the statistical chances of a repetition must be small unless there are other factors, including mental disorder, which might influence the prediction. A risk assessment is done by identifying both static and dynamic risk factors. It is essential to take a detailed psychiatric history from the patient and to ensure that, as far as possible, the information given by the patient can be validated. There are no short-cuts to risk assessment and information about infancy, childhood behavioural problems, socio-economic status of the family, racial and cultural background, parental separation, involvement of social services, parental violence, physical and sexual abuse, offending—particularly violent offending—substance abuse, physical and mental health, sexual preferences and attitudes, educational achievement, work record, and the patient's personality, must be obtained before any weight can be given to individual risk factors. This information is largely static, historical, and cannot be changed. Mental disorders are dynamic risk factors and individuals with an antisocial personality disorder may be more or less dangerous depending on whether they are drinking alcohol, at a football match, or abusing illegal drugs. Environmental factors are particularly important when assessing risk in personality disordered patients.

Serious mental illness is associated with an increased risk of violence. However, most violence is perpetrated by people who are not mentally ill. Antisocial personality disorder should be given a much higher weighting for recidivist violence than mental illness. The life-time prevalence of substance-misuse (including alcohol) disorders is

80% in antisocial personality disorders and 40% in schizophrenia. Substance-misuse is the main risk factor in predicting violence, and those with mental illness who also misuse substances are three times more likely to be violent.

Risk management is the manipulation and modification of identified risk factors. The aim of treatment is to minimize the risk. The challenge to care teams is to identify risk and make reasoned judgements about what action to take. What should be done when a mentally ill patient refuses to take medication? Is the care team aware of the pattern of this individual's illness? How soon can a violent outcome be predicted? Is the patient also abusing alcohol or drugs? What effect is the patient's poor housing and social isolation likely to have on the illness or on the assessment of risk? What degree of violence is predicted? Do they use a weapon? Has the patient a named victim? Does the diagnosis predict a high risk, for example pathological jealousy? Do they demonstrate threat/control override symptoms? Do they have insight into their illness? These are some of the questions that arise when clinicians try to manage risk.

The following examples highlight the importance of threat/control override symptoms in the first case, and the use of a knife, in the second case. In both cases there was social isolation and no evidence that the illness was under control. Both patients suffered from paranoid schizophrenia and neither had insight into the nature of their illness.

Example: A 26-year-old man with a history of admission to psychiatric hospitals had a diagnosis of paranoid schizophrenia. Following his last admission he remained rather solitary and was unemployed. He lived with his mother and sister, and had never shown any violence. On the day of the offence he was watching his sister peel potatoes and suddenly became convinced that she was stealing his brain. He got up, walked into the kitchen, picked up a knife, and stabbed his sister to death. Following this he could give no other explanation for killing than that he felt an uncontrollable urge to stab her. This patient did recover to some extent, but because of the unpredictable nature of his violence he will be difficult to supervise.

Example: A 25-year-old woman was diagnosed as suffering from paranoid schizophrenia at the age of 16. During the previous nine years she had spent several months each year in hospital. Following discharge from hospital she had not taken her medication and her illness had relapsed. Each admission to hospital was precipitated by some form of violence involving her stabbing or attempting to stab her family or strangers. As she had not caused any serious harm she was not considered to be particularly dangerous. This was an error of judgement: a patient suffering from schizophrenia who attacks or threatens people with knives is a considerable danger to the public. She was admitted to Broadmoor Hospital after stabbing a stranger in the street. Following treatment in Broadmoor Hospital she has made an excellent recovery, but while it may be appropriate to recommend her transfer from conditions of maximum security, caution must be exercised before recommending her discharge to the community.

Treatment and management

The treatment of mental disorders is given in hospital, and in the community, and the model of care is the Care Programme Approach and Case Management. Most patients are treated informally, and compulsory assessment and treatment cannot be given in the community. Treatment is co-ordinated by multidisciplinary teams who work together to deliver care that is regularly reviewed. Teams are composed of psychiatrists, social workers, psychiatric nurses, and occupational therapists. A key worker is responsible for ensuring that there is a care plan and for arranging regular reviews.

All those concerned with the care of the mentally disordered in hospital and in the community are conscious of their need to protect the public. The supervision of psychiatric patients is of the utmost importance, and social workers, psychiatrists, families, and in some case the Home Office work together to minimize the risk to the public by providing adequate support, close supervision, and regular assessments of the patient's mental state. Psychiatrists and others who are asked to make predictions about dangerousness have no reliable scientific tools to help them. At best, predictions are made on the basis of statistical evidence, for example, the reconviction rate of sex offenders, but statistics will not give an accurate prediction in any individual case.

Example: A 30-year-old man had convictions for indecent exposure during his early teens, and at the age of 17 indecently exposed himself to a woman, who retaliated by attacking him with a rake. He claimed he lost his temper, pushed her to the ground, put his hands around her throat until she lost consciousness, and after undoing her trousers ran off. He was convicted of attempted rape and after serving a 3-year prison sentence committed no further offences for 5 years. He then committed a series of offences involving breaking into houses where young women were asleep on their own, indecently exposing himself to them while wearing a mask, and then waking them up by indecently assaulting them and masturbating over them. He could give no explanation for this behaviour and did his best to distance himself from any sexual motive. This man had been committing similar offences since the age of 16, which is evidence that he does have serious sexual psychopathology. There is certainly a risk that he will offend when released from prison, but it is impossible to make an accurate prediction. It is also difficult to know whether treatment for his sexual deviation can be expected to minimize the risk, or over what period. Sex-offender treatment programmes have been widely used in prisons and follow-up studies seem to suggest a reduction in re-offending in the short-term. We await the results of controlled trials and longer term follow-up studies.

People who care for disturbed and sometimes violent members of society need support and respect. They put themselves at risk and are responsible for the safety of others. This responsibility is easier to shoulder if the professional can feel confident that their work is being scrutinized by their peers and by other disciplines. They must always be aware of the dangers of professional isolation and the need to work in collaboration with other disciplines.

Further reading

Mitchell, E.W. (1999). Does psychiatric disorder affect the likelihood of violent offending? A critique of the major findings. *Med. Sci. Law*, **39**, (1).

(1997). Risk assessment and management in psychiatric practice. *International Review of Psychiatry*, **9**,(2/3).

Royal College of Psychiatrists Special Working Party on Clinical Assessment and Management of Risk (1996). *Assessment and clinical management of risk of harm to other people.* Council Report CR53. Royal College of Psychiatrists, London.

Wessely, S. (1997). The epidemiology of crime, violence and schizophrenia. *British Journal of Psychiatry,* **170**, Supplement 32, 8–11.

References

Appleby, L., Shaw, J., Amos, T. *et al.* (1999). *Safer services: report of the national confidential inquiry into suicide and homicide by people with a mental illness.* Department of Health, London.

Beck-Sander, A., and Clark, A. (1998). Psychological models of psychosis: implications for risk assessment. *Journal of Forensic Psychiatry,* **9**, (3), 659–67.

Buchanon, A. (1999). Risk and dangerousness. *Psychological Medicine,* **29**, (2), 465–73.

Coid, J. (1996). Dangerous patients with mental illness: increased risks warrant new policies, adequate resources, and appropriate legislation. *British Medical Journal,* **312**, 965–6.

Department of Health (1992). *The health of the nation.* (Cm1986). HMSO, London.

Department of Health (1994). *Guidance on the discharge of mentally disordered people and their continuing care in the community.* NHS Executive HSG(94)27 and LASSL(94)**4**, 10 May 1994.

Department of Health (1995). *Building bridges. A guide to arrangements for inter-agency working for the care and protection of severely mentally ill people.* HMSO, London.

Department of Health, Home Office (1992). *Review of health and social services for mentally disordered offenders and others requiring similar services. Final summary report.* (Cm2088). HMSO, London.

Gunn, J. (1993). Dangerousness. In *Forensic psychiatry: clinical, legal and ethical issues* (ed.), J. Gunn and P.J. Taylor, pp.624–45. Butterworth–Heinemann, Oxford.

Hedderman, C. (1995). The supervision of restricted patients in the community. *Research findings No. 19.* Home Office Research and Statistics Department, London.

Johns, A. (1997). Substance misuse: a primary risk and a major problem of co-morbidity. *International Review of Psychiatry,* **9**, 233–41.

Link, B.G., and Stueve, A. (1994). Psychiatric symptoms and the violent/illegal behaviour of mental patients compared to community controls. *In Violence and mental disorder. Developments in risk assessment* (ed. J. Monahan and H.J. Steadman), pp.137–59. University of Chicago Press, Chicago.

Link, B.G., and Stueve, A. *et al.* (1998). Psychotic symptoms and violent behaviours: probing the components of 'threat/control-override' symptoms. *Soc. Psychiatic Epidemiology* **33**, 55–60.

Marshall, P. (1994). Reconviction of imprisoned sexual offenders. *Home Office Research and Statistics Department: Research Bulletin,* **36**, 23–29.

Monahan, J. (1996). The MacArthur Violence Risk Assessment Study. An executive summary of the research of the working group. Proceedings of the MacArthur Foundation Research Network. *Violence, competence and coercion: the pivotal issues in mental health law.* Wadham College, Oxford 3–4 July 1996.

NHS Management Executive (1994a). *Guidance on the discharge of mentally disordered people from hospital and their continuing care in the community.* HSG (94)27 (Leeds, NHSME).

NHS Management Executive (1994b). *Introduction of supervision registers for mentally ill people from 1 April 1994.* HSG (94)5 (Leeds, NHSME).

Noble, P., and Rodger, S. (1989). Violence by psychiatric in-patients. *British Journal of Psychiatry,* **155**, 384–90.

Ritchie, J.H., Dick, D., and Lingham, R. (1994). *The Report of the Inquiry into the care and treatment of Christopher Clunis*. HMSO, London.

Roth, D.L., and Coles, E.M. (1995). Battered woman syndrome: a conceptual analysis of it's status *vis-à-vis* DSM IV mental disorders. *Medicine and Law*, **14**, (7–8), 641–58.

Swanson, J.W. (1994). Mental disorder, substance abuse, and community violence: an epidemiological approach. In *Violence and mental disorder. Developments in risk assessment* (ed., J. Monahan and H. Steadman), pp.101–36. Chicago University Press, Chicago.

Swanson, J.W., Holzer, C.E., Ganju, V.K., and Jonjo R.T. (1990). Violence and psychiatric disorder in the community: evidence from the Epidemiologic Catchment Area Surveys. *Hospital and Community Psychiatry*, **41**, 761–70.

Swanson, J, Borum, R., Swartz, M., and Monahan, J. (1996). Psychotic symptoms and disorders and the risk of violent behaviour in the community. *Criminal Behaviour and Mental Health*, **6**, 309–30.

Taylor, P.J., and Gunn, J. (1984). Violence and psychosis I—Risk of violence among psychotic men. *British Medical Journal*, **288**, 1945–9.

Taylor, P.J., and Gunn, J. (1999). Homicides by people with mental illness: myth and reality. *British Journal of Psychiatry*, **174**, 564–5.

Taylor, P.J., Mullen, P., and Wessely, S (1993). Psychosis, violence and crime. In *Forensic psychiatry. Clinical, legal and ethical issues* (ed. J. Gunn and P.J. Taylor), pp.329–72. Butterworth–Heinemann, Oxford. *Working for patients. Provision for mentally disordered offenders*, Home Office Circular 66/90. Home Office, London.

Chapter 4

Non-accidental injury of children

Alan Emond

Historical and cultural background

Children have been victims of violence since ancient times, and in all societies (Finkelhor and Dziuba-Leatherman 1994). Violence has been perpetrated against them in every conceivable manner: physically, emotionally, by sexual exploitation, through neglect, and by enforced labour. Exposure and infanticide have been near universal forms of child abuse over the years, allowing many societies to ensure that only healthy newborns survive. This freedom for parents to kill defective or unwanted babies continued in some parts of Europe until the nineteenth century. In 1885, the Society for the Prevention of Cruelty to Children reported the ways in which London children were battered: by boots, crockery, pans, shovels, straps, ropes, thongs, pokers, fire, and boiling water. Severe physical chastisement was regarded in Britain as an acceptable form of disciplining children until well after the Second World War. The introduction of the term 'battered child' in 1962 was thus a new name for a very old problem, but marked the beginning of increasing awareness and concern about violence towards children (Helfer and Kempe 1987). Physical abuse is still, however, often underestimated as a cause for childhood fatalities (Committee on Child Abuse and Neglect, American Academy of Paediatrics 1993).

The most fundamental change that has taken place in society's attitude towards children in the last 40 years has been the acceptance (and now enshrinement in UK law under the Children Act 1989) that children are not the possessions of their parents, but have rights of their own (Department of Health and Social Security and Welsh Office 1988). In addition, it is now accepted that children require special protection because of their dependency on adults for care, and parents and society have a responsibility to meet their needs. However, violence towards children remains an enormous problem in Britain, and takes many forms. Non-accidental injury is merely the physical and most obvious manifestation of violence; but sexual abuse, emotional abuse, and neglect have equally damaging effects on children in the long-term (Malinosky-Rununell and Hansen 1993). Although it is probable that violence towards children occurs in all societies, cross-cultural variability in child-rearing beliefs and practice make it difficult to define a universal standard for good child-care, abuse, and neglect. While cultures differ in their definitions of child maltreatment, all societies have criteria for what constitutes acceptable behaviour towards children (Belsky 1993). In a society like Britain, which is changing and becoming more multicultural, the boundaries of acceptable behaviour towards children in areas like discipline are also changing. Professionals who work with children require both a sensitivity to different rearing practices in families from different cultural and religious backgrounds, and also a clear understanding of the consensus of what is acceptable adult behaviour towards children.

Non-accidental injury in the family

The vast majority of non-accidental injuries take place within families. The family is paradoxically both the most physically violent group or institution that a typical citizen will encounter and also a group that children look to for love, support, and gentleness. Violence towards children cannot be separated from violence in families on a wider scale. The caretakers who abuse and injure children are most often biological parents, but may be step-parents, adoptive or foster parents, grandparents, siblings, or other relatives. Violence towards children is often linked to other violent behaviour in families, and is particularly associated with wife-battering. A study in Bristol UK (Ward et al. 1993), compared an Accident and Emergency department register of adult victims of violence with the Child Protection Register of children who had been physically abused. Women who had been the victims of domestic violence were shown to be significantly more likely to have their children registered for physical abuse. This research emphasized the importance of ensuring protection of the children of women who seek treatment for injuries sustained in assault.

The origins of violence in the family, and of its manifestations as non-accidental injury to children, are complex. The risk factors for physical child abuse are multi-causal, and are illustrated in Table 4.1. For example, it is common for abusive parents to give a history of experiencing neglect or violence in their own childhood. Inconsistent, unsympathetic care in childhood, with unrealistic demands, excessive criticism, and punishment for failure results in adults with poor self-esteem, poor basic trust, and a poor understanding of how to provide for a child's needs (MacMillan et al. 1995). Violent behaviour will manifest in such adults at times of stress, and if directed at children in the family will lead to patterns being transmitted from parent to child and so the potential for physical abuse, neglect, and sexual exploitation is transferred to another generation (see Chapter 9).

Table 4.1 Risk factors for child physical abuse

Young maternal age

Social isolation

Single parent

Large family size

Psychotic illness in a parent

Violence between spouses

Parents own experience of abuse

Unplanned pregnancy

Disabled child

Physical injury to children is usually perpetrated by a caretaker who has a tendency to be violent, which is related to his or her early life, and this is often directed at a child who is perceived in some way to be unsatisfactory. The child may be unwanted, or the wrong sex, or have the wrong facial features. The precipitant to the violence is often a crisis of some sort, placing extra stress on a caretaker who is poorly supported and externalizes inner conflict and frustration as violent behaviour. The stress and conflict that characterizes certain families is a major factor in the non-accidental injury of children (Belsky 1993). However, violence is only one response to stress. The male predominance in perpetrators of violence to children reflects not just man's physical strength, but also his typical behavioural response to stress, while women tend to respond to stress by depression rather than violence, and may neglect their children's needs.

Fathers who are physically violent to their children are more likely to have observed their own fathers hit their mothers. Higher rates of child abuse are found in families where adults believe that physical punishment and slapping a spouse are acceptable behaviour.

Certain groups of infants and children are at risk of being physically abused and neglected. Included in this group are normal infants who are the product of a difficult pregnancy or delivery, or are born from an unplanned pregnancy, of the wrong sex, of an unloved father, or during a period of severe family stress and crisis. Infants who are perceived as 'abnormal' are particularly at risk, and these include infants born significantly pre-term, those with congenital abnormalities, and those who have chronic illnesses or physical disability. A further group of children who can be particularly at risk of non-accidental injury are those who are described as 'difficult'. These children tend to be hyperactive, fussy and difficult to feed, have abnormal sleep patterns, cry excessively, and are perceived by their parents to be unresponsive to loving care. However, although it is true that some children are extremely difficult and push their caretakers beyond their ability to cope, it is important not to stress the provocative behaviour of the child at the expense of disregarding the parent's own difficulties and deficiencies in caretaking (Wolfner and Gelles 1993).

Presentation of non-accidental injuries in children

Fractures

The original description of the battered baby syndrome by Kempe recognized the importance of any discrepancy between the parent's history and the child's clinical injuries, and highlighted the significance of multiple injuries in different sites and of different ages (Kempe *et al.* 1962). Fractures to infants and young children should be treated with particular suspicion. Most accidental fractures in infants and toddlers result from falls from more than three feet, and are single, linear, or green-stick fractures of the child's long bones, or narrow parietal skull fractures. One study from Nottingham (Worlock *et al.* 1986) showed that all abused children with fractures were under 5 years of age, and 80% were under 18 months. In contrast, 85% of accidental fractures in children occurred after the age of 5 years. Abused children are much more likely to have associated soft-tissue bruising of the head and neck, or to have multiple injuries. Other indicators of child abuse, such as failure to thrive or facial bruising, may be important cues in distinguishing non-accidental from accidental fractures.

Fractures following physical abuse occur in almost any bone, and child abuse cannot be diagnosed on the pattern of fractures alone. A careful history, including risk factors for abuse in the family, followed by a full examination, is essential for a correct diagnosis. When the injury, or the history, suggests physical abuse, or if the child is less than 18 months old, a skeletal survey will be necessary. This should be a complete radiographic survey of the child's skeleton, and should be reported by an experienced radiologist, as many cases of abuse have been diagnosed from fractures that are not clinically obvious (American Medical Association 1992). Such fractures may be old or healing, or the sites may be hidden (e.g. in the ribs, pelvis, or skull).

Metaphyseal and epiphyseal fractures are the classic injuries of child abuse; caused by pulling and twisting forces from shaking the child by the arms and legs. Fragments of bone become separated from the ends of long bones, usually as a chip or as a whole plate. Although they only account for 10% of fractures resulting from abuse, they are virtually diagnostic, as they are such uncommon accidental fractures (Ludwig and Barman 1984).

Rib fractures strongly suggest physical abuse unless there is a clear history of trauma (e.g. crush injury). Deliberate rib fractures are caused by chest compression, which often occurs during the shaking of babies, or through punches or kicks delivered to older children. Rib fractures are often multiple, and occur posteriorly. Careful and expert radiological examination is required to detect some rib fractures. Recent fractures are especially difficult to identify, particularly at the costo-vertebral junction, and an isotope bone scan may be necessary to confirm them (Haller *et al.* 1991).

Accidental fractures of the shaft of long bones usually result from direct trauma, which causes a transverse break. Non-accidental fractures, however, often arise from indirect trauma: for example, being swung by the legs leads to spiral fractures. However, there is no clear distinction between long-bone fractures arising from accidents and those arising from abuse. Other factors in the history, or the presence of other injuries, must be taken into account when considering the cause of long bone fractures (Worlock 1986).

The discovery of multiple long-bone fractures, fractures of different ages, or injuries that are not reported by the carers, should raise suspicion of abuse. Thickening or elevation of the periosteum may be a pointer to a previously unrecognized fracture.

Sub-periosteal haemorrhage lifts the periosteum from the shaft of the bone, and this process often takes 10–14 days to appear radiographically. An experienced radiologist may be able to date fractures, as healing takes place through recognized stages of periosteal new bone formation, soft callus, hard callus, and remodelling. A radiologist will also be helpful in confirming that the rest of the skeleton is radiologically normal, excluding uncommon but important genetic, metabolic, or bone diseases (e.g. osteogenesis imperfecta).

In all cases of fracture where abuse is suspected, good communication is essential between the various professionals involved — casualty staff, radiologists, orthopaedic surgeons, paediatricians, and social workers — so that mistakes are not made in diagnosis. It is very important to avoid conflicting messages being given to the family, and to ensure that clear evidence is given to the police and to the courts. The child will need follow-up, not just to ensure that the fracture has healed satisfactorily, but also to consider his or her growth, development, and emotional needs.

Head injuries

Young children frequently sustain minor injuries, often to the forehead, when learning to walk or from bumping into furniture. Most of the injures to children under 5 who fall out of bed, prams, and couches do not result in skull fractures. Although fractures of the skull can occur after fairly minor falls, most accidental fractures have been shown to result from moderate falls of between 3 and 6 ft, e.g. falling from a standing adult's arms. Skull fractures resulting from such accidents are usually linear and narrow, and characteristically affect the parietal bone. They are rarely associated with other intracranial injury (e.g. subdural haematoma). The parent may only realize that significant damage has been sustained when a hard swelling appears on the child's scalp one or two days later, and sometimes may have forgotten the original injury. Such late presentation may be viewed with suspicion, and requires careful evaluation by experienced paediatricians and radiologists to avoid a mistaken diagnosis of non-accidental injury (Billmire and Myers 1985).

Although parents who have abused their children often give a history of a minor fall or accident, the force actually used in physical abuse (violent shaking or hitting the child's head against a wall) is so much greater than that in common accidents that the pattern of injury is different. After abuse, skull fractures tend to be complex or multiple, involve more than one cranial bone, and cross more than one suture line (Carty and Ratcliffe 1995). Fractures of the temporal and frontal bones, and the thick bones at the base of the skull, are also much more likely to be due to violent abuse rather than an accident.

A useful indicator of abuse in young children is a measurement of the maximum width of the fracture. If the fracture is more than 5 mm wide, it is very likely to have been the result of child abuse, whereas accidental fractures are usually less than 1 mm in width. Growing or expanding skull fractures occur in infancy, and are associated with a dural tear and brain injury beneath the fracture. Such fractures are the result of a more serious blow to the head, and are much more likely to be associated with abuse. Subsequent enlargement of the fracture may form a cranial defect that requires surgical repair. The presence of a growing fracture, when the explanation given is a minor fall, should therefore raise suspicion of abuse.

Depressed fractures are very uncommon in young children, and indicate abuse unless a history is given of a fall on to a sharp object. A particularly characteristic injury is a depressed fracture of the frontal bone caused by hitting the child's head against the wall, the floor, or furniture (Wilkins 1997).

Children who develop irritability, vomiting, or impaired consciousness after a seemingly trivial injury are likely to have been violently abused, and should be investigated by CT or MRI scanning (Alexander *et al.* 1986). This may demonstrate a subdural haematoma, cerebral contusion, or cerebral oedema resulting from violent shaking. The presence of any of these signs is a reflection of the severity of the head injury, and is indicative of abuse (Salman and Crouchman 1997). Subdural haematomas may occasionally arise after birth trauma, but usually present within the first few days of life, and do not result in chronic signs or symptoms. Subdural haematomas presenting outside the perinatal period indicate severe head injury, and in the absence of an adequate history are diagnostic of abuse (Jayawant *et al.* 1998).

However, children may suffer serious head injuries from abuse without there being any history of trauma or external signs of physical injury (Alexander *et al.* 1990). The shaken infant syndrome is due to whiplash and rotational injury to the brain, resulting in intracerebral and subdural bleeding (Caffey 1972). Children who have sustained intracranial injury may present with unexplained neurological deficit, irritability, seizures, apnoeic attacks, or non-specific symptoms, such as feeding problems (Hadley *et al.* 1989). A careful history, neurological examination, skull X-ray, lumbar puncture, and a CT scan may be helpful in the diagnosis (Carty and Ratcliffe 1995). It is important to exclude bleeding disorder (O'Hare and Eden 1984).

Infants with head injuries, or those suspected to have been abused, should have a retinal examination after the pupils have been dilated. The presence of retinal haemorrhages without adequate explanation is strongly indicative of abuse, and is usually the result of shaking (Kaur and Taylor 1992). Violent shaking causes cerebral oedema, and the underlying increase in intracranial pressure leads to increased pressure in the central retinal vein resulting in multiple retinal haemorrhages (Duhaime *et al.* 1992).

Cerebral contusion, haemorrhage, and oedema lead to many of the deaths and much of the long-term disability resulting from physical abuse (Bonnier *et al.* 1995). Haemorrhage within the brain can directly damage cortical pathways (e.g. those concerned with vision), lead to infarction and cerebral atrophy, or result in post-traumatic hydrocephalus (Green *et al.* 1996). It is thus particularly important to identify and protect children who are subject to violent abuse to the head.

Burns and scalds

Accidental burns and scalds of young children are unfortunately far too common, and reflect inadequate supervision or lack of awareness of the dangers that common domestic appliances pose to children. It is often difficult to distinguish between careless or ignorant parenting (which is a temporary lapse in the usual protection afforded to a child) and deliberate neglect (which is a deliberate failure to protect the child).

Deliberate burning or scalding of children can cause very significant injuries, and is usually used as a punishment or to provoke fear in the child. Such injuries may also be sadistic and inflicted by an adult for excitement or sexual arousal. The separation of deliberate from accidental heat injuries is best made on the history and the behaviour of the parents. Parents whose children have accidentally burnt themselves will be anxious and guilty, and will want urgent treatment for their child. Abusive parents may lack concern, delay presentation of the injury, or tell a vague or changing story, or may be hostile and angry towards staff and refuse admission for treatment. Mothers who burn their children deliberately may themselves be depressed or seeking help, or have been themselves the victims of abuse. Children who have been deliberately injured may be withdrawn and passive, or excessively angry and rebellious.

Accidental burns and scalds are most common during the second year of life when toddlers become more mobile, whereas the peak age for children being deliberately burnt is during the third year. The reported incidence of deliberate heat injury is low (1–2% of children admitted to hospital), but this form of violent abuse is almost certainly under diagnosed and under reported.

A hospital-based study in Leeds (Keen *et al.* 1975) that compared accidental with deliberately inflicted burns and scalds found that all the abused children were under 6 years of age, and that nearly half had additional injuries or were failing to thrive. Deliberate injuries typically affected the backs of the hands, the buttocks, the feet, and the legs. The injuries were incompatible with the history given, and scalds accounted for the majority of accidents, usually following spillage from kettles or saucepans. In these accidents the hot liquid usually scalds the front of the child's body, affecting the face, trunk, shoulders, or upper arms. In contrast, the most common way of deliberately scalding children is forced immersion in a bath or a sink. This form of violent injury typically affects the soles of the feet and the lower legs or the hands and arms in a stocking or glove distribution, without splash marks. A clear tide-mark confirms that such scalds have been caused by forced immersion (Keen *et al.* 1975).

Dry contact burns from household appliances are common after both accidents and abuse. The usual site for accidental burns in the palm and tips of the fingers. Contact burns in unusual sites, showing the clear outline of an object, should give rise to suspicion of abuse. Deliberate cigarette burns are usually inflicted as punishment on the back of the hands, the arms, or the legs. Accidental brushing against a lighted cigarette causes a very superficial eccentrically shaped burn, and not the well-defined circular mark of a deliberate cigarette burn.

An improvement in the recognition of deliberate injury by burning or scalding requires increased awareness by all who deal with children, and good liaison between hospital, primary care team, social workers, and police. Visits to the home will be necessary to assess the circumstances of the injury, and to support the parents. The characteristics of the children and their interaction with their parents may give useful insight into the dynamics that lead to violent abuse. Gaining the child's confidence may lead to a disclosure of what really happened.

Bruising

Careful examination of the bodies of most children who have learned to walk is likely to reveal some small bruises of different ages. These are typically found on the bony extensor surfaces, such as the shins, knees, and elbows, and the forehead. In exploring the world, and in normal play, healthy children frequently suffer minor injuries, and these usually heal without any sequelae or disability.

Children who have been physically abused often have minor soft-tissue bruises that have been dismissed or not noticed, and these may be the early warning of much more serious injuries. The most important rule when assessing bruises and scratches, and other injuries of the skin, is not to confuse the severity of the injury with its significance in terms of child abuse. For example, small round bruises on a baby's cheek may be trivial injuries that will quickly heal, but they could be highly significant if they are finger-marks from violent gripping and shaking. Some forms of bruising are characteristic of physical abuse, e.g. finger-marks, slap-marks, and bilateral black eyes (Meadow 1989). In most cases, a careful evaluation is needed of the history, the parents' attitude, and the whole child in terms of growth, development, and behaviour, as well as of the actual injury. Checking the Child Protection Register every time a child is seen with a suspicious injury may be a time-consuming process, but will help to identify children with repeated injury, and prevent the escalation of violent abuse leading to serious injury.

The site of injury may also be critical in determining whether or not a bruise is accidental. Bruises to the head and neck are particularly significant, and would support a non-accidental diagnosis if they affect soft tissues like the cheeks or the eyelids, or if they are multiple and of different ages.

Grip-marks are commonly seen at the angle of the jaw or on the cheek. Slap-marks are found on the face or the ears, often including fine haemorrhages. Black eyes may be acquired accidentally during playtime fights or by bumping into furniture, in which case the child can usually give an account of what happened. Bruising inside the bony rim of the orbit, bruising of different ages, or eye bruising for which no explanation can be given should arouse suspicion that the injury may be the result of adult violence.

In babies and toddlers, injuries inside the mouth (a torn frenulum or bruising to the gums) may result from forced feeding, with a bottle or a spoon being rammed into the mouth — though again, such injuries alone are not diagnostic. In older children, dislodged or broken teeth may be the result of accidental falls, but can also be caused by punches to the mouth, or by being pushed down the stairs. A high index of suspicion is required to identify cases of non-accidental injury in casualty departments and dental surgeries.

Violent sexual abuse

Sexual abuse is part of the spectrum of violence towards children. In one large group of children proven to have been sexually abused, 15% initially presented with bruising or other injury (Hobbs and Wynne 1990). Doctors who examine children as part of the assessment of non-accidental injury need to be aware of the overlap between physical and sexual abuse. However, most sexual abuse in childhood does not result in physical injury, or in abnormal physical signs on genital examination.

Bruising of the buttocks, the genital area, and the breasts may be associated with sexual abuse. Grip marks on the thighs and symmetrical bruises around the knees, suggest sexual abuse with forceful gripping by the abuser. Bite marks or burns of breasts, abdomen, buttocks, or genitalia are often associated with sexual abuse. Laceration or scars in the hymen or loss of hymenal tissue are virtually diagnostic of forceful penetration. An enlarged hymenal opening, labial bruising or oedema, or vaginal discharge are supportive signs of, but are not diagnostic on their own, of violent sexual abuse (Royal College of Physicians 1991).

Similarly, abnormalities of the anus should be interpreted with caution, and other supportive evidence is required to make a diagnosis of abuse. Fresh lacerations with swelling, bruising, and congestion are strongly supportive of blunt penetrating trauma to the anus. Reflex anal dilation, anal laxity, chronic anal fissures, and 'funneling' of the anus are also seen in conditions not associated with abuse, and should be evaluated in conjunction with other evidence from a joint investigation with social services and the police.

Children suffer cognitive, emotional, and social impairments in addition to physical damage (Malinosky-Rununell and Hansen 1993). Although injuries associated with sexual abuse may be horrific, the most long-term damage caused by such violence is emotional and psychological. Many studies from around the world have shown the long-term psychiatric and sexual morbidity suffered by women and men who have been sexually abused in childhood.

Intervention and treatment

The identification of a non-accidental injury to a child is only the first stage in a process that needs to be founded on co-operation between different agencies. The first priority is to ensure that the child is protected in a 'place of safety', in hospital, in foster care, or in a safe family situation in the community. The period of separation of mother and child should be kept as short as possible whilst further investigations are carried out into the cause of the non-accidental injury and the underlying domestic situation. It may be necessary to apply to a family court for an Emergency Protection Order, which lasts for 8 days (and may be challenged in court after 72 h).

Once the child's protection is assured, a case conference will need to be convened at the earliest opportunity, with an independent chairman not involved in the case. Representatives from social work, health, the police, and education will be invited, and have to provide written reports if they cannot attend. Good practice in multi-agency working in child abuse is described in *Working together* (DHSS and Welsh Office 1988).

Good communication between the various agencies is essential, and should be combined with a respect for each other's differing roles in the assessment and management of the child and the family. The case conference is the forum to share concerns, in confidence, and to make a joint action plan that will be carried out by a 'core group' containing key workers from lead agencies involved with the family. The conference will also decide on whether to recommend that the child should be placed on the Child Protection Register (CPR), a decision that is usually ratified by an area-based review panel. It is now regarded as good practice to include one or both parents in the case-conference discussions, and it is very important to ensure that only matters of substantiated fact are placed before the conference. The parents should also have the decisions of the conference confirmed in writing.

As part of the action plan, the case conference may wish to seek legal advice on the necessity of applying to the court for a further legal order. Under the terms of the Children Act, the court may only make such an order if it is concerned that the child is at risk of significant harm, and that the child's interests are better served by making an order than by not making one.

If the order involves further assessment of the child or of the parents, the court is empowered to set a timetable for the assessment and a review date in court. The aims of the Children Act legislation are to encourage good multidisciplinary assessment with the minimum delay, to promote goal-directed treatment work with child and parents, and to keep 'out of home' placement as short as possible.

In the majority of cases of violent abuse, treatment of the child can begin as soon as the diagnosis is first suspected. Once the child's safety is secured, a treatment programme should be devised to replace what has been missing at home, and to modify behaviour patterns developed as a response to violent and unpredictable parenting (Brayden et al. 1993). If the child is placed in temporary foster care, the foster parent will need advice, guidance, and support to deal with developmental delay and disturbed behaviour. If the abused child is kept in his or her own home, regular monitoring and support will be needed from social worker and health visitor. Pre-school children who have been abused often benefit from a structured day-nursery environment, which helps their development, behaviour, and relationships with peers, as well as with other adults. The imposition of a consistent structure offers the child the opportunity to reduce anxiety, to develop impulse control, and to mature in behaviour. School-age children will need encouragement to talk about their experiences, and structured 'life history' counselling may help children come to terms with what has happened to them.

However, in order for the child's treatment to be effective, the parents must receive treatment as well (Wolfe and Wekerle 1993). First, the abuser must acknowledge responsibility for the abuse and its impact on the child. Second, the extent to which family members have not adequately provided protection for each other is an important aspect of the acknowledgement process, and families may need help to move away from blaming one member for the violence. Third, the individual who perpetrated the non-accidental injury will need help in recognizing his or her violent response to stress, and in establishing new patterns of parenting. All this takes time, appropriate help from committed and well-trained professionals, and the necessary resources (e.g. family centres). Unfortunately, adequate resources for treatment and rehabilitation of families in which violent abuse has occurred are lacking in most parts of the UK, and hard-pressed social service departments are forced to prioritize limited funds and manpower into child protection, rather than into treatment or rehabilitation.

The prevention of child abuse is an even more challenging task, which cannot be achieved by statutory provision alone (MacMillan et al. 1994). The Child Protection Registers (CPR) that are now held by every local authority in the UK are designed to facilitate the recognition of children who are at risk of abuse. The effectiveness of these registers depends on the awareness of all professionals who come into contact with children and effective communication between them. However, preventing child abuse within families requires changing parenting behaviour and interrupting the trans-generational pattern of violent responses to stressful situations.

A comprehensive preventive service would include: all new parents receiving parenting education and support; all children receiving preventive education in schools; all parents under stress having access to self-help groups and other supportive services; and all victims of abuse having access to supportive help. Such preventive services are available only in skeleton from in many areas.

Although media coverage has resulted in increasing public concern about child abuse, more education and informed discussion is required to increase awareness of non-accidental injury of children, its causes, and its implications. Violent abuse of children will ultimately only be prevented if violent behaviour within families is reduced—and this requires fundamental changes in society.

References

Alexander, R.C., Schor, D.P., and Smith, W.L. (1986). Magnetic resonance imaging of intracranial injuries from child abuse. *Journal of Pediatrics*, **109**, 975–9.

Alexander, R., Crabbe, L., Sato, Y., Smith, W., and Bennett, T. (1990). Serial abuse in children who are shaken. *American Journal of Diseases of Children*, **144**, 58–60.

American Medical Association (1992). Diagnostic and treatment guidelines on child physical abuse and neglect. *Archives of Family Medicine*, **1**, 187–97.

Balmire, M.F., and Dyers, I.A. (1985). Serious head injury in infants: accident or abuse. *Pediatrics*, **75**, 34.

Belsky, J. (1993). Etiology of child maltreatment: a developmental — ecological analysis. *Psychology Bulletin*, **114**, 413–34.

Billmire, M.E., and Myers, S.A. (1985). Serious head injury in infants: accident or abuse? *Pediatrics*, **75**, 340–2.

Bonnier, C., Nassogne, M., and Evrard, P. (1995). Outcome and prognosis of whiplash shaken infant syndrome; late consequences after a symptom-free intervals. *Developmental Medicine and Child Neurology*, **37**, 943–56.

Brayden, R.M., Altemeier, W.A., Dietrick, M.S. *et al.* (1993). A prospective study of secondary prevention of child maltreatment. *Journal of Pediatrics*, **122**, 511–6.

Caffey, J. (1972). On the theory and practise of shaking infants. *American Journal of Diseases of Children* **124**, 161–9.

Carty, H., and Ratcliffe, J. (1995). The shaken infant syndrome. *British Medical Journal*, **310**, 344–5.

Committee on Child Abuse and Neglect and Committee on Community Health Services, American Academy of Pediatrics (1993). Investigation and review of unexpected infant and child deaths. *Pediatrics*, **92**, 734–5.

Department of Health and Social Security and Welsh Office (1988). *Working together. A guide for inter-agency co-operation for the protection of children from abuse*. HMSO, London.

Duhaime, A.C., Alamo, A.J., Lewander, W., Schut, L., Sutton, M.D., Seidl, T.S. *et al.* (1992). Head injury in very young children: mechanism, injury types and ophthalmologic findings in 100 hospitalised patients younger than 2 years of age. *Paediatrics*, **20**, 179–85.

Finkelhor, D., and Dziuba-Leatherman, J. (1994). Children as victims of violence: a national survey. *Pediatrics*, **94**, 413–20.

Green, M.A., Lieberman, G., Mitroy, C.M., and Parsons, M.A. (1996). Ocular and cerebral trauma in non-accidental injury in infancy: underlying mechanisms and implications for paediatric practice. *British Journal of Ophthalmology*, **80**, 282–7.

Hadley, M.N., Volkes, K., Sonnteg, H., Rekate, H.L., and Murphy, A. (1989). The infant whiplash shake injury syndrome: a clinical and pathological study. *Neurosurgery*, **24**, 536–40.

Haller, J.O., Kleinman, P.K., Merten, D.F., Cohen, H.I., Cohen, M.D., Hayden, P.W. *et al.* (1992). Diagnostic imaging of child abuse. *Pediatrics*, **87**, 262–4.

Helfer, R.E., and Kempe, R.S. (1987). *The battered child*, (4th edn). University of Chicago Press, Chicago.

Hobbs, C.J., and Wynne, J.M. (1990). The sexually abused battered child. *Archives of Disease in Childhood*, **65**, 423–7.

Jayawant, S., Rawlinson, A., Gibbon, F. *et al.* (1998). Subdural haemorrhages in infants: population based study. *British Medical Journal*, **317**, 1558–61.

Kaur, B., and Taylor, D. (1992). Fundus haemorrhage in infancy. *Survey Ophthalmology*, **37**, 1–17.

Keen, J.H., Lendrum J. and Wolman, B. (1975). Inflicted burns and scalds in children. *British Medical Journal*, **i**, 268–9.

Kempe, C.H., Silverman, F.N., Steele, B.F. *et al.* (1962). The battered child syndrome. *Journal of the American Medical Association*, **181**, 17–24.

Ludwig, S., and Barman, M. (1984). Shaken baby syndrome. A review of 20 case. *Annals of Emergency Medicine*, **13**, 104–7.

MacMillan, H.L., MacMillan, J.H., Offord, D.R., Griffith, L., and MacMillan, A. (1994). Primary prevention of child physical abuse and neglect: a critical review. part 1. *Journal of Child Psychology and Psychiatry*, **35**, 835–56.

MacMillan, H.L., Niec, A.C., and Offord, D.R. (1995). Child physical abuse: risk indicators and presentation. In: *Recent Advances in Paediatrics* (1). Churchill Livingstone, Edinburgh.

Malinosky-Rununell, R., and Hansen, D.J. (1993). Long-term consequence of childhood physical abuse. *Psychology Bulletin*, **114**; 68–79.

Meadow, R. (ed) (1989). *ABC of child abuse*. British Medical Journal, London.

Royal College of Physicians (1991). *Physical signs of sexual abuse in children*. The Royal College of Physicians, London.

O'Hare, A.E., and Eden, O.B. (1984). Bleeding disorders and non-accidental injury. *Archives of Disease in Childhood*, **59**, 860–4.

Salman, M., and Crouchman, M. (1997). What can cause subdural haemorrhage in a term infant? *Pediatrics Today*, **5**, 42–5.

Ward, L., Shepherd, J.P., and Emond, A.M. (1993). Relationship between adult victims of assault and children at risk of abuse. *British Medical Journal*, **306**, 1101–2.

Wilkins, B. (1997). Head injury — abuse or accident. *Archives of Disease in Childhood*, **76**, 393–7.

Wolfe, D.A., and Wekerle, C. (1993). Treatment strategies for child physical abuse and neglect: a critical progress report. *Clinical Psychology Review*, **13**, 473–500.

Wolfner, G.D., and Gelles, R.J. (1993). A profile of violence toward children: a national study. *Child Abuse and Neglect*, **17**, 197–212.

Worlock, P., Stower, M., and Barbor, P. (1993). Patterns of fractures in accidental and non-accidental injury in children: a comparative study. *British Medical Journal*, **293**, 100–2.

Chapter 5

Domestic violence: a health-care issue

Debbie Crisp and Betsy Stanko

Domestic violence has recently begun to work its way onto the health-care agenda. The BMA has published a report that reviewed the health-care implications of domestic violence. A number of the Royal Colleges have produced guidelines for practitioners working with domestic violence cases: these were consolidated in the Department of Health's publication *Domestic violence: a resource manual for Health Care Professionals* (2000). Since people experiencing this type of abuse are as likely to get in touch with a GP or other medical professional as they are to come into contact with the police, it is vital that health-care workers be informed about domestic violence. This chapter aims to:

- look at definitions of domestic violence;
- come to some understanding of its prevalence and incidence;
- identify who is affected by this type of abuse, and who are its perpetrators;
- explore individuals' help-seeking behaviours and needs;
- examine how domestic violence impacts on health-care workers.

Definition

Despite the increase in the amount of research and other work from the past twenty-five years, which has served to problematize violence within intimate relationships, the nature, frequency and extent of this type of abuse remain under debate. The term domestic violence is itself currently without a universally agreed definition, but is instead used generically to define a number of factors involved in serial abusive relationships. The intimacy of the parties involved, the nature of the abuse, and the wide range of its impact combine to make 'domestic violence' an important social problem.

Each of these aspects can be examined in turn:

1. *The parties involved.* The most common form of domestic violence is male partner or ex-partner against female. The BMA report *Domestic violence: a health-care issue?* (Radford *et al.* 1998) defines this type of abuse as behaviour 'from an adult perpetrator directed towards an adult victim in the context of a close relationship', and goes on to state that 'most often this will mean domestic violence from a man to his wife, ex-wife, female partner or ex-partner'. This is not to say that other sorts of violence do not exist within the home. Indeed, research has uncovered a high degree

of overlap between abuse of partners and abuse of children (see Hester *et al.* 1998). Further, a study undertaken for NCH Action for Children (Abrahams 1994) suggested that where women experiencing violence are mothers, three-quarters of their children will have witnessed at least one abusive incident. This in itself can be viewed as abusive to the child. The focus of this chapter, however, will be on inter-partner and ex-partner violence, with recognition that in many of these situations, children may also be involved.

2. *The behaviours comprised.* Domestic violence encompasses physical, sexual and psychological abuse, along with the threats of these forms of violence. As Harwin (1997) demonstrates, the array of behaviours included within any definition can be wide.

- *Physical abuse* ranges from the more commonplace hitting, punching, and choking all the way through to actual or attempted murder. Two women a week are killed by their partner or ex-partner in England and Wales alone. This accounts for half of all women murdered each year (Smith and Stanko 1999).

- *Sexual abuse* can refer to rape, sexual assault with objects, refusal to have sex, and even enforced prostitution. Mirrlees-Black (1999) found that 12% of women subjected to regular and repeated domestic assaults reported being forced to have sex in the last incident of abuse.

- *Psychological abuse* includes restriction of a person's movements or contact with others, criticism and belittling, possessiveness and the destruction of property. Studies have shown that physical and sexual violence are often accompanied by psychological abuse (see, for example, Dominy and Radford 1996), which can have a 'pronounced impact' upon an individual's 'general mental health, well being and sense of worth'. This psychological harm can be long-term in nature, as this quote in Stanko *et al.* (1998a) shows:

> *I was in a violent relationship fifteen years ago. No-one will ever do that to me again and walk away. I have constant panic attacks and most men who know me are wary of me as I tend to be aggressive. Really I'm just scared.*

3. *The impact of the abuse.* Stanko *et al.* (1998a) highlighted the fact that 'what constitutes domestic violence varies from individual to individual, as do the legal, economic and psychological consequences which serve to keep people entangled within abusive relationships'. The fact that there is (or was) a relationship between the parties creates especial pressures. It also goes some way to explain why domestic violence is more likely to involve *repeat* victimization than other types of violence (Mirrlees-Black *et al.* 1998). It is not uncommon for a health-care provider to come into contact with many women and some men in the course of their professional lives, who need advice about and treatment for the consequences of domestic violence.

The reason for requiring a wider understanding of domestic violence is linked to the diversity of its impact on different individuals. Lloyd (1997) made a distinction between the terminology used by the people experiencing violence, and that used by professionals and experts. In both cases, it is important to 'name' the behaviour as abusive:

- so that the person who is being abused is not treated as responsible for the *perpetrator's* behaviour;
- so that those working in the field ensure that the assistance they offer in these cases is appropriate and supportive. In health-care provision, for instance, treating wounds or depression could easily be accompanied by reassurance and the offer of referral to other agencies for relevant support.

Lloyd (1997) also drew attention to legal definitions of violence. These she described as being 'usually the most narrow and they tend to carry the most authority since they determine whether agencies such as the police, social services or the courts of law can intervene or prosecute'. However, it should be remembered that a large proportion of domestic violence does *not* currently come to the attention of criminal justice agencies (Mirrlees-Black *et al.* 1998). The majority of incidents are not reported to the police, others do not fit within the existing classification of criminal offences, or do not comprise behaviours that have been criminalized (Stanko *et al.* 1998a). Moreover, of the incidents that are reported to the police, only a relatively small proportion are recorded (just over a quarter, as opposed to nearly two-thirds of burglaries; Mirrlees-Black *et al.* 1998), with an even fewer number resulting in arrest (Kelly *et al.* 1999). Domestic violence is not just a matter for criminal justice agencies. Research shows that a comparable proportion of women who experience domestic violence consult their GPs as come into contact with the police (Mirrlees-Black 1999).

We have reviewed what we mean when we refer to domestic violence. We know that domestic violence exists, and that unfortunately such behaviours are likely to continue to exist for some time to come. We also know that those experiencing this type of abuse have a legitimate claim to access public service provision for a variety of reasons—including their health-care needs. We now move on to explore the extent of the problem.

Prevalence and incidence

Much relevant research work to date has focused on capturing the prevalence and incidence of domestic violence. There are variations between studies, depending on the methodology used, the behaviours that a questionnaire classifies as abusive, and the categories of people who are included as perpetrators. With few exceptions, the majority concentrate on women's experiences of men's violence. This work has shown that women may be subjected to abuse that they would not refer to as domestic violence, but which would fall within many studies' definitions of abusive behaviour (Dominy and Radford 1996). When differences in definition and methodology are accounted for, however, the findings of studies of domestic violence appear more compatible (Stanko *et al.* 1998b): estimates centre around one in ten women in any given year reporting various forms of domestic violence. There is even greater parity between women's reported lifetime prevalence levels, including research from other countries, e.g. Canada (Johnson and Sacco 1995) and Finland (Heiskanen and Piispa 1998). These estimates generally seem to fall somewhere between one in five and one in three (20–33%).

Larger scale studies, such as the British Crime Survey (BCS) have also examined the levels of prevalence of violence against men by their partners and ex-partners. The domestic violence self-completion supplement to the 1996 BCS (Mirrlees-Black 1999), found that women and men were equally likely to report having experienced this type of physical assault within the last 12 months, but that lifetime prevalence rates were higher for women (26% as opposed to 17%). The number of incidents within the previous year was also lower for men—in other words, women were more likely to experience a pattern of abuse as opposed to a one-off event. The 1998 BCS estimated that there were 835,000 domestic assaults during 1997: *more than one incident every 40 seconds*, 24 hours a day, 365 days a year. Over two-thirds of these (70%) were against women.

While it is clear that some men are abused within their relationships, in general there are differences in the types and the amount of violence to which men and women are subjected by their partners or ex-partners. There are also differences in the impact the abuse has: men are less often upset by violence, less often frightened, less often injured, and less likely to seek medical help (Mirrlees-Black 1999). These disparities cannot be fully understood from existing research, but we know that women experience violence in a different way to men (Nazroo 1995). We also know that domestic abuse looms larger for women as a proportion of the violence they encounter: the 1998 BCS (Mirrlees-Black *et al.* 1998) found that abuse of this sort accounted for 42% of all contact crime reported by women, but only 11% of that reported by men.

Who experiences domestic violence?

From the discussion above, it is clear that domestic violence impacts on the lives of a large proportion of the population. Using data from the Office of National Statistics (1999) and extrapolating from the 1998 BCS (and remembering that the survey itself acknowledges that it underestimates the extent of domestic violence), approximately 8 million adults in England and Wales would report experiencing this type of abuse at some point in their lives. Studies have examined the demographic characteristics of those experiencing domestic violence, and whilst there are some patterns, it is true to say that individuals are abused regardless of their age, sex, sexuality, marital status, ethnicity, religion, geography, class, wealth, employment status, and whether or not they have a disability or illness. As we note below, levels of abuse are higher for those with dependants and for those with a history of depression, self-harm, or addictions. Any service provision designed for those experiencing abuse must be sufficiently flexible to cover this broad spectrum of need. However, there are a number of 'risk factors' which are worth highlighting:

• For both men and women, those aged under 25 are most likely to experience domestic violence. For women, the level of reported abuse does not substantially reduce until they are in their mid-40s (Mirrlees-Black *et al.* 1998).

• Those who describe their status as 'separated' are the most likely to report having experienced domestic violence (Mirrlees-Black *et al.* 1998). It is hard to say whether this finding is misleading: for both women and men, where they were still living with the perpetrator, they were less likely to have told someone about their experiences (Mirrlees-Black 1999): this may also mean that they are less willing to disclose to a researcher. In some cases, ending a relationship may see the start of the abuse. Other work has shown that as many as one in three marriages that end in divorce involve domestic violence (Borkowski *et al.* 1983). Women are more at risk from their ex-partners than are men: many women are abused even after they no longer live with their violent partners (Kelly *et al.* 1999). Violence may also escalate post-separation (Binney et al. 1981).

• The risk of domestic violence is higher in homes where there are children (Mirrlees-Black 1999); it may begin and/or escalate during pregnancy (Bewley and Mezey 1997). Perpetrators may also target children either directly, or indirectly to reinforce control over the parent, and after a relationship has broken down, child-contact arrangements can be used by perpetrators to continue their abuse (Hester and Radford 1996). As a result of the abuse at home (or post-separation), children may have behavioural difficulties at school or may come to the attention of social services or the criminal justice process (Saunders *et al.* 1995).

• People in same-sex relationships also report experiencing abuse (Mirrlees-Black 1999). It is unclear whether these proportions are similar to those for heterosexual couples.

• The relationship between household income and domestic violence is a complex one. Some studies suggest that rates of abuse are higher in poorer households (Mirrlees-Black *et al.* 1998). Local studies in affluent areas, however, have uncovered similar prevalence levels to those in less privileged locations. Figure 5.1 compares the findings from two small-scale surveys in very different locations: Surrey and Hackney (Dominy and Radford; 1996; Stanko *et al.* 1998a). The former is one of the wealthiest counties in England, whereas (at the time of the research) just under half the population of the latter were in receipt of income support. The similarities in the nature of the abuse reported are, however, far more conspicuous than the differences. We know that this type of violence cuts across all income brackets, and that the financial abuse that some experience within their relationships can keep them in dire straits, however comfortable their circumstances might appear to the outside world (Glass 1995). We do not yet have enough information to say whether the level of domestic violence experienced is related to income, or whether this has any impact on an individual's willingness to access services and/or disclose their experiences (Radford *et al.* 1998). We know that those who describe themselves as having financial difficulties are significantly more likely to report having experienced domestic violence in the past year (Mirrlees-Black 1999) but we do not know the extent to which the abuse has precipitated this situation.

• There may be some geographical variation in the levels of domestic violence (Mirrlees-Black *et al.* 1998) but we are unclear whether this is because people in urban areas are more likely to report experiencing abuse, have easier access to services, or have a heightened recognition of their situation due to local public awareness campaigns. We do not know whether those in rural areas are more likely to remain silent about their experiences.

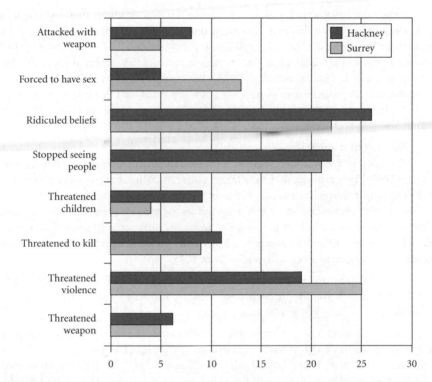

Fig. 5.1 Abuse experienced by women at some point in their lives (proportions shown are percentages of all respondents. Individuals may have experienced more than one type of abuse).

• People who report experiencing domestic violence have higher levels of drug or alcohol dependency (Radford *et al.* 1998). These dependencies may in fact be coping strategies to abuse.

• Those who report being abused are more likely to suffer from a limiting illness or disability (Mirrlees-Black 1999) or to have mental health problems (Campbell *et al.* 1997). We are unclear as to how violence affects mental health.

• A proportion of suicide and self-harm is known to be attributable to experiences of domestic violence (Williamson 2000).

The bulk of the above information has been collected directly from those reporting experiencing violence. There may be some overlap between the risk factors identified — for instance, younger women are more likely to be in households where there are children, and many women who have been abused report being prescribed psychotropic drugs by their GPs: the domestic violence that they experience may well be at the root of their depression. Campbell *et al.*'s (1997) work suggests that women's depression eases when they are no longer being abused.

By far the clearest indicator that someone is 'at risk' of experiencing domestic violence is that they have *already* been abused by their partner or ex-partner (Walby and Myhill, 2000). In other words, *the strongest predictor of future violence is not the characteristics of the person experiencing abuse, but the previous behaviour of the perpetrator*. This means that if we are to find ways to disrupt patterns of abuse and the accompanying consequences for health, we must look to find ways to support the people who are being or have been abused.

Who are the perpetrators?

Interestingly, in contrast to the large amount of data available on people who report experiencing domestic violence, surprisingly little is know about the abusers (Crisp and Stanko 2000). Most of the material available comes from evaluations of perpetrator programmes, but since in most cases acceptance on these schemes follows on from a conviction for abuse, it is not possible to assume that those attending are necessarily representative of perpetrators within the population as a whole.

- We know from the people experiencing violence that 'their' perpetrator tends to be of a similar age to themselves (Hanmer *et al.* 1999).

- There is speculation, but only some evidence to confirm that a proportion of perpetrators have witnessed their parents experiencing violence or have been abused themselves (Johnson and Sacco 1995). We know that there are many raised in violent families who would never be abusive themselves; conversely there are those raised in non-violent households who later go on to become perpetrators. The theory that there is a 'cycle of violence' in some ways offers the perpetrator an excuse not to take responsibility for their actions.

- Some perpetrator programmes may intervene in men's abusive behaviour towards their female partners and ex-partners. Evaluations of these programmes suggest that 'some men can change in fundamental ways' as a result of their participation (Burton *et al.* 1998). Some of this change also makes women feel better (Dobash *et al.* 1999). However, despite the small proportion of perpetrators attending these programmes, few men end up completing them. These programmes vary widely. Research suggests that those programmes based on cognitive behavioural models have a better chance of altering men's behaviour (Mullender and Burton 2000).

We know something about the prevalence and incidence of domestic violence (see above) but we know much less about the proportion of people who are abusive. Mooney (1994) found that nearly one in five men admitted to having used violence against their partner or ex-partner at least once, with only 37% claiming that they would *never* act violently.

Considering the number of women who report experiencing violence at some point in their lifetimes, this figure of one in five has some resonance, but it makes the paucity of data on the abusers somewhat harder to justify. Innovative use of information from the police or Accident and Emergency records could give a more holistic view of perperators. They currently manage to disappear from the picture, leaving any stigma from the abuse — and even the responsibility for the violence — attached to the person who is being abused.

The relationship between the abused, the abuser and the abuse

The widely recognized Duluth model of violent behaviour describes the perpetrator's use of coercive and controlling actions as a mechanism for maintaining a position of superiority or power within the relationship (see the discussion in Radford *et al.* 1998). This model offers a helpful framework for the purposes of this chapter, as it allows us to view domestic violence as a continuum of abusive behaviours. Its diverse nature, extent, and impact will necessarily vary according to the individuals involved and the power balance within their relationship. It also helps us to understand why violence may begin or escalate with the end of a relationship, as one party tries to re-establish 'control' over the other. It is therefore important to understand how power and personal control work in situations of domestic violence.

Patterns in the way coercion is used in intimate or family contexts show up in the descriptive data about domestic violence. For example, the 1996 BCS (Mirrlees-Black *et al.* 1996) found that where women reported incidents of domestic violence, over four-fifths of these involved their partners or ex-partners; for men, the comparable proportion was just under half (the remaining assaults involved other relatives or household members). Stanko *et al.* (1998a) found that 88% of the incidents dealt with by a police domestic violence unit involved partners or ex-partners, and 95% of these were against women. Several studies have shown that the pattern of abuse within relationships is generally established at an early stage, often within the first six months (Tayside Women and Violence Working Group 1994). Dominy and Radford (1996) found that the average length of time that women said that they remained in violent relationships was just over seven years (although the range was from a matter of weeks through to most of a lifetime). These observations, though, demonstrate that we need to ask the client themselves to provide details of how abuse affects their lives.

Not all domestic violence is in 'in-tact' partner or family relationships. In her report on the domestic violence self-completion component of the 1996 BCS, Mirrlees-Black (1999) examined the relationship between respondents who had experienced inter-partner or ex-partner abuse and the perpetrator at the time of interview:

- ◆ a third of those reporting one or more incidents of domestic violence in the previous year were no longer in a relationship with their abuser, with women roughly twice as likely as men to report that they were not still with this partner;
- ◆ nearly three-fifths of those reporting at least one incident of domestic violence at some point in their lives were no longer with the partner in question: again women were more likely than men to indicate that the relationship was over.

This survey failed to specify whether the separation referred to happened before or after the violent incident, or to clarify the extent to which the violence was ongoing in the cases where the abuser and abused had remained together as a couple. However, the higher levels of separation for those reporting lifetime prevalence suggest that it can be assumed that people do leave violent relationships (even though, in some, abuse may start or escalate post-separation). It is perhaps harder to understand why people stay.

Most health professionals use cues to try to establish proper treatment for particular medical conditions. Our information on domestic violence often manages to mask its pattern (its frequency, escalation, and so forth) but also its particular connections to other health needs. For instance, Mirrlees-Black (1999) suggests that 2% of incidents of domestic violence result in broken bones. Using the 1998 estimate that there were 835,000 incidents in the previous 12-month period in England and Wales, this means that there were at least 16,700 broken bones during the course of the year (equivalent to one every half-an-hour, 24 hours a day, 365 days a year). These bones belong to people, a significant proportion of whom will have had the same or other bones broken in a similar way on other occasions. Many of these injuries result in treatment by the National Health Service, costing tens of thousands of pounds each year. As service providers, it is important to remember that a large proportion of those using health and other agencies do so as a result of domestic violence and think about the possible implications this has for our working lives.

Research has shown that people who are being abused will often under-report the amount of violence that they are experiencing or have experienced. A study of male perpetrators found that they too were likely to minimize the extent and the seriousness of their actions (Dobash *et al.* 1998). Since most of the data generated on the nature and extent of abuse is collected via victimization studies of those experiencing violence, this means that we will always have a partial picture. Partial pictures arise from the particular perspective of health professionals as well. An A&E department may put an arm in plaster, but it rarely records how or why the arm was broken in the first place. There is a context to any individual incident of domestic violence and to remove that incident from that context is to impair our understanding of appropriate health response. Mooney (1994) found that women experiencing violence would on average have had a physical injury inflicted on them four times during the course of a year. Health personnel need to find a way to monitor the various forms of domestic violence that come to their attention, so that when interventions happen we are better informed about its realities, its regularities, its premeditation, its duration, the overlap between types of abuse, their impact on people experiencing violence, as well as on those around them, and on the public services to whom they turn for help.

Health-care provision and help-seeking strategies

From victimization studies we have information about the key agencies — including health — that people contact when they are looking for support and assistance in relation to domestic violence. Information about client usage — and the efficient and effective delivery of services — has been virtually untapped for its insights into the scope of the problem domestic violence, and its impact on the public and voluntary sector. There are variations between studies, but research has shown that somewhere between two- and three-fifths of those experiencing violence will disclose what has happened to them either to friends and family, or to within a more formalized help-seeking context (see, for example, McGibbon *et al.* 1989). The public services most likely to be contacted are the police, nurses or doctors, solicitors, the Housing Department, and Women's Aid. Table 5.1 compares a number of local studies of the agencies contacted by women who have experienced domestic violence at some point in their lives.

On comparison of these local studies, there do appear to be some regional differences in the agencies contacted, but it is unclear the extent to which this is due to the amount of available local provision or perceived quality of services. Women experiencing violence are more likely to contact service providers than are men Both women and men are less likely to tell someone about their situation if they were either still married to or living with their assailant (Mirrlees-Black 1999). From a trawl through a variety of service-providers' case files, Stanko et al. (1998a) found that a number of 'crisis' contacts were recorded for domestic violence. We know that abuse may escalate post-separation, but we do not know the degree to which the increased levels of disclosure, once a relationship is over, intersect in with this escalation.

The failure by the majority of agencies to monitor the proportion of their caseload that is domestic violence related means that we can only estimate the overall amount of contacts that are made, the reason for contact, and the degree to which multiple contacts are as a result of practitioners making referrals on to other service providers. Some agencies are able to account for the number of domestic violence contacts, but these tend to be the ones that deal specifically with a domestic violence caseload. Yet the numbers involved are substantial. Roughly one in six of the 105,640 homelessness applications each year come as a result of domestic violence (London Research Centre 1999). This is equivalent to more than two applications, every hour, 24 hours a day, 365 days a year. Women's Aid Federation of England runs a national domestic-violence helpline, which handles 20,000 calls each year. This is equivalent to more than 11 calls for every hour that the helpline is open, and does not include the many calls that are unable to get through (WAFE 1999).

Table 5.1 Women's contact with key service providers

	Hammersmith[a]	Surrey[b]	Islington[c]
Police	24	15	22
Solicitor	12	20	22
Housing Department	10	10	*
Women's Aid	6	6	5
Social Services	6	17	9
GP 14 21 22 Hospital	7	*	*
Health Visitor	3	9	*

*Indicates that data were not collected.

[a]McGibbon et al. (1989).

[b]Dominy and Radford (1996).

[c]Mooney (1994).

The contention has previously been that domestic violence was 'hidden': that as it took place 'behind closed doors' it was difficult to gain a detailed picture of what was deemed to be a 'private' situation. However, an examination of any relevant service-providers' files would clearly reveal that people — overwhelmingly women — who are being or have been abused by their partners or ex-partners are making contact with key agencies to try and get assistance. Paradoxically, the dearth of data from service providers may to some extent be explained by the large number of cases presenting as a result of domestic violence. We suggest that domestic abuse is not hidden so much as normalized.

The individual experiencing domestic violence is the unit of analysis by which the majority of data on help-seeking are collected. We know individuals contact a variety of agencies for a variety of purposes, but since the order of, and reasons for, these contacts are currently not well documented, it is hard to interpret patterns of help-seeking. Research has shown that where people do get in touch with formalized help-seeking networks, they are likely to be in contact with more than one service provider. It is unclear whether this is because they are being referred on to appropriate agencies, or whether they have to make a number of contacts before being able to find someone who is able to offer them the support that they require.

Studies examine the levels of satisfaction with the support by the different agencies contacted (e.g. McGibbon *et al.* 1989), but the findings are complex. It appears that those who are experiencing a repeated pattern of abuse are more likely to be satisfied with the service that they receive from key agencies (Mirrlees-Black 1999). This could be said to reinforce the findings of Stanko *et al.* (1998a) that practitioners recognize that there are 'crisis' contacts within their caseload. Kelly (1999) shows that women want support: if the health service took a different, more proactive approach to trying to recognize domestic violence cases, then these women might be prepared to disclose their experiences earlier. Other work has found that an unsupportive contact can discourage future help-seeking (Dominy and Radford 1996).

We do know something about the reasons why people remain silent about the abuse they suffer. For example, two out of three BCS 1998 respondents who said that they had not reported an incident of domestic violence to the police indicated that they avoided doing so because they felt that the matter was private, or that they were able to deal with it themselves. Roughly one in six did not report the matter as they thought that the police could not or would not do anything, and one in seven feared reprisals from their assailant if they did so (Mirrlees-Black *et al.* 1998). Not all women want involvement with the criminal justice process; but most may want support. The Home Office document *Supporting families* (1999) drew attention to the fact that, in cases of domestic violence, health-care practitioners are often the first point of contact with formalized help-seeking networks. Mirrlees-Black (1999) found that those experiencing abuse will seek medical attention after 1 in every 11 domestic assaults: in other words, *every 7 minutes, 365 days a year, 24 hours a day someone will contact a health-care worker for support in relation to domestic violence.* Since two out of every five domestic assaults result in some form of injury, it would appear that in three-quarters of cases where a person is hurt in this way by their partner or ex-partner, they do *not* seek medical attention. Mirrlees-Black also found that women who are being subjected to a repeated pattern of abuse are more likely to contact a health-care worker after a domestic assault — they will get in touch after one in every five incidents. However, these women are also more likely to have been hurt, and their injuries are more likely to have been serious: contact is still only made in one in every three cases where such an injury has been sustained.

The abuse itself can also have an impact on whether or not the person experiencing violence feels able to contact people for help in the first place, as this quote in Dominy and Radford (1996) shows:

> . . . you can't dial a telephone number on a telephone, you can't do anything because when you've been put down so much you believe what they tell you, you believe them, you look at yourself and you think well I'm nothing, I don't exist.

Research has found that in a large proportion of cases where women experience domestic violence, the perpetrator is very controlling over their movements, limiting their contact with other people — even on occasion keeping them physically under lock and key (Stanko *et al.* 1998a). Where this is the case, help-seeking is made even more problematic, as such restrictions can make it difficult to either make or keep appointments with key relevant agencies. This is all the more reason to include domestic violence within the wider remit of health service response.

Informal support networks: another intersection with health service providers

Whether or not they also contact a service provider, almost all of those who choose to disclose that they are experiencing violence will tell at least one relative or friend: on a lifetime prevalence estimate, these friends and family represent in excess of 3.6 million people or one in twelve of the adult population (this assumes only one such disclosure per person and so is almost certainly an underestimate). Domestic violence affects not just the person experiencing abuse, but also their friends and family. The existing work here — except perhaps in relation to the children concerned — is limited, especially given the significant number of the population who fall into this category.

In general, the relative or friend will offer the abused person information or advice. Usually they will find this support helpful (Mirrlees-Black 1999). We are, however, unclear as to the nature of this advice and information, or about the practical backup that relatives or friends might feel that they need themselves. The relatives and friends of people experiencing violence represent a mainly unexplored opportunity for advice about health. They are often the first port of call in an abused person's help-seeking. Due to the ongoing nature of their relationship with the person experiencing domestic violence, they can offer an enhanced understanding of the abused person's needs (both shorter and longer term), and of the types of crises that may be faced. They can also give useful insight into the barriers and triggers that exist to any formalized help-seeking. Health practitioners can offer indirect support to people experiencing abuse by offering support or making information available to their friends and family.

The role of health-care workers

Put simply, the reason that domestic violence is a health-care issue is because when they are abused by their partners or ex-partners, people get hurt. In some cases the harm can be extreme: research has estimated that as many as 10% of women will be knocked unconscious by their partner at some point in their lives, 2% will suffer an internal injury, and 2% will miscarry as a result of domestic violence (Stanko *et al.* 1998a). There is also growing evidence to suggest that there are serious long-term health implications for the survivors of domestic abuse: the American Medical Association (as quoted in the Scottish Needs Assessment Programme (SNAP) report on domestic violence, 1998) drew attention to the possible links with arthritis, hypertension, and heart disease. The SNAP (1998) report indicated how, in domestic-violence cases involving sexual abuse, women may suffer from a range of health problems including sexually transmitted diseases or vaginal bleeding. There are also emotional and mental health issues, such as an increased likelihood to be in general poor health, or to be drug or alcohol dependent.

The fact that health-care workers may be the first person to whom someone experiencing domestic violence turns for help means that primary health-care workers (including GPs, nurses, health visitors), hospital practitioners (including A&E services, psychiatrists, psychologists, obstetrics, and gynaecological services) and other medically trained staff (e.g. dentists) all have a vital role to play in offering much needed support and validation in these cases.

Stevens (1997) reviewed the literature in relation to the proportion of A&E attendances that are domestic-violence related. She found that very little work had been done in the UK and that estimates from other countries varied widely: 2–12% of all female attendances, and 25–30% of all female trauma-related attendances. The SNAP (1998) report uncovered similar variations for other health-care workers. The report emphasized that the health problems relating to domestic violence 'are potentially consuming large quantities of scarce health service resources'. Stanko *et al.*'s (1998a) study of the financial implications of domestic violence estimated that selected health-care costs for one year for one London Borough were in excess of £580,000 (including consultations with GPs, health visitors, and A&E visits; excluding hospitalization and medicines).

The WHO technical paper on *Gender and Health* (1998) estimated that rape and domestic violence together accounted for 19% of the total disease burden for women in developing countries. Yet at present there is no routine monitoring of domestic violence related cases and that as a result no data exists as the proportion of health-care practitioners' workloads that relate either directly or indirectly to this type of abuse. Stevens (1997) identified a number of indicators within the A&E, which might lead practitioners to suspect that the reason for contact is domestic-violence related. These include:

- delay in presentation;
- inappropriate history;
- the attitude of the person attending or the person accompanying them;
- deliberate self-harm;
- the fact that the person is a frequent attender.

These factors may raise the suspicions of a health-care worker that a patient may be experiencing abuse from their partner or ex-partner, but in and of themselves they do not guarantee this to be the case. Perhaps the most straightforward way to find out whether or not the reason that the person has made contact is domestic-violence related is to *ask them directly* if this is the case. This may seem somewhat simplistic, especially as there are many reasons why practitioners currently do not routinely screen for this type of abuse:

◆ fear that it is inappropriate to intervene in a private matter (The Women's Unit 1999);

◆ failure of training to help practitioners identify domestic-violence related cases, e.g. child-protection cases where the mother is also experiencing abuse;

◆ uncertainty about how to raise the issue: not asking the relevant questions because of uncertainty about how to do so appropriately (Jones 1997);

◆ concern that any intervention may in fact exacerbate harm due to lack of understanding of the issues relating to domestic violence, or how to make appropriate referrals (Jones 1997);

◆ reluctance to intervene in the shorter term, as to do so may add to an individual's workload — even though non-intervention may well result in repeat victimization and therefore additional work in the longer term;

◆ personal issues relating to domestic violence.

The SNAP report (1998) strongly recommended initiating discussion about domestic violence by asking direct questions in a sympathetic and non-judgemental way. Feder and Richardson (1999) made some suggestions about how best this might be done — either by more general questions such as: 'Do you think you have ever experienced domestic violence?', 'Have you ever felt *afraid* of your current partner or any previous partner?', or alternatively by more specific questions such as, 'How often has your current or any previous partner ever done any of the following things [show list] *so that you have had to be careful about what you said or did?*'. If in these cases, a patient chooses to disclose that they have in fact experienced domestic violence, it is very important that the person asking the question acknowledges that they believe what they are hearing and that they wish to be supportive: it may be the first time that the patient has ever told *anybody* about what has happened to them.

In their research based in primary care settings, Feder and Richardson (1999) identified a gap between the willingness of health professionals to ask women patients whether or not they have experienced abuse and the extent to which women felt it was acceptable to *be* asked. Although 83% of the health-care workers surveyed agreed with the statement that domestic violence against women was a health-care issue, only 31% of health visitors, 15% of practice nurses, and 14% of GPs felt that patients should routinely be asked. Conversely, 77% women in a GP waiting-room survey thought that such routine questioning was acceptable.

Stanko *et al.* (1998a) included a series of composite case studies as part of their report to demonstrate the diversity of individuals' experiences within one geographical area. We have included some of these case studies here to give examples of why and how people experiencing domestic violence may come into contact with health-care workers. They are also useful to demonstrate the context of abuse, and to emphasize that, if practitioners do not ask patients about their experiences, it is all too easy for them to become removed from this context.

Case study 1

Dela is 64, Turkish, and despite having lived in this country for 40 years, speaks only limited English. She married Mehmet, 70, just before coming to England. They have three adult children: two daughters and one son who still lives home. The house is only in her husband's name. Mehmet has always been physically violent to Dela, as well as very restricting (he wouldn't let her go out very often, didn't let her have friends round to the house, didn't give her very much money). Dela called the police out to an incident once, about fifteen years ago, but afterwards was beaten so severely she needed medical attention; she has not called them out again since. When they were younger, he bullied the two girls — one one has now moved well away from the area and refuses to have any contact with her father.

Recently Dela went into hospital for a hysterectomy. The hospital had arranged for a home help to come to the house daily after her release to do the majority of the cleaning. On returning home, Dela found that Mehmet had cancelled the home help, and expected her to immediately go back to doing all the housework. Dela was still in considerable discomfort, and despite his repeated threats, instead went to move in with her daughter who lives around the corner. Mehmet has taken to phoning the daughter's house at all hours, and being abusive: this is proving upsetting to all who live there (including his two grandchildren). Mehmet continues to cash, and spend, Dela's pension as well as his own. He has also succeeded in alienating her son from her, which is causing her a good deal of distress.

Dela has decided that she does not wish to go back to her husband and has contacted the Housing Department to discuss the idea of sheltered accommodation in the area. She is currently sharing a bed with her daughter, while her son-in-law sleeps on the sofa. This is proving quite stressful, and it is hoped she will be able to find her own flat soon. She is considering taking out an injunction against her husband to stop him harassing her (and her daughter's family).

Case study 2

Karen, 35, was born in Hackney and is now in council accommodation there. She has been in a wheelchair most of her life due to a bone condition. She has been with Alec (also 35, originally from Manchester) for seven years. He is her main carer and works part-time in a pub.

Recently, Alec's alcohol intake has started to cause her some concern: he has started to drink very heavily, and is often verbally abusive to her when drunk. She has discussed his drinking with her sister. Two weeks ago, Alec came back from a night out with some friends, and an argument developed between them. He started to hit her repeatedly about the arms and head. She contacted the police by phoning 999. Two uniformed officers attended and arrested Alec on the spot. The case was then picked up by the police domestic violence unit, who suggested that she visit her GP. The GP found her arms to be badly bruised, and Karen has found it hard to use the wheelchair.

Alec has never been violent before and is remorseful about the incident. Karen wants the relationship to continue, and so did not want the police to pursue the case. She is trying to persuade Alec to go for alcohol counselling.

Case study 3

Rachel met Sam at the Jewish Society at college in Bristol, and they are now active in their local synagogue. They are both 29 and work in the computer industry. They have been together as a couple for five years and married three years ago, buying a house in Stoke Newington. Rachel's career has proved somewhat more successful than Sam's, and this has created quite a lot of tension between them. Rachel has slowly cut herself off from her group of university friends, as seeing them invariably led to a row between her and Sam. She also avoids social events at work, as these tend to make Sam very jealous. She does not discuss her relationship with anyone. During this time, they started to discuss the possibility of starting a family, but discovered that Rachel was not ovulating properly. This put added strains on their relationship.

Sam has been violent to her on a number of occasions, but only once has she required medical treatment. He broke her jaw. She told the hospital that she had been late for an appointment, and in her hurry to get out had fallen downstairs. She refused to discuss any more details; although no one in the A&E believed her, no one pressed her. To try and patch things up, they decided to go on an extended foreign holiday together. When Rachel went to the GP for her injections, she did not say anything about her jaw.

On returning from their holiday, Rachel approached her GP to find out about IVF treatment. She disclosed that her jaw had been broken by Sam during an argument, but did not want to say anything further about her injury.

Case study 4

Vera (53) and Bill (50) live with their two adult sons in a former council house, which they bought six years ago. The three men are undermining towards Vera — telling her that she is stupid and ordering her around. They reinforce their instructions with threats or physical violence. This situation has been going on for over ten years. Vera has suffered from depression and other problems related to stress and anxiety. She has taken five overdoses in the past. The last overdose resulted in the Mental Health Locality Team becoming involved: Vera was threatening to kill herself if she was discharged. She then spent an additional five months in hospital.

Vera has been offered housing and counselling, but she has not been able to decide what she wants to do. She has just found a part-time job.

For the most part, the violence highlighted in the above case studies is not the most extreme in nature. As with Dela, however, abuse can be long term without necessarily involving escalation. The person experiencing domestic violence may still have health-care needs and these, along with other needs they might have, may change over time (Kelly 1988). As with Vera, having some information about a patient's background can help to give some insight into the reasoning behind their decision-making: the reluctance to go home appears less quixotic once the nature of her home-life is understood. Karen's case serves as a reminder that people experiencing domestic violence may have a variety of other specific needs. Rachel's case demonstrates that it should not be assumed that that the best way not to increase harm is simply not to ask. A quote in Langley (1997) underscores this point:

> I wish I'd been asked what had happened. I was so ashamed but I really wanted to tell them. They didn't ask me though and I didn't have the courage to tell them myself. Even though he wasn't there I lied for him just like I always did. They just gave me some painkillers and sent me home. It wasn't any good though, because he thought I'd told them anyway and hit me even though I hadn't. No-one seemed to believe me.

A final word

A notable and consistent proportion of the population will experience domestic violence. These people have health-care needs, and substantial health service resources are already required to meet those needs. By reaching a better understanding of the issues surrounding this type of abuse, health-care workers can make patients feel more comfortable about disclosing their experiences. It is also in the interest of best clinical practice for practitioners to become knowledgeable about domestic violence: in the case of a patient who presents repeatedly for depression of unspecified origin, it would not be good medicine to ignore the context of the illness. Direct, non-judgemental questioning can help to uncover whether or not a case is domestic-violence related. Routine monitoring can ensure that such cases are catered for supportively, with due regard to individual patients' specific needs and personal safety. Inaction, as the Women's Unit (1999) report restates, is no longer an option: 'it is time to act to change attitudes and make sure that women are not subject to violence in their own home or anywhere else'.

References

Abrahams, C. (1994). *The hidden victims — children and domestic violence*. NCH Action for Children, London.

Bewley, S., and Mezey, G. (1997). Domestic violence and pregnancy. *British Medical Journal*, **314**, 1295.

Binney, V., Harkell, G., and Nixon, J. (1981). *Leaving violent men*. WAFE, Leeds.

Borkowski, M., Murch, M., and Walker, V. (1983). *Marital violence: the community response*. Tavistock, London.

Burton, S., Regan, L., and Kelly, L. (1998). *Supporting women and challenging men: lessons from the Domestic Violence Intervention Project*. Joseph Rowntree Foundation, York.

Campbell, J.C., Kub, J., Belknap, R.A., and Templin, T.N. (1997). *Predictors of depression in battered women*. In *Violence against women*, Vol. 3(3), pp. 271–93.

Crisp, D., and Stanko, E. (2000). *Reducing Domestic Violence . . . What Works?* Monitoring Costs and Evaluating Needs. Home Office PRCU Briefing Note http://www.homeoffice.gov.uk/domesticviolence/moncost.pdf

Department of Health (2000). *Domestic Violence: A Resource Manual for Health-Care Professionals*. http://www.doh.gov.uk/domestic.htm.

Dobash, R.P., Dobash, R.E., Cavanagh, K., and Lewis, R. (1998). *Separate and intersecting realities: a comparison of men's and women's accounts of violence against women. Journal of Violence Against Women*, **4** (4), 382–414.

Dobash, R.P., Dobash, R.E., Cavanagh, K., and Lewis, R. (1999). *A research evaluation of british programmes for violent men. Journal of Social Policy*, **28**, (2), 205–33.

Dominy, N., and Radford, L. (1996). *Domestic violence in Surrey: developing an effective inter-agency response*. Roehampton Institute, Surrey County Council.

Feder, G., and Richardson, J. (1999). http://www.domesticviolencedata.org/5_research/health/fed_nc1.htm

Glass, D. (1995). *All my fault: why women don't leave abusive men*. Virago, London.

Hanmer, J., Griffiths, S., and Jerwood, D. (1999). *Arresting evidence: domestic violence and repeat victimisation*. Police Research Series Paper 104. Home Office, London.

Harwin, N. (1997). *Understanding women's experience of abuse.* In *Violence against women* (ed. S., Bewley, G., Mezey, and J. Friend, Royal College of Obstetricians and Gynaecologists, London. pp. 59–75.

Heiskanen, M., and Piispa, M. (1998). *Faith hope and battering: a survey of men's violence against women in Finland.* Statistics Finland and the Council for Equality.

Hester, M., and Radford, L. (1996). *Domestic violence and child contact arrangements in England and Denmark.* The Policy Press, Bristol.

Hester, M., Pearson, C., and Harwin, N. (1998). *Making an impact.* NSPCC.

Home Office (1999). *Supporting Families.* http://www.homeoffice.gov.uk/cpd/fmpu/ofamr.pdf

Johnson, H., and Sacco, V. (1995). Researching violence against women: statistics canada's national survey. *Canadian Journal of Criminology,* **37**, (3), 284–304.

Jones, R.F. (III) (1997). *Domestic violence—a physician's perspective.* In *Violence against women* (ed. S., Bewley, G., Mezey, and J. Friend,) Royal College of Obstetricians and Gynaecologists, London. pp. 76–82.

Kelly, L. (1988). How women define Their experiences of violence. In *Feminist perspectives on wife abuse* (ed. K. Yllo, and M. Bograd) Sage, Newbury Park, California. pp. 114–132.

Kelly, L., Bindel, J., Burton, S., Butterworth, D., Cook, K., and Regan, L. (1999). *Domestic violence matters: an evaluation of a development project.* Home Office Research Study No. 193. Home Office, London.

Langley, H. (1997). *An overview.* In (ed. S. Bewley, G. Mezey and J. Friend) *Violence Against Women.* Royal College of Obstetricians and Gynaecologists, London. pp. 147–156.

Lloyd, S. (1997). Defining violence against women. In *Violence against women.* (ed. S. Bewley, G. Mezey, and J. Friend) Royal College of Obstetricians and Gynaecologists, London. pp. 3–12.

London Research Centre (1999). *Relationship breakdown: a guide for social landlords.* Department of the Environment, Transport and the Regions, London.

McGibbon, A., Cooper, L., and Kelly, L. (1989). *What support?* Hammersmith and Fulham Council Community Police Committee Domestic Violence Project. Hammersmith and Fulham Community Safety Unit, London.

Mirrlees-Black, C. (1999). *Domestic violence: findings from a new British crime survey self-completion questionnaire.* Home Office Research Study No. 191. Home Office, London.

Mirrlees-Black, C., Mayhew, P., and Percy, A. (1996). *The 1996 British Crime Survey.* Home Office Statistical Bulletin Issue 19/96. Home Office, London.

Mirrlees-Black, C., Budd, T., Partridge, S., and Mayhew, P. (1998). *The 1998 British crime survey.* Home Office Statistical Bulletin Issue 21/98. Home Office, London.

Mooney, J. (1994). *The hidden figure: domestic violence in North London.* Middlesex University, London.

Mullender, A., and Burton, S. *Reducing Domstic Violence . . . What Works?* Perpetrator programmes. Home Office PRCU Briefing Note. http://www.homeoffice.gov.uk/domesticviolence/perpprog.pdf

Nazroo, J. (1995). Uncovering gender differences in the use of marital violence: the effect of methodology. *Sociology,* **29**, (3). pp. 475–494.

Office of National Statistics (1999). http://www.statistics.gov.uk/ukinfigs/pop.htm

Radford L., Richardson, J., and Davies, L. (1998). *Domestic violence: a health care issue?* British Medical Association, London.

Saunders, A., Debbonaire, T. Keep, G., and Pahl, J. (1995). *It hurts me too.* WAFE, Bristol.

Scottish Needs Assessment Programme (1998). *Domestic violence.* Scottish Forum for Public Health Medicine, Glasgow.

Smith, J., and Stanko, E. (1999). *Femicide: the killing of women in England and Wales 1986–96.* Unpublished paper, Centre for Criminal Justice, Brunel University.

Stanko, E., Crisp, D., Hale, C., and Lucraft, L. (1998a). *Counting the costs: estimating the impact of domestic violence in the London Borough of Hackney.* Crime Concern, Bristol.

Stanko E., Marian, L., Crisp, D., Manning, R., Smith, J., and Cowan, S. (1998b). *Taking stock: what do we know about violence?* ESRC Violence Research Programme, Brunel University.

Stevens, K.L.H. (1997). The role of the accident and emergency department. In *Violence against women* (ed. S. Bewley, G. Mezey, and J. Friend). Royal College of Obstetricians and Gynaecologists, London. pp. 168–178.

Tayside Women and Violence Working Group (1994). *Hit or miss: an exploratory study of the provision for women subjected to domestic violence in the Tayside region.* Tayside Regional Council.

Walby, S., and Myhill, A. (2000). *Reducing Domestic Violence . . . What Works?* Assessing and Managing the Risk of Domestic Violence. Home Office PRCU Briefing Note. http://www.homeoffice.gov.uk/domesticviolence/accman.pdf

Williamson, E. (2000). *Domestic Violence and Health: the response of the medical profession.* Bristol: Policy Press.

Women's Aid Federation of England (1999). *Annual Report 1998–99.* WAFE, Bristol.

World Health Organisation (1998). *Gender and health: technical paper.* Women's Health and Development, Family and Reproductive Health, WHO.

The Women's Unit (1999). *Living without fear: an integrated approach to tackling violence against women* Cabinet Office, London.

Chapter 6

Limiting violence through good design

Susan Francis

Introduction

The relationship between space and human behaviour is an issue that has been explored in various disciplines over time. Whilst now widely accepted that there is a relationship between them, the extent to which the environment can actually determine behaviour is more debatable. Some have tried to link environment and behaviour in a determinstic way, suggesting that physical space can direct behaviour. Many people acknowledge that the design of the environment can influence how people react and how they feel. Indeed, it can support certain work patterns and make others more difficult to achieve. So, the idea that the environment can play a part in limiting violence has currency both in literature and practice.

There is increasing concern about violence in health buildings and recently a particular emphasis on making the workplace environment safe and secure. Whilst in the recent past the approach to design had been to find fortified solutions using grills, cameras and enclosures, more recent ideas have taken a more sophisticated approach. This involves the use of passive design that provides a calming and controlled environment, supported by minimal and unobtrusive measures for safety and security.

New ideas emerge for design from both theory and practice, and this chapter draws ideas both from published literature and built projects. Three areas of consideration emerge:

- the design of spaces, including the arrangement of rooms, relationship of the building to the surroundings, and the detailed design of finishes and furniture within;
- the use of technical devices such as the provision of security hardware and controls;
- the training and management of people, namely how people manage space through observation and training by detecting signs of possible violent behaviour and managing the consequences.

The literature includes studies relating to the design of spaces that address crime, violence, and the notion of the therapeutic environment. Information on technical devices is regularly published and updated in the technical and building press. Improving work conditions and training staff to manage violent incidents has become an issue for health and safety, and risk management regulations. A review of built examples demonstrates how unobtrusive design can deal with violence in a variety of settings including hospitals, primary and community locations, and psychiatric facilities.

Some general principles about reducing opportunities for violence

Designing health-care buildings involves the synthesis of many variables, some of which may be at odds with one another. The design may address the conflicting needs of various users such as managers, professionals, and patients; or be the result of matching preferred arrangements to the physical site-constraints of any specific location. Many of the most inventive designs have sought to find a resolution to reduce violence and fear of violence, not by devising an overtly secure and fortified solution but rather one that aims to create a calming environment with unobtrusive devices to ensure safety and security.

Other chapters in this volume give more detailed explanations and definitions of violence and it is not the purpose of this contribution to duplicate them. But it may be useful to sketch out some design principles that are highlighted in literature about crime and violence. Key themes that emerge from the literature in relation to issues of designing spaces to address crime, for example, include:

- making clear and observable routes;
- restricting entry to specific spaces and zones;
- avoiding culs-de-sac where people can become trapped;
- creating barriers to avoid physical attack;
- making spaces visible by good lighting and visual surveillance.

Those design issues that are highlighted in the literature on psychiatric care relate to principally to violence and include:

- making sufficient space to avoid crowding;
- providing adequate security;
- minimizing opportunities for self-harm.

The literature about the therapeutic nature of health environments does not specifically address issues of violence or crime. Some general ideas for designing buildings that positively contribute to healing and therapy are articulated, such as making social spaces and creating visual links between indoor and outdoor spaces. But these studies demonstrate a general trend and interest in designs that respect privacy and dignity, and seek to articulate humane interpretations for the design of spaces.

Technical literature has concentrated not so much on space planning as equipment and installations that help to control and monitor spaces. The kinds of devices that are illustrated include, for example, alarms, shutters, and cctv monitors.

The third source of information, from a health and safety perspective, covers issues such as the training of staff to deal with incidents and development of policy to manage both patients and staff.

Literature review

There is no comprehensive or single source of design literature on this topic that relates specifically to health buildings. However, theories about human behaviour and the design of the environment, particularly in relation to security and crime, have been developed for housing estates since the 1960s. At least one of these theories has been tested in relation to hospital planning. Within the literature on health buildings, research studies on environments for psychiatric care offer a source of information and theories about designing-out violence. These mostly address issues of physical safety and psychological security in relation to a particularly extreme care group but some principles may be transferable to more general environments for health care. Research on the therapeutic contribution of design has been developed mainly in relation to hospital buildings and does not address specifically issues of violence but draws out ideas for creating calming and controllable spaces to reduce stress and irritation.

Crime

An interest in the impact of the environment on crime developed in the 60s and 70s, and a number of theories emerged. One of the most notable was the concept of 'defensible space' articulated by Oscar Newman (1972). He placed great faith in the determinism of design, believing that if the design of the environment provides opportunities for crime, then making changes to the design can reduce or eliminate crime. This has been challenged in various critiques (Steventon 1996) and it is now more widely accepted that, although the design of the environment cannot determine peoples behaviour, it can influence by hindering or helping. So, it may be that some of the design features intended to increase the risk for offenders may actually make other users more confident and less fearful. In this way the design may provide a deterrent to the offenders. One of the key ideas in Newman's theory is that isolated routes are underused and unsafe. He proposes to attach these spaces to specific buildings in order to generate a sense of belonging to these spaces. In this way, he suggests that these spaces become part of someone's territory and will therefore be perceived as being more risky places for potential perpetrators. In effect he proposes making private the common spaces and in doing so reduces space that is part of the public domain.

An earlier theory was that of Jane Jacobs (1961) who suggested that feeling safe relies on places being in continuous use and that the design and arrangement of the spaces therefore becomes critical in determining the vitality of areas and their safety. Her proposition is the exact opposite of Newman's in that she suggests keeping space in the public domain with clear definitions of public and private places, orienting buildings or parts of buildings to overtook places, and using people to provide informal surveillance and observation.

Alice Colman's *Utopia on trial* (1985) is one of the studies most explicit in asserting that the design of the environment determines social behaviour. Colman 'puts on trial' the ideal environment, in this particular case, social housing, and suggests that design can have a disadvantaging effect on social structures. The conclusions drawn identify 15 design variables in blocks of flats that affect behaviour; six test measures include lift graffiti, vandal damage, children in care, urine pollution, and faecal pollution. Amongst the recommendations are that no more flats should be built. The direct and singular link between design and behaviour has been fiercely criticized and questioned by academics and practitioners. The critics point out, not only the narrowness of the problem definition but also that the link between behaviour and design is more complicated than this study suggests. Ravetz (1988) points out that 'it is difficult and unwise to be dogmatic about the exact connections between environments and behaviour, let alone to impute causal relationship . . . Over and above physical attributes, buildings and environments are endowed with symbols and meanings, which are held not only in the minds of the providers and designers, but also of the users — and also, incidentally, of any researchers'.

A study by Van der Voordt and van Wegen (1993) sought to integrate the findings of many research studies into a practical method. The result was the 'Delft Checklist', a tool for mapping crime and environmental design, which distinguished between two types of measures to combat crime, namely:

♦ *socioprevention*: protection with the aid of visible or tangible presence of people who may be expected to intervene if necessary — aims to raise the psychological threshold through 'natural surveillance';

♦ *technoprevention*: protection of objects or spaces through technical means, such as burglar-proof locks on doors and windows, alarm systems, etc. — aims to raise the physical threshold by restricting access.

Five key design variables are identified which may be summarized as:

♦ *Protective eyes*: visual contact and supervision.

♦ *Visibility*: this is important for preventing crime but also for reducing the sense of fear; it increases personal control; it relates to public spaces inside and outside.

♦ *Involvement and responsibility*: this not only encourages people to care for their environment but also actively discourages potential perpetrators. There need to be clear transitions between public and private responsibilities so that it is obvious who is responsible for what. There is an implied involvement in design and management.

♦ *Attractiveness of the environment*: helps to reduce the extent of vandalism and feelings of insecurity; it is related to form, colour, materials, and the need for maintenance.

♦ *Accessibility and escape routes*: ease of access is important for formal and informal surveillance; there needs to be a balance between giving possible victims escape routes and enabling perpetrators to escape.

This study demonstrates a shift in emphasis from protection (technical) to natural surveillance (socio) and introduced the concept of the attractiveness of the environment as a key feature, namely that the quality of the design and ambience of a space can contribute.

Hospitals and crime

Bill Hillier (1986) has developed a further theory known as 'Space Syntax' in which he suggested that places are more likely to be unsafe as a result of not forming a legible and well-used network of routes. He proposed that the organization of the space and their relationships are essential to generate, sustain, and control patterns of movement. This theory was developed, like many others, in relation to housing estate planning and in 1994, Hillier's theory was applied to a series of studies of hospitals to inform the planning and design of routes. The studies (Hillier 1994) sought to establish the impact of space and people on crime and security, rather than security hardware and control systems. They tested whether three factors, identified in housing studies as having a bearing on space, applied to hospital planning, namely:

+ accessibility: perpetrators of all categories of planned crime like to keep their means of escape clear — they want to be able to make a quick exit;

♦ presence of others: violent crimes are prevented if someone is present or potential offenders feel someone can walk in, whereas pick-pockets operate in busy places;

♦ attacks tend to occur in spaces just off the main route or its approach.

The findings suggested that it was necessary to distinguish between day and nighttime use, protocols to limit entry to certain areas, such as wards or departments, were useful and that there were certain areas of high risk. The study pointed out that the organizational concept of planning the hospital in villages or clusters of departments was good from a security point of view. This enabled control of the entrance and could be supplemented with clear observation of the public waiting room by the reception desk or staff base. The study recommended making clear the separation of public and private spaces in order to effect control. One of the limitations of the research was that it did not specifically address issues of violence and the behavioural relationships in attacks in Accident and Emergency departments. But it did introduce the notion of a tool for mapping behaviour, for use to support design proposals.

Violence

The most common source of literature on violent behaviour and design is covered by studies of psychiatric facilities. One feature of this work, which distinguishes it from studies of other buildings, is the additional concern for the safety of patients who may harm themselves as well as others. Many of the earlier studies and texts in this area reacted to the design for custodial care. Remen (1987) calls for consideration to be made of the perception of psychiatric patients and points out the contrasts between those who perceive the environment 'as clear, ordered, predictable, and peaceful' and others for whom it is 'chaotic, confusing, and agitating'. The author goes on to say that psychiatric patients may experience both in rapid succession. Conditions that will enhance mental health, provide for the personal safety of patients and staff without relaying that any negative aspects of that protection are desirable. Patient security should therefore be aimed at preventing self-harm or harm to others. Remen called for windows to be designed without grills and for seclusion rooms not to look like padded cells.

The issue of social density is addressed in a paper published in the early 1990s that suggested that 'crowding increases the likelihood of aggressive behaviour, especially in schizophrenic patients' (Palmstierna *et al.* 1991). This anticipated one of the key design issues for in-patient care for all health buildings: the trend for an increase in privacy and personal space is challenging the provision of shared bedrooms for short-stay patients. It is now generally accepted that for those who are resident in continuing care homes or long-stay facilities, single rooms are essential. Concepts of good nursing practice in the UK relying on close personal observation of patients by staff raise the issue about whether single rooms are appropriate for high-dependency patients who require more nursing observation.

This also raises issues about public areas and day rooms. Many articles and reviews point out the dull and institutional nature of day rooms and call for a more sophisticated understanding of the potential for social interaction in the public realm. The question about opening day rooms at night for those who cannot sleep is also raised. Another response has been to suggest that variety and distraction should be sought: first, by the organization of spaces, for example, by visually differentiating between building parts, creating a variety of spaces to support social interaction, and clearly indicating room use; second, by considering the interior decor, with ideas about the use of distinct colours to enhance activities and space, light to define space, and materials to provide different tactile and visual experiences (Gulak 1991).

In a survey of the quality of care in acute psychiatric wards entitled *Acute problems* (Sainsbury Centre for Mental Health 1998), special consideration is called for in relation to the needs for safety and privacy of women patients. Whilst it is acknowledged that mixing genders is a relatively recent phenomenon, which was considered a social and therapeutic advance, concerns about the high level of sexual harassment of women has led to government policy to eliminate mixed-sex wards. This report suggests that this is not enough and should be extended beyond day rooms to include bedrooms, washing, and toilet areas.

Therapeutic environments and the control of violence

A shift to a positive emphasis on the therapeutic environment began to emerge in the 1990s. The emphasis is on linking principles that positively improve the relaxing and calming influence of the environment to those ensuring that safety is clearly articulated.

A paper published by the Royal College of Psychiatrists (1998) sets out guidelines for the design and management of imminent violence in psychiatric facilities. This study draws on evidence from selected research studies, national guidance and consensus documents, and reports from user and carer discussion groups. The review of research studies concludes that the quantitative evidence base is insufficient to support the hypothesis that 'characteristics of the human and physical environment have a powerful effect in mitigating and preventing, or exacerbating and precipitating the manifestations of violence'. Nevertheless, the report calls for a well-planned environment: one that allows adequate space, reasonable comfort, privacy, and safety. A checklist of features for ward design and organization is articulated under two headings: calming features and those ensuring a secure environment. Key aspects of the calming environmental include: privacy; control of noise, heating, and ventilation; access to activity areas inside and outside; adequate space and perception of space; and safe and accessible place for personal effects. Those listed under security include: safe room for severely disturbed people; good observation; exits within sight and accessible; alarms for one-to-one working spaces; and furniture of safe size, weight, and construction.

A guideline for community-based mental health facilities addressing safety and security by design suggests that 'if a pleasant domestic environment can be supplemented by supportive but unobtrusive management and care assistance the likelihood of violent, anti-social or disruptive behaviour by residents can be considerably reduced' (WLH Estates, undated). The report provides a checklist of design and technical guidance covering general planning and design issues, highlighting those that relate to safety and vandalism in particular. The need for good observation is mentioned, as well as the benefits of attack alarm systems for the protection of staff.

In a manual for nurses and health-care workers (1999) a wide range of environmental factors are cited as having an effect on behaviour, including: charges from electromagnetic fields; noise levels; temperature; ozone levels; and the invasion of personal space. The manual suggests that safety can be at odds with issues of choice and dignity. Environmental factors such as the structure of the building, layout of rooms, decor, disrepair, available space, neatness, setting, and location, as well as philosophy of organization and management, can have a bearing on how people feel and react.

The notion that the environment can play a positive role in the healing process is one that has been gaining interest in recent years. Ulrich (1997), in a paper summarizing theories on the therapeutic potential of the environment, proposes three guidelines for supportive design: a sense of control, social support and access to nature and positive distractions. Scher (1996) identifies 10 key aspects for consideration in developing 'patient focused architecture' that include privacy, social support, comfort, choice and control, variety and wayfinding. Some of these ideas have caught the imagination of clients and designers, and are published in advisory guidance documents such as *Better by design* (NHS Estates 1994a) and *Environments for quality care* (NHS Estates 1994b) However, the fact that it is difficult to capture and measure the precise nature of these characteristics means that there is little substantial scientific evidence to support the propositions. Nevertheless there is growing interest in creating designs that are non-confrontational, calming, stress-reducing, and attractive, and as well as respect for the idea that the planning and design of spaces can make a contribution to the feelings and behaviour of people.

Technical devices

The protection of the environment by the use of technical devices, such as security grills, locks, and cameras, is an approach that is increasingly regarded as one that can assist in specific locations but is not sufficient as a design and planning measure by itself. The Department of Health and the Welsh Office (1980) give guidance on planning and design and address the issues of violence and security. The note emphasises the need to minimize hazards by ensuring observation and good communication. It then suggests incorporating further technical options that include the appointment of alarm systems connected to other departments and main switchboard; the fitting of security glass screens at reception to protect staff; the possible provision of separate security measures to deal with difficult situations; the supervision of the department to prevent those with no valid reason from entering; and the fitting of locks to the department at night to stop unauthorized access. However, in a survey of 310

Accident and Emergency departments in the UK (Jenkins 1998), it was noted that panic buttons and video cameras were the most common security measures.

Numerous articles in the technical and construction press review the potential and usefulness of technical equipment, such as pagers, cctv, and specialist ironmongery. More recent reports suggest that installations have become more sophisticated and less obtrusive: for example, the use of pagers gives individuals the ability to call without restricting mobility. In fact, there may be lessons to learn from other sectors, such as the precautions taken by security vans carrying money fitted with delayed opening devices and shops that advertise empty tills to deter thieves from breaking in after hours. In banking, the distinction between the secure cash counter and the open enquiry desk in more open foyers gives clues for the design of health-care buildings that meet security needs without fortification.

Risk management

Concerns for staff safety through improving training and work conditions have been endorsed through regulatory frameworks concerned with health and safety issues and risk management. This has been backed by health and safety legislation for staff with support from the Trade Unions. The TUC strategic appraisal of health and safety *Better Jobs for better people: a millennial challenge* (1999) calls for a National Health and Safety Partnership and Audit to raise standards and the profile of this issue with employers.

Several organizations have recently published guides to raise awareness amongst staff on this topic such as the guide for nurses and managers on improving work conditions in hospitals and community published by The Royal College of Nursing and supported by the Department of Health (1998) entitled 'Dealing with violence against nursing staff: an RCN guide for nurses and managers.'

A Health and Safety Executive Report (1997) *Violence and aggression to staff in health services* suggests a systematic approach to risk management using five steps. These are: identify the hazards using records of incidents/potential assailants; consider who might be harmed; assess whether existing precautions are adequate; record findings; and review/revise the assessment. The report suggests that design applications, which include easily identifiable reception desks and give a clear route to treatment rooms, can help to put patients at ease. It discusses the need for personal space, quiet rooms, subdued interior decor, and clear information to enhance patient satisfaction and staff security in waiting rooms. It also suggests that solutions, such as wide reception desks, may be preferable to glass screens in that they are less alienating.

In a survey of 450 GP practices (Chambers 1998), on attitudes to workplace health activities, two key issues that were identified as priorities were minimizing stress and violence in the workplace. Practical advice on design for handling aggression and violence in primary care is offered in an article by Hodgson (1998), which relates to both spaces and technical devices. It raises issues about isolation and observation, the use of furniture as weapons, the installation of panic buttons, video surveillance, security and car parking, lighting and locks, and intercom systems to secure external doors. But it also questions whether the building is pleasant to visit and includes a quiet area.

The Audit Commission report on Accident and Emergency services (1996) suggested segregating patients, particularly psychiatric patients and children, from the general department. The report suggested that the risk of violent incidents in such depart-ments would be reduced if separate psychiatric crisis intervention services were pro-vided for patients. Comments from a patient satisfaction survey showed a greater concern for comfort than security, although adequate car park security and safe access to public transport at night were mentioned. It is widely accepted that incidents of violence are higher in urban areas.

Although Accident and Emergency, learning disabilities, and psychiatric services are traditionally associated with greater risk of violence a study reported in the Nursing Standard (Pattenson 1999) suggests that incidents have been reported in almost all services. The article calls for an environmental audit to provide benchmarking tools for health and safety, and identifies four factors that could be measured: physical assaults, security devices, incidents, and vandalism.

In summary, the literature that relates to the design of environments for health care to combat crime and violence is drawn from three sources: that which relates to the planning and designing of spaces, that which is concerned with technical devices, and lastly, that which addresses risk management — particularly from the point of staff working conditions. Whilst each of these focuses on different aspects of violence and safety, there is at present a convergence of approach. Greater emphasis is being put on passive measures for calming patients, on good observation and communication, on better training for staff to anticipate incidents, supported by less intrusive security measures to identify and record incidents. This same trend is evident in recent designs for health-care environments and a selection of exemplary projects for different health building services is now reviewed.

Design review

It is widely recognized that there are many different kinds of health buildings that are developed for different care groups and in contrasting locations. Some are on sites specifically for health care, such as hospitals, whilst others are in community loca-tions. There is another distinction in relation to violence that leads to two main cate-gories. First, the design of environments for general health use where violence may sometimes occur, commonly in Accident and Emergency departments, GP surgeries, waiting and reception areas, interview and consultation rooms; and second, the design of environments for people who are violent: specifically, psychiatric facilities.

Hospitals

A number of hospitals have upgraded Accident and Emergency departments recently and some have adopted approaches based on the design of space as a passive deter-rence. Poole Hospital in Dorset is one such example. It is affiliated to the Planetree movement, an organization committed to empowering patients, giving information about health, and involving patients and carers in their treatment. In the recently upgraded Accident and Emergency department, the design incorporates a low but wide reception desk that is more welcoming to patients and yet protects staff who are out of direct reach of patients. The waiting room furniture is also arranged as clusters of chairs rather than rows, to divert attention away from reception. Although not considered essential, cctv was installed in the department. This was more to give staff the confidence that they were not alone and were well-connected to other staff in the hospital in case of a violent incident.

A similar approach to reception was taken at Great Ormond Street Hospital. The reception desk is divided into two parts: one that is low and informal to suit small children and the other that is higher for more formal transactions. An informal desk for volunteers, who help orient patients and provide more general information, also overlooks the waiting area. Staff are trained to call for security help if they anticipate the need. But greater emphasis has been placed here on distracting young patients and their carers, making a place for play with toys and equipment, and social contact, which is consistent with the family-centred approach of the hospital.

At Conquest Hospital in Battle, Hastings, the re-organization of the hospital into villages or care centres has limited the circulation of patients to the part of the hospital relevant to their treatment or appointment. This relies on local control and supervision of entrances and waiting areas, which is proving easier to manage. It is also more convenient for patients who do not have to negotiate the whole building to arrive at the specific area that concerns them. Whilst this means that there are many entrances requiring security, once patients are inside the building their movement is limited to one area. At night, entry to the hospital is further restricted to one entrance and controlled by entry locks. Certain departments, such as maternity, have become targets for baby-snatching and here entry to the wards is restricted and controlled by cctv and touch pads.

Primary and community care

In primary care buildings the need to provide a welcoming reception area for patients has to be reconciled with maintaining a degree of confidentiality between patient and receptionist, as well as ensuring staff safety. The conflicting requirements of ease of access, confidentiality, and safety present a considerable design challenge throughout the building but are especially significant at reception. This is the first place that the patient meets staff and where staff have to be able to deal with anyone who walks in.

The design of reception desks plays a key role in creating a welcoming approach without compromising staff safety. The desk at Iveagh House Surgery, designed by Penoyre and Prasad Architects, for example, resolves these conflicting requirements in an elegant way (Figs 6.1–6.3). It enables good observation of the entrance and waiting area from the reception desk, so that trained staff can anticipate problems. The height of the desk is designed to deter patients from jumping onto or over it and the bulkhead fitting above both assists with this and gives cheerful and practical lighting over the desk. Space behind the desk enables receptionists to withdraw from the desk and to escape to the room behind. At the same time a section of the desk is low enough to be used comfortably by people in wheelchairs. Also some patients may want to have confidential conversations at reception without having to speak loudly, risking being overheard by others in the waiting room. This has been achieved without resort to barriers, grills, and glass screens at reception by giving space between the waiting room and the desk. From the reception desk, staff are able to see and generally hear people in the waiting room and the entrance.

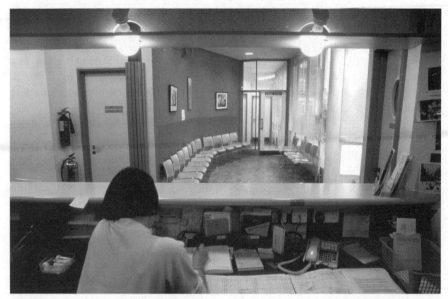

Fig. 6.1 Iveagh House Surgery. Photograph showing the view of the waiting-room from behind the reception desk.

At Herne Hill Group Practice, designed by Stock Woolstencroft Architects, the desk is designed along similar principles. In this building special attention has been paid to creating good observation by the receptionists of the waiting room (Fig. 6.4). This has been done by the use of two visual devices. First, a decorative glass screen divides the waiting room so that one part may be used for clinics and the other for waiting. Second, a window at the end of the desk means that the receptionist can overlook the waiting room and corridor, even when the shutters to the reception desk are closed. Making the public areas, such as the entrance, reception, waiting-room, and corridors to the clinical areas, more easily overlooked supports visual surveillance of the spaces without recourse to technical devices.

Clinical areas for consulting, interview, and treatment may require an alarm system for staff. In primary care premises it is most common for these activities to be provided in separate rooms rather than cubicles and for the rooms to have doors without vision panels. For clinical staff who feel vulnerable, a simple alarm call system may be installed to alert a receptionist if help is required. These can be fitted in a discrete way to the underside of the desk so that the devices are generally not visible. Layouts for consulting rooms for Iveagh House Surgery have presumed that the doctor does not come between the patient and the door.

Planning the building into separate zones is another effective way to minimize risk: this enables, for example, staff areas and offices to be planned adjacent to one another, so that entry can be limited and better controlled.

Few primary care buildings open at night except for meetings or community events. But a recently refurbished building in Kings Cross specifically planned to provide services to alcohol and drug-dependants, sex workers, homeless people, and local

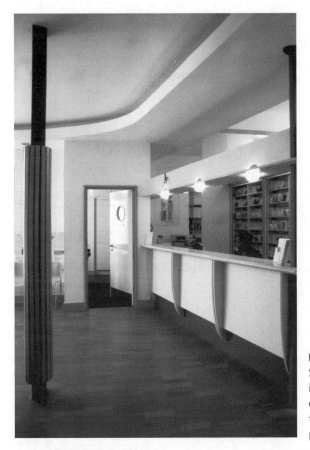

Fig. 6.2 Iveagh House Surgery. Photograph showing the design of reception desk, which is welcoming to patients whilst offering protection to staff.

hostel communities, opens at night for health-care services whilst operating as an office base during the day (Figs 6.5–6.7). Issues of safety and security are paramount and include safety of staff, security of stored drugs, and supervision of clients. The design by Monahan Blythen Architects (Rogers 1997) adopts many of the same principles as other primary care buildings: patient spaces on the ground floor; administration and staff facilities on the first floor; general offices for the trust to use during the day on the top two floors.

Since the site is very restricted, the entrance and reception is shared by the general office users and the care services. Specific issues generated by the hostile location and nature of the patient group for whom services are intended have led to a number of innovative design solutions. Externally, sound-insulated opaque glass makes the façade to a busy traffic congested street. Whilst this allows light into the waiting area it also prevents overlooking from the street and retains privacy for those waiting. The entrance is marked by tight security in the form of a lobby between the entrance door and waiting room. Access through the inner door of the lobby is only possible when the electronically controlled street door is closed. This lobby connects to the reception desk via a special hatch.

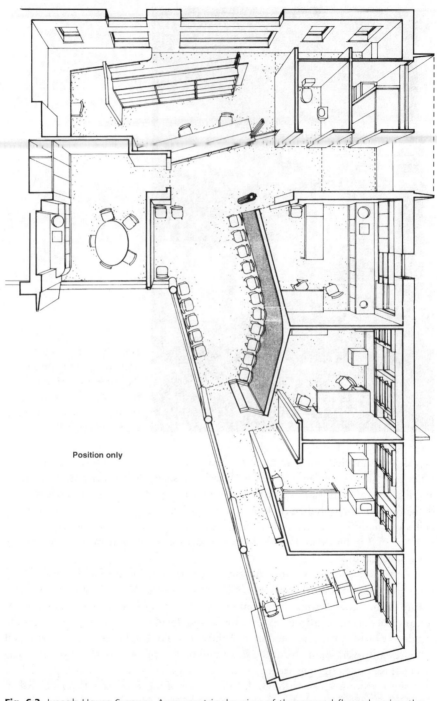

Position only

Fig. 6.3 Iveagh House Surgery. Axonometric drawing of the ground floor showing the relationship between the reception desk, the entrance, and the waiting room.

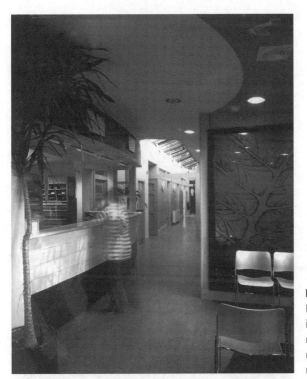

Fig. 6.4 Herne Hill Group Practice. Photograph showing the reception desk in relation to the waiting-room and consultation rooms.

The curved reception desk makes a long surface joining together, spatially, the lobby and waiting room. At the same time it protects staff and overlooks the waiting room. A door from the area behind the desk affords an escape route for staff into the corridor near to the treatment rooms. During the daytime a security shutter protects access to files and computers whilst giving access for staff to reception.

Psychiatric facilities

Detailed design consideration has to be given to environments where patients are detained against their will and staff require safety measures for their own protection. These buildings pose perhaps one of the most challenging design problems for those seeking a humane and calm resolution.

Foque-Denkens-Adriaenssens's medium secure unit in Belgium is exemplary in this respect (Figs 6.8 and 6.9). The pavilion building accommodates 54 beds in two units of 24 and 30 beds, with some shared therapeutic facilities. The pavilion is located in the parkland of an existing hospital site shared with a general hospital. Patient disorders are characterized by temporary adaptations to normality and skillful ability to disrupt treatment systems. Many patients are unable to control or suppress temper, anger, desires, and sudden impulses. There is a tendency for self-mutilation and suicidal behaviour, as well as being aggressive or threatening. The client brief described a fully closed controlled ward, offering a suitable environment for optimum treatment and, where possible, re-socialization taking account of the specific and complex disorders of the patients. Special emphasis was placed on three aspects:

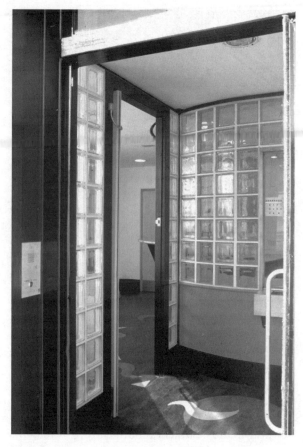

Fig. 6.5 Kings Cross Health Centre. Photograph showing the entrance lobby to the health centre.

- a protective function accentuating individual and group security, safety devices, and controlled shelter;
- a residential function in groups of eight patients in individual rooms, emphasizing individual privacy, possibilities for social contact, outdoor life, and self-development;
- a therapeutic function through structured settings, socio-therapeutic environment, and treatment spaces.

It was well-recognized that within these three factors there were conflicting demands: such as the need for patient privacy versus permanent control involving protection against self-destructive activities and aggression to others. For staff there was a conflict between the need for an open therapeutic environment and the permanent threat of unpredictable aggression. Defining the limits of privacy and protection were key to the design resolution. The design was based on the concept of the safety belt, which encloses the whole building. The zoning distinguishes seven main safety areas, each with its particular features: the entire pavillion, the patios, the unit, the staff desk, individual rooms, sanitary rooms, and seclusion room. Apart from one centrally controlled entrance, the ring is fully closed with no doors or opening

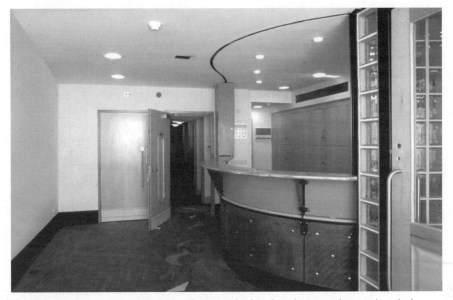

Fig. 6.6 Kings Cross Health Centre. Photograph showing the curved reception desk overlooking the waiting-room.

windows. Three residential units and one sports/therapy facility are arranged around an enclosed courtyard. The residential units provide a systematic gradation of privacy and social interaction.

The design seeks to articulate these security needs in a way that avoids the building looking fortified. For example, shatterproof glass enables large windows to sustain views of the outside and mirrored glass prevents people from seeing inside. The courtyard walls are designed with an elegant cove at high level, which both visually lowers the height of the external wall whilst also preventing patients from escaping. The use of angled corners internally makes the appearance of the building softer and less aggressive, whilst diminishing the danger of injuries and helping observation and visual control. To meet the stringent safety regulations the doors to the patient rooms open outwards but these have been positioned and detailed to ensure that staff cannot be trapped by violent patients as they move around. Materials and finishes have been selected for durability and low maintenance, and for resistance to fire damage and vandalism. In order to protect patients from self-harm and from destroying their personal space, the rooms have been thoughtfully detailed: controls for lighting, heating, window blinds in the bedrooms can be individual and centrally operated. Most of the furniture is built-in, including a wooden couch on a fixed concrete base. The television is protected by a synthetic screen, the writing desk has a concrete base and all cupboards are fully fixed. *En suite* bathrooms are fitted with sanitary ware that is fully built-in and the window glazing consists of three layers of fireproof security glass. It would be absurd to suggest that the result is an environment resembling normality but it would also be unreasonable to expect such for this care group. It does not give

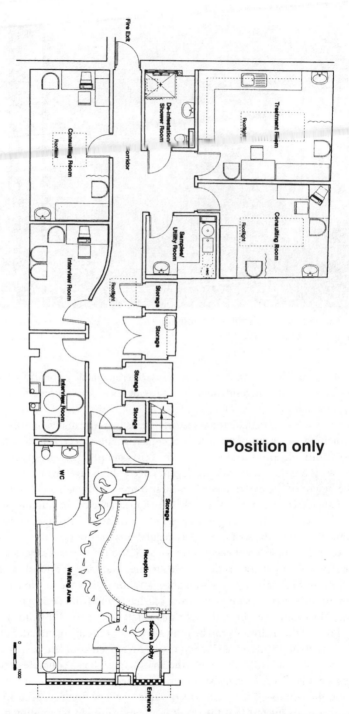

Fig. 6.7 Kings Cross Health Centre. Ground-floor plan showing the entrance into the secure lobby and the curved reception desk overlooking the waiting room.

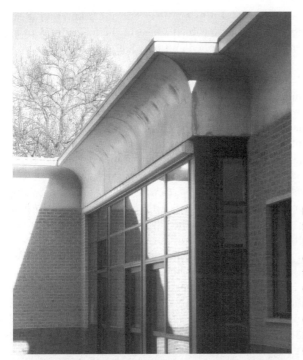

Fig. 6.8 Handelsei Medium Secure Unit, Belgium. Photograph showing the elegant cove at high level to the internal walls of the courtyard, which visually lowers the height of the external wall whilst also preventing patients from escaping.

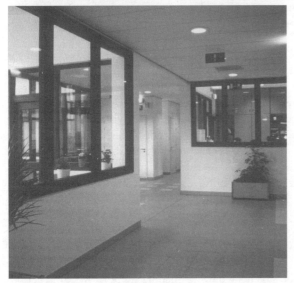

Fig. 6.9 Handelsei Medium Secure Unit, Belgium. Photograph showing an interior view of the unit with the glazed panels that give a sense of space and afford good observation.

the appearance of a fortified enclosure, although it addresses and provides for physical security and psychological security.

David Morley Architects have recently completed a secure mental health unit in Luton (Fig. 6.10). The linear planning is in contrast to many earlier such schemes built in the UK based on highly articulated layouts, such as racetrack plans and culs-de- sac, that are now regarded as confusing, disorienting and present ideal opportunities for concealment. This issue was highlighted in the major incident at a centre where a member of staff was trapped and murdered in a corridor by a patient.

The master plan for the Luton secure unit is based on a series of courtyard spaces defined by simple linear buildings that provide the boundaries to the external spaces and so reduce the need for security fencing. The design of the roof is a monopitch in which the high side faces the patient courtyards. There are two other zones between the secure courtyards and the public street. One of these is a 'buffer zone' accessible to public and patients, and the other is along the front of the complex where the main entrance and car park are located.

The unit has 36 beds divided into two 16-bed wards with a small four-bed linking ward. Each ward is further subdivided into eight beds with shared bathrooms. Each of these has its own day and activity areas that open directly onto the secure courtyards.

The internal planning of the ward areas recognizes the conflicting needs for observation and informality to facilitate staff control and patient dignity. Three devices have been used to achieve this in the design: first, the open plan social spaces at the centre of each T- shaped wing create a place for patients to gather and from which staff can observe; the corridors are lit by clerestorey glazing, which provides natural light and ventilation and is positioned to give emphasis to the entrances to two sets of adjacent bedrooms; the doorways to these bedrooms are recessed to give further emphasis to this space whilst avoiding marking hiding places. The intention of the architects is to transform the corridors into pleasant places by marking the hierarchy of spaces from public to social to private and giving identity to significant places along the route.

The landscaping of the spaces around the buildings is designed to make clear the entrances to the building, which are through air-locked doors and lobbies. At the same time, a sunken garden off the main forecourt offers patients with visiting privileges an opportunity to meet their visitors in a secure outdoor garden. The patient spaces on the wards have been designed to overlook the gardens and so create strong visual and functional links between the inside and outside of the building. This design aims to provide for a high standard of security and observation, whilst creating a friendly environment without resorting to overt features of control.

The Canning Crescent Health Centre in North London, designed by MacCormac Jamieson Pritchard, is an exemplary building for community mental health care services. The project was conceived as part of the programme of moving services from Friern Barnet Hospital, a large and austere psychiatric hospital that was closed under the 'Care in the Community' initiative. The centre provides counselling, treatment, and support for people who would otherwise have to attend hospital. As a service with an open-door policy for patients requiring ongoing support over long periods of time, the design needed to be accessible, robust, and safe, as well as friendly and calming.

The centre is part of a network of community facilities across the Borough of Haringey. One of the key intentions behind the programme was to remove the stigma and institutional nature of mental health care and to make it more accessible. This is

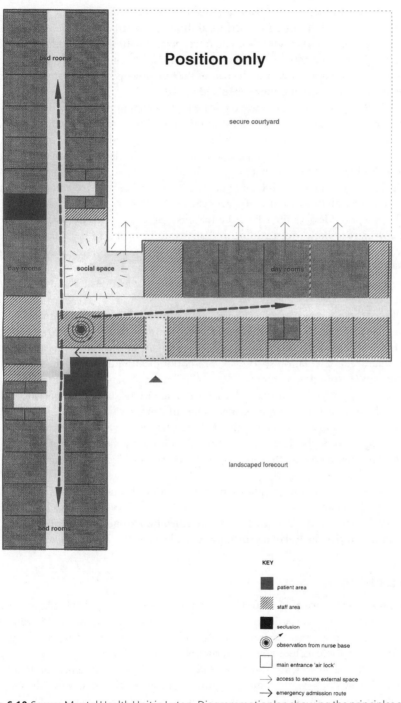

Fig. 6.10 Secure Mental Health Unit in Luton. Diagrammatic plan showing the principles of the layout indicating observation lines from the nurse base and the secure external courtyard.

reflected in both the service organization and building design. The site is on a main road and is a short distance from the local shopping centre, a deliberate decision to make it part of everyday activities. The introspective nature of the building and the need for privacy for patients has resulted in a somewhat austere and closed public façade along the street. However, the rear of the building opens onto a small, enclosed garden and this elevation is more open and glazed.

The building accommodates two day-care units, a community mental health centre and an adult day hospital. These units require autonomy from each other but share staff, catering, and administrative facilities. The L shaped plan was developed to respond to these needs. The main entrance to the building is at the corner and opens onto a double-height space that is light and open. The two wings radiate from this reception giving a clear and legible plan. The clinical spaces are arranged on the ground floor with offices and staff spaces above.

The reception desk to the left of the main entrance doors overlooks the entrance and corridors to both wings. Although designed to be open, the desk has been fitted more recently with a glass screen to give staff improved reassurance and security. They had expressed concern that the office behind the desk did not lead onto any other rooms and were afraid of becoming trapped if someone attacked them at the desk.

The general ambience of the building is cheerful and bright with treatment rooms taking best advantage of natural lighting and ventilation. The corridors have been skillfully manipulated in plan and volume to relieve the merely functional and institutional nature of circulation spaces, so common in health buildings. The set-back of rooms on the ground floor, for example, makes informal waiting areas and a place for incidental meetings. Social spaces have been made on the first-floor corridors that relieve the narrow routes and make places for informal exchange between staff, often working in stressful and over committed circumstances. Daylight and natural ventilation from the rooflights passes down through voids in the floor to the ground floor, giving a positive quality to the internal corridors around which the essentially cellular rooms are planned.

The specification of high-quality materials and well-crafted detailing creates a friendly and calm ambience. Natural wood finishes have been used for floors, cupboards, ceilings, and doors. These are matched by a limited palette of colours and furnishings to give the feel of a subtle, warm, and supportive environment.

Conclusion

There is a convergence of ideas and intentions to make buildings that are humane and dignified rather than curative or custodial. This approach is supported in research studies, technical and professional journals, and built projects. The three sources of literature for this topic include texts concerned with design of spaces, more specific issues around technical devices, and those addressing issues of risk management and training of staff. Reviews of recently completed building projects show that these ideas about calming environments with unobtrusive security measures are being put into practice, resulting in some innovative and attractive designs for health-care buildings.

A checklist of key issues for consideration in relation to designing to limit violence is drawn from the issues highlighted in the literature, from built projects, and by designers' experiences in this fascinating and challenging arena. It does not attempt to be comprehensive or exhaustive.

Issues to consider include:

- approach car parking/entrance: make these visible and legible both at night and day;
- use the landscaping and the buildings to provide security and thus avoid additional barriers and fencing;
- inside/outside space: views can be usefully distracting and calming;
- waiting rooms
  - reduce stress and boredom
  - provide good observation by staff
  - make the desk welcoming and non-confrontational
  - make the space information rich;
- provide escape routes to outside or other spaces
  - apply this to outside and within the building
  - avoid the cul-de-sac and places where people can be trapped;
- define visually the nature of private, social and public spaces
  - limit access to spaces
  - make clear the delineation between spaces;
- address the conflicting requirements of the reception desk
  - consider in particular the height, depth, bulkhead
  - make it possible for staff to withdraw safely from the desk
  - provide an escape route from the room behind the desk;
- consider the density of space— avoid the sense of personal invasion of space;
- create a comfortable ambience
  - select lighting fittings and heating systems to suit
  - avoid unnecessary and distracting noise;
- fit technical devices for added safety and security where appropriate and ensure these are unobtrusive, where possible, e.g. alarms, cctv, locks.

Special considerations for psychiatric care include:

- consider designs that minimize opportunities for self-harm and causing harm to others;
- provide, where possible, a sense of control that fosters ownership and territoriality.

Finally, the question posed in this chapter is to review whether design can make a contribution. The answer is undoubtedly that it can, but not perhaps in ways that are obvious and directly to do with security or safety. Creating designs that are calming with unobtrusive measures for dealing with security and safety is believed to be more effective than fortified solutions. The evidence base for this is yet to be fully developed through further evaluation studies of buildings in use, although there is a consistency of ideas from both theory and practice. Current thinking may enable us to benefit from the added value of design by developing buildings for health care that are essentially humane, dignified, and caring.

References

Audit Commission (1996). *By accident or design: improving A&E services in England and Wales.*

Chambers, R. (1998). *Survey of general practices: health at work in primary care research study.* Health Education Authority, London.

Colman, A. (1985). *Utopia on trial: vision and reality in planned housing.* Hilary Shipman, London.

Department of Heath and the Welsh Office (1980). *Accident and Emergency department heath building note* 22. HMSO, London.

Gulak, M. (1991). Architectural guidelines for state psychiatric hospitals. *Hospital and Community Psychiatry,* **42**, (7).

Health and Safety Executive Report (1997). Violence and aggression to staff in health services. *Hospital Development,* March.

Hillier, B. (1986). *The social logic of space.* CUP, London.

Hillier, B. (1994). *Estates design against crime — a strategic approach to hospital planning.* Health Facility Notes NHS. HMSO, London.

Hodgson, M. (1998). Handling aggression and violence in primary care. *General Practice Manager,* Special Report, 18th May, 16.

Jacobs, J. (1961). *The life and death og the great American cities: the failure of town planning.* New York: Random House.

Jenkins, M. (1998). Violence and verbal abuse against staff in accident and emergency departments: a survey of consultants in the UK and the Republic of Ireland. *Journal of Accident and Emergency Medicine,* **15**, (4), July.

Mason, T. (1999). *Managing violence and aggression: a manual for nurses and health-care workers.* Churchill Livingstone, Edinburgh.

Newman, O. (1972). *Defensible space: people and design in the violent city.* Architectural Press, London.

NHS Estates (1994a). *Better by design — pursuit of excellence in healthcare buildings.* HMSO, London.

NHS Estates (1994b). *Environments for quality care.* HMSO, London.

Patterson, B. (1999). Violence at work. *Nursing Standard,* **13**, (21), 43–6.

Palmstierna, T., Huitfeldt, B. and Wistedt, B. (1991). The relationship of crowding and social aggressive behaviour on a psychiatric intensive care intensive care unit. *Hospital and Community Psychiatry,* **42**, (12), December.

Parker, J. (1998). Mean Streets. *Hospital Development,* **29**, (3), March.

Ravetz, A. (1988). Malaise, design and history: scholarship and experience on trial. In *Rehumanising housing* (ed. N. Teymur, T.A. Markus, and T. Wooley), p. 154.

Remen, S. (1987). Planning psychiatric hospitals — human design considerations. *The Psychiatric Hospital,* **18**, (1), 11–6.

Rogers, L. (1997). Streetwise lifeline interior study. *RIBA Interiors,* June.

Royal College of Nursing (1998). *Dealing with violence against nursing staff: an RCN guide for nurses and managers.* Royal College of Nursing.

Royal College of Psychiatrists (1998). *Management of imminent violence. Clinical practical guidelines to support mental health services.* Occasional Paper OP41. London.

Sainsbury Centre for Mental Health (1998). *Acute problems, a survey of quality care in acute psychiatric wards.* London.

Scher, P. (1996). *Patients focused architecture for health care.* Faculty of Art and Design. Manchester Metropolitan University.

Steventon, G. (1996). Defensible space: a critical review of the theory and practice of a crime prevention strategy. *Urban Design International*, 1, (3), 235–45.

TUC (1999). *Better jobs for better people: a millenium challenge.* TUC strategic appraisal of health and safety.

Ulrich, R. (1997). Research on healthcare building design and medical outcomes. In *Human centred design for health care buildings.* Proceedings of International Conference and Workshop. Sintef, Trondheim, Norway, pp. 42–50.

Van Der Voordt, T., and Van Wegen, H.B.R. (1993). The Delft Checklist on safe neighbourhoods. *Journal of Architectural and Planning Research*, 10, (4), 344–5.

WHL, Estates. *Safety and security by design. Community-based mental health facilities.* London.

Chapter 7

Attacks on doctors and nurses

Stefan Cembrowicz, Sue Ritter, and Steve Wright

Violence in the UK is widespread. A rate of 667 violent offences per 100 000 population was recorded by police in England and Wales in 1997 (Home Office 1998). The British Crime Survey (BCS) found that just over 5% of survey respondents had been victims of violent crime in the previous year (Mirlees-Black *et al.* 1996). Both of these figures are likely to under-represent the true prevalence of violence. Violence is clearly a major public health problem (Golding 1996; Shepherd and Farrington 1993), and health-service workers are not immune.

Violence is usually defined as 'the use of physical force which is intended to hurt or injure another person' (e.g. Megargee 1982; Siann 1985). In the health-service context it has been defined as 'any incident where (doctors or staff) are abused, threatened, or assaulted in circumstances related to their work, involving an explicit or implicit challenge to their safety, well-being, or health'.

Verbal threats and abuse, which can be traumatic and damaging, are frequently encountered in health-care settings. Adams and Whittington (1995) found 29% of a sample of hospital- and community-based psychiatric nurses reported verbal aggression over a 10-week period, which often provoked high levels of anxiety and traumatic stress. McNeil and Binder (1989) suggest that verbal aggression is not separate from physical aggression, but forms a continuum with it.

In Britain, medical sites have been found to have the greatest risk of all workplaces for verbal abuse and threats to staff. The Health Services Advisory Committee (HSAC) survey in 1987 found that 73% of staff on medical premises had suffered abuse, compared to 63% for transport and public administration; 5% of NHS staff reported having been threatened with a weapon. Hobbs (1991) reported that 63% of a sample of GPs in the West Midlands had experienced abuse or violence, and that 3% had sustained minor injuries from assaults by patients in the previous year.

Fear of violence to general practitioners has led to the quality of service offered to patients suffering, with some GPs being anxious about home visits to the extent of abandoning night visits (Anonymous 1995). In general hospital settings, Whittington *et al.* (1996) found that 21% of a sample of staff reported having been assaulted in the previous year. Victims were predominantly nurses and staff working in medical wards. Mental health was found to be significantly worse among staff exposed to threats.

Violence is also common in Accident and Emergency (A&E) departments. Cembrowicz and Shepherd (1992) found that a total of 407 violent assaults were recorded in the A&E department of the Bristol Royal Infirmary by A&E and hospital security staff over a 10-year period, although this is likely to be an underestimate because of inconsistent reporting. Of the 283 assaults recorded by these A&E staff, just over 11% involved the use of a weapon.

There is particular concern about assaults on staff in mental health services. Gournay *et al.* (1998) found that on average there was an assault every three days per ward in a sample of inner-London adult acute wards and psychiatric intensive care units. Approximately two-thirds of these were directed at nurses. Ryan and Poster (1993) found that 26% of a sample of psychiatric nurses reported having been a victim of violence in the preceding month. Few nurses (8%) reported never having been assaulted in their career.

Kidd and Stark (1992) found that 35% of a sample of psychiatric senior house officers and registrars (median experience = 30 months) had been assaulted at least once, and over 90% reported experiencing incidents where they had felt in imminent danger. The risk of violence has also been found to deter junior doctors from choosing a career in psychiatry. Davies and Schlich (1999) found that out of a sample of 1093 senior registrars who responded to a survey of career choices and their determinants, 257 respondents rejected the idea of a career in general adult psychiatry. Of these, 49 (19%) cited the high risk of violence as a reason for their rejection of the speciality.

Action points:

- violent incidents are an issue for all health staff:
- see that training and support is built in to your work.

Causes of violence

Possible causes of violence range from reductionistic neurologic explanations to more holistic social and contextual ones, with different types of explanation coming into vogue at different times. These various explanations are not necessarily mutually exclusive. Certain explanations may be more appropriate than others for different situations, and various factors may feature in the same assault.

Another problem is that research into the causes of assault is often carried out in different settings and on different populations. Factors relevant to assaults in in-patients psychiatric settings, for example, may not be relevant to assaults in A&E.

Remember that:

- violence is a complex phenomenon, with no single explanation for it;
- multiple levels of intervention are therefore necessary;
- research on violence in particular contexts or populations may not be widely generalizable, but may have useful heuristic value. Some approaches to understanding causes of violence are outlined below.

Social and contextual factors

Social structures and cultural norms influence the expression of a wide range of behaviour, including violence. Social and contextual factors can exert a general effect on rates of violence at a certain point in time, as well as locally, in certain sections of society and locations.

Historically, tidal waves of crime have occurred in Europe and the USA during periods where social, economic, and political changes have been coupled with decline of cultural values (Cohn 1961; Graham and Gurr 1979; Tuchman 1978). Violence may therefore be the result of social anomie, when the power of social institutions has weakened. Under such conditions, respect for traditionally authoritative social institutions — including medicine and nursing — has declined. Their staff may be vulnerable, either because any protection formerly afforded by their status as practitioners of a socially valued service has become null and void, or because they are seen as representing the Establishment.

Besides more general social disorganization, certain characteristics of neighbourhoods may affect the risk of violence and other crime. Empirical studies since the earliest days of social science research have demonstrated that various forms of deviance are more frequently encountered in conditions of poverty and social disorganization (Bottoms and Wiles 1997; Hiday, 1995). This may be because of a general community effect, due to the concentration of high-risk people in certain neighbourhoods. Particular forms of community relations, which lead to high rates of offending, and other social problems such as poverty, income inequality, and deprivation, may also be involved (Hope 1998). For example, the 1996 BCS (Mirrlees-Black *et al.* 1996) reported that nearly 5% of adults surveyed who lived in non-inner city areas had been victims of contact crime (woundings, common assaults, robberies, and snatch thefts) in 1995, compared to just over 7% of adults surveyed in inner city areas.

It appears that violence is mediated by a neighbourhood's level of social cohesion (Sampson *et al.* 1997). The relatively high levels of violence known to occur in disadvantaged neighbourhoods may therefore make it more likely that that residents will choose aggression as a means of resolving interpersonal disputes.

The expression of violent behaviour may be an important norm within certain subcultures. Wolfgang and Ferracutti (1967) proposed the existence of an actual *subculture of violence* — part of a more general pattern of attitudes favouring excitement, status, honour, and masculinity, with violence being the response when these are threatened. Wolfgang and Ferracutti also suggested that because the highest homicide rates are to be found in young, male, non-white, and lower-class groups, then these groups support violent subcultural values, which conflict with those of the dominant culture. This hypothesis has not fared well when tested empirically (e.g. Ball-Rokeach) 1973; Erlanger 1974). Marsh's (1985) study of the social rules governing the aggressive behaviour of British soccer fans suggested that the occurrence of violence is governed by shared conceptual schemata, which specify when it is appropriate. Similarly, Anderson (1997) reports that within inner-city neighbourhoods, while interpersonal violence does not appear to be valued as a goal in itself, it has become an accepted and tolerated means of resolving conflicts. A 'code of the streets', a set of informal rules governing displays of interpersonal violence, has emerged.

Social and contextual explanations may help us to understand why violence may be more prevalent in certain periods and among certain groups of people, but they cannot explain why all people in such circumstances are not violent.

The important lesson for doctors and nurses is that at certain times and in certain social settings they may be at increased risk of violence, either because violence is generally more prevalent, or because of what they might be thought of as representing. For example, health-care professionals working in neighbourhoods where physical aggression is commonly used to resolve disputes are at increased risk, not only because of the overall prevalence of violence, but also if they are trying to persuade a patient to comply with treatment or desist in unusual or health-threatening behaviour.

Vulnerable patients (particularly if suffering from mental disorders) may also be attractive targets for bullying in such physically aggressive environments (Estroff and Zimmer 1994). This may lead to hypersensitivity to possible threat and an expectation of mistreatment by others. Medical and/or nursing follow-up may then be interpreted as intrusive, irritating interference.

Individual factors

Psychology and psychiatry have predominantly sought to explain violence by factors within the individual. The extent to which these factors apply to an individual affects their likelihood of being violent. The MacArthur Risk Assessment Study conceived of risk factors for violence by psychiatric patients as falling into the four domains of dispositional, clinical, historical, and contextual factors; the first three being explicitly individual. Commonly described individual risk factors are presented below.

Neurobiologic traits

Violent behaviour has been linked to brain injury since classical times, although the extent to which brain damage is a sufficient explanation for violence generally, as opposed to an explanation for violence in those who have received a brain injury, is debatable. For example, as recently as the 1970s brain damage has been blamed for violence that might ostensibly be seen as caused by predominantly social and political factors (i.e. urban rioting in the USA), and psychosurgery was hailed as the answer to this problem (Mark and Ervin 1970). The literature of this period also included the intriguing proposal that criminals have electrodes planted in their brains to enable their mood and behaviour to be monitored and altered by remote control if necessary (Delgado 1971). This argument proposes two related ways in which brain damage can lead to violent behaviour. Brain damage may either impair inhibitory control of violent behaviour or, if it occurs in early life, it may impair the development of functions necessary for cognitive development or socialization, which ordinarily lead to the development of such inhibitory control in the first place.

Violence has been associated with several different types of brain pathology. These include frontal lobe damage (Bryant et al. 1984; Yeudall and Fromm-Auch 1979), temporal lobe damage (Brickman et al. 1984), temporal lobe epilepsy (TLE), 'episodic dyscontrol syndrome' (Mark and Irving 1970), and left hemisphere dysfunction (Nachson 1988; Yeudall and Fromm-Auch 1979; Yeudall et al. 1982).

Although some people who have brain damage or dysfunction are undoubtedly violent, the extent to which such trauma is the actual cause is often unclear. Even when violence can be confidently attributed to brain damage or dysfunction, this explanation can only apply to people who suffer from such conditions, and does not explain all violence. Many studies do not distinguish between angry aggression (aggression as an expression of an emotional state), which has a neurologic substrate in the hypothalamus, and instrumental (goal-directed) aggression, which does not need a neurologic substrate. Second, these studies tend to be based upon the examination of court-referred patients undergoing neuropsychiatric assessment, who are likely to have high rates of violence irrespective of brain trauma. Finally, experimental and control groups are seldom matched for confounding variables such as social class and intelligence.

Even where violence and brain injury coexist, the violent behaviour may actually predate brain injury (Jamieson 1971; Miller 1992). For example, because the location of the frontal lobes renders them vulnerable to damage in fights, frontal lobe damage may be a result of violence, rather than its cause.

Research findings can also contradict expectations. Gunn and Bonn (1971) found that epileptic prisoners were no more likely to have committed violent offences than non-epileptic prisoners, and that prisoners with idiopathic epilepsy (which has no identifiable neurologic focus) were more likely to have committed violent offences than prisoners with TLE. Furthermore, Gunn and Fenton (1971) found that few offences were committed at around the time of a seizure.

Finally, neurologic conditions that have been associated with violence can be poorly defined. The concept of 'episodic dyscontrol syndrome' assumes that temporal lobe and limbic lesions cause violence (although adjustment is adequate between episodes). This syndrome has been criticized on the grounds that it amounts to a vaguely defined behavioural syndrome correlated with signs of brain pathology with no clearly established validity. Fenton (1984) argues that the syndrome merely represents a convenient label for impulsive and aggressive antisocial tendencies, which may be more understandable in terms of the patient's damaging early life experiences.

While brain damage and dysfunction may often be an insufficient causal explanation of a person's violence, health-care professionals may be wise to bear in mind the association between violence and brain damage (irrespective of the direction of causality) when treating patients with a history of such injury.

Action point:

♦ consider the patient's past medical history.

Personality traits, social learning, and cognitive factors

While a person may behave in an uncharacteristically violent way because of situational factors or because of a temporary mental state, a tendency towards aggressive resolution of conflict may be influenced by personality factors, learning history, and the ways in which he or she interprets situations. Aggression appears to be substantially stable over time and across different situations (Feshbach and Price 1984; Huesmann *et al.* 1984; Olweus 1980), and is linked to criminal aggression (Farrington 1978; Robins 1978).

Learning theorists reject the idea of a specific aggressive drive (as proposed in psychoanalytic and ethnological approaches). They propose that aggression is acquired and maintained by successfully obtaining a desired reward and by removing a threat or aversive stimulus. Social learning theorists (e.g. Bandura 1983) emphasize the role played by the social context within which learning occurs. According to this view, people learn by experience and observation that aggression can achieve concrete aims or satisfy emotional ends, and they develop expectations regarding the likely positive and negative outcomes and consequences of aggression, and adjust their behaviour accordingly. However, if a person has developed few or no alternative means of achieving their needs besides aggression, or has come to view aggression as an appropriate and effective way of resolving conflict, aggression becomes their typical response.

Cognitive distortions about situations, appropriate and expected behaviour, and the intentions and actions of others can also lead to aggressive reactions, as can emotional states such as anger. While anger, as an emotional state, is often considered to exist in a separate psychological realm to cognition, cognitive theorists have been particularly interested in the relationship between anger and its behavioural expression, and how cognition mediates this.

Beck (1976) views anger as resulting from the appraisal of an assault on one's domain (which includes values, moral code, and protective rules). The experience and expression of anger is also described by Beck as being mediated by evaluating the infringement as serious and negative, and as not representing immediate or continuing danger (primary concerns with safety would be more likely to provoke anxiety rather than anger).

Another important mediating factor is an externalized appraisal of the infringement, focused towards the wrongfulness of the offence or the offender, rather than on injury or harm sustained. Novaco (e.g. 1994) presents a model of the determinants and consequences of anger, in which environmental cues affect both cognitive interpretations of the situation and physiological arousal (which influence each other), which lead to anger and behavioural reactions, which feed back upon both the environmental circumstances and anger itself.

Action points:

- your own behaviour may be misinterpreted, which may increase anger;
- your behaviour can also reduce angry arousal;
- can you present the patient with alternatives to confrontation or violence as a means of resolving conflict?

Historical factors

Certain events in a person's history may also increase risk of violence. This has already been alluded to in the earlier discussion of the effect of substance abuse and head injury on later violence, but other factors also exist. Childhood exposure to violence, either in the form of direct child abuse, or witnessing violence between parents, is commonly associated with later violent behaviour. Harsh parental attitudes and discipline, and separation from parents have also been implicated in later violence (e.g.

Farrington 1978). While empirical evidence does tend to suggest the existence of such a 'cycle of violence', not all abused children go on to become violent (Falshaw *et al.* 1996; Widom 1989).

Clinical and situational factors

Very often health-care staff must deal with people whose history they do not know, and who are often in pain, anxious, and uncertain about what is happening and what the future holds. Staff have to attempt to provide help in the context of a relationship between strangers, perhaps intruding into private areas of patients' lives.

The anxiety, uncertainty, and discomfort that accompany both symptoms and clinical interventions, and the frustration and resentment at loss of autonomy and becoming subject to institutional routines, can all find expression in aggression. Long waiting times for medical treatment, and anxiety among patients and relatives are also described as causes (Hobbs 1991).

Sex differences

Physical violence is generally far more commonly found in men than in women. In 1984, women constituted only 7% of those convicted of violent offences (Walmsley 1986). It has been argued that this figure is inaccurate, and that women are in fact responsible for more violence than official statistics might suggest (Pearson 1998). In-patient studies consistently find that male patients do not necessarily pose a greater level of risk, either finding no difference in assault rates between men and women (e.g. Hodgkinson *et al.* 1985), or that a disproportionate number of assaults were caused by women (e.g. Convey 1986 Larkin *et al.* 1988). Convey (1986) attributes this to staff underestimating the risk of violence in female patients (particularly younger patients), making them more likely to confront female patients alone, thereby exposing themselves to greater risk.

Aggressive elderly people

Perhaps the most useful and well-known demographic predictor of violence is age, since younger patients seem to present a higher risk than other age groups (e.g. Acquilina 1991; Noble and Roger 1989). However, older patients may also present a significant risk. Aggression may result from misperception caused by clouding of consciousness as a result of dementia or delirium.

Both Noble and Roger (1989) and Hodgkinson *et al.* (1985) found that patients in their seventies were involved in a disproportionate number of assaults. The HSAC survey (1987) found that over a fifth of staff working with geriatric patients reported receiving physical injury from assault by a patient over the previous year. Brain damage caused by dementia may reduce the person's ability to inhibit violent impulses or cope with provocation or frustration by other means, and the attention given to such behaviour (or the removal of aversive attention) may maintain it. Large numbers of staff can appear particularly threatening to the elderly, and elderly patients may not understand that informal clothes can be worn by qualified staff. Once again, because the risk of violence in this client group is often underestimated, staff may expose themselves to unnecessary risk by not treating such patients with due caution.

While elderly patients do cause some unique concerns, it should be remembered that they are basically just people who have been around for longer than the rest of us. Any considerations regarding reducing the risk of violence by improving the general quality of patient care therefore apply equally to this client group. The following general considerations may be helpful in working with all client groups:

- Always demonstrate non-possessive warmth and positive regard.
- Do not stereotype, or force patients to fit in with your routine.
- Never force attention on a patient who is irritable or hostile towards you.
- Establish rapport prior to each intervention. Violence may erupt when unprepared patients are suddenly required to comply with an instruction.
- Helpful calming influences for particular patients may include photographs of young children or babies.
- Religious and spiritual beliefs are as important to some patients as they are to some staff. The opportunity to visit the chapel, to pray, or to share the sign of the cross can be calming.

Action points — prediction of violence, and assessment of dangerousness:

- the best predictor of violent behaviour is a history of violent actions;
- some patients with a dual diagnosis (especially substance-misuse and psychosis) give particular concern;
- aggression can occur at all ages — the risk of violence by the very old should not be underestimated;
- the risk of violence in female in-patients should not be underestimated.

Action points — how managers can reduce the risks of violence:

- consider environmental and organizational factors in preventing violence;
- train staff to intervene as rapidly and as effectively as possible when a violent incident occurs;
- provide comprehensive support for staff who may be stressed both by the need to maintain high standards, and the feelings of self-blame, which often result from involvement with a violent person.

What to do if ...
A patient or relative becomes agitated and distressed:

- Are they in pain? Re-assess and deal with the cause of the pain if necessary. They may be frightened or overwhelmed by their surroundings (e.g. a noisy or crowded room). Remove sources of noise if possible. Move the person to a quieter place if you can.
- Ensure that patients and relatives can make telephone calls, use the lavatory, and obtain refreshments without fear of losing their place in any queue.

A patient becomes hostile and resistive during a procedure:

- Think: 'Because this is an uncomfortable or painful procedure, it is difficult for this person to be calm'. Stop what you are doing, if possible, and say 'Tell me what is wrong and I will try to put it right'.

♦ Encourage the patient to use words to express his or her feelings, rather than to act.

♦ Before and during any procedure, explain clearly and fully to the patient what is involved, how long it will take, and whether it will hurt.

Staff-related factors

Staff experience, behaviour, and attitudes may contribute to the risk of violence. While the characteristics of assault-prone staff have been particularly explored in mental health-care settings, the lessons learned have implications for the training and supervision of health-care staff in general.

Morrison (1990) describes two patterns of staff victims, *tough men* and *vulnerable others*; although the evidence base regarding this typology can be contradictory. Research has tended to show that trainees and young and inexperienced staff across specialities have been found to have an increased risk of victimization (e.g. Bernstein 1981; Carmel and Hunter 1989; Davies and Burgess 1988; Whittington *et al.* 1996), although this finding is by no means unqualified. Lanza *et al.* (1991) found no relationship between youth, inexperience, physical size or gender and assault, while the HSAC survey (1987) found high levels of victimization in both trainee nurses and charge nurses. Inexperienced staff are probably at risk because of a relative lack of skills, confidence, and experience. Staff who are experienced but new to a particular service might therefore be at risk because they are unfamiliar with their patients. For example, James *et al.* (1990) found increased levels of violence to be strongly associated with an increased level of temporary staff. Finally, charge nurses might have a higher level of risk because they are more frequently involved in giving bad news to patients or are more likely to refuse requests (Turnbull 1999).

The effects of staff personality traits and attitudes on risk of assault have also been studied. Ray and Subich (1998) found that, although nurses with high levels of trait anxiety and an external 'locus of control' (i.e. a tendency to blame patients for assaults rather than to reflect on the possible role played by their own attitudes and behaviour) were more likely to be assaulted, nurses scoring highly on measures of authoritarianism were not. However, authoritarianism was found to be associated with external locus of control. There is clearly a fine line between the firm, direct interactions with patients and strong leadership skills that are associated with low assault frequency (James *et al.* 1990; Katz and Kirkland 1990) and the authoritarian attitudes associated with increased assaultativeness (Cooper and Mendonca 1990). Specific staff attitudes that are unhelpful in attempting to manage potentially violent situations are described by Davies (1988, 1989). Counter-productive attitudes that are inflexible, confrontational, and unrealistic, expressed by health-care workers attending violence-prevention workshops facilitated by the author, include the following:

♦ 'They must not be allowed to get away with anything.'

♦ 'If you give them an inch they take a yard.' (Often followed by 'I know these people'.)

♦ 'I must stand up to him/her.'

♦ 'I must never run away.'

- 'I must not show that I am afraid.'
- 'I personally must be able to deal with everyone.'

Many health-care interventions, while performed for the patient's benefit, may be aversive in some respects. This may also increase the risk of violence (especially if the patient is aroused or has some temporary or more long-lasting impairment of cognition). In mental health-care settings, violence has been found to be preceded by aversive stimulation by staff in the form of imposing limits, frustrating patients' demands, or unwelcome physical contact (Powell *et al.* 1994; Whittington and Wykes 1996). This implies that attention should be paid to non-aversive means of setting limits in nurse training, and evidence suggests that such interactions can be effective in imposing limits without generating anger. Lancee *et al.* (1995) examined the effect of six different limit-setting styles (belittlement, platitudes, solution without options, solution with options, affective involvement without options, and affective involvement with options) used by nurses in role plays with patients. Belittlement was found to be the least effective strategy, and while platitudes and offering solutions generated less anger, some anger was still generated. Offering a solution with options, affective involvement, and affective involvement with options were effective in setting limits without generating anger. The care and concern, attention to the patient's experience, and tailoring of the solutions offered to the patient's experience that such interactions embodied did not cause the patients to feel defensive or at the mercy of the hospital system.

Patient and staff characteristics clearly interact. Whittington and Wykes (1994a) propose a model (which has received a degree of empirical support, e.g. Whittington and Wykes 1992, 1994a, 1994b), whereby verbal and physical aggression on the part of patients increases the stress and anxiety experienced by nurses. This leads to nurses avoiding interactions with patients, expressing hostility, and behaving in an overly-controlling manner, which feeds back into the level of verbal and physical aggression expressed by patients.

Action points:

- one's own mood, attitudes, and behaviour (irrespective of intentions) may contribute to assaultativeness;
- training and practice in ways of imposing limits and managing other potentially conflict-laden situations with patients and visitors in non-confrontational, face-saving ways are vital;
- there is a fine line between being firm and direct, and being authoritarian and controlling;
- authoritarian attitudes, belittling, and platitudes can generate anger;
- the patient's experience must be attended to and respected, and solutions you offer must be tailored to it.

Service-related factors

The explanations of violence that have been considered so far, primarily view its causes as located within the violent person and the situation in which he or she is placed, and within the attitudes and behaviour of staff victims. However, work-related violence can also be viewed as a health and safety issue. As such it should be approached though an integrated organizational approach, which aims to prepare for and prevent violence as well as to react to it effectively, legally, and safely.

Environmental factors

Physical environment

Safety starts at the drawing board and is never an add-on feature. The outside of premises should be well lit, without dark corners and illumination. Car parks attract crime, and bright lighting and camera surveillance help reduce this. Many older health-service premises present particular risks to staff, who may find themselves working alone or visiting isolated areas out of hours. Security patrols, police presence, electrically controlled door locks, panic buttons, and CCTV may need to be considered (Paterson et al. 1999a). However, while security cameras can deter casual crime, they may be ignored by the intoxicated or psychotic. Resolution is also too poor on some CCTV cameras for ready identification. Architectural 'blind spots' are another obvious risk factor, and the need for clear lines of sight in psychiatric wards was specifically highlighted by Blom-Cooper et al. (1995).

The general quality of the physical environment exerts a powerful influence on expectations of appropriate behaviour. Comfortable, well-designed, well-lit, and clean surroundings show patients that the environment is valued and hence that they too will be treated with respect. Aggression has been linked to shabby or ill-maintained environments (White et al. 1987). The physical safety of the environment is also important, with such features as the absence of potential weapons and outward-facing office doors (to minimize the risk of being barricaded inside) being essential. Safe, private areas for rest and for confidential interviewing should be provided, and expert advice should be taken on the design of reception areas. For example, rather than 'bandit glass', today's reception areas use high open desks. Patients can lean on these in a confiding way and speak quietly across them.

Panic buttons and alarms will only give protection if staff are trained to react appropriately to them. Designing and practicing an agreed drill for violent incidents is vital.

Social environment

Unsupportive staff, lack of planned rather than demand-driven contact with staff, lack of structure, and predictability in ward routine in general, and factors that increase noise and stimulation (such as the presence of large numbers of staff and patients) have all been found to be related to the level of violence in mental health care settings (Friis and Helldin 1994; Lanza et al. 1994).

At one extreme is the situation described by Prins (1993) on Abingdon Ward in Broadmoor Hospital. The inquiry team reported finding little evidence of empathy among the nursing staff, and that while nurses were typically uninvolved with patients between incidents, the first hint of a problem was treated with massive overkill. On the other hand, Katz and Kirkland's (1990) description of a ward where violence was rare describes staff members as being consistently observed interacting with patients during the day.

Working practices

On the ward

Common sense suggests that we should plan working practices to minimize the risk of violence, and establish contingency plans to manage incidents before they occur. However, this can be a complex process, because a range of emergencies may arise in most settings, and there may be many ways in which a task can be performed safely. Some evidence-based suggestions are presented below.

On wards and similar units, different shifts must be approximately matched for experience. As we have seen, relatively inexperienced and unskilled staff tend to be at higher risk of violence, and so competent and experienced staff are needed on all shifts.

Staffing levels are also important, although findings (predominantly from studies of psychiatric settings) can be contradictory. Lanza *et al.* (1994) found an inverse relationship between assault frequency and number of staff, but high levels of violence can also occur where staffing levels are adequate (Binder and McNeil 1994). The presence of large numbers of staff at certain times, especially if coinciding with the presence of large numbers of patients (e.g. during mealtimes), might be overstimulating, and appear provocative. This seems to reflect Depp's (1982) finding that violence occurred more frequently in public areas of the ward at times when many patients and staff were present, rather than in architectural 'blind spots'. While sufficient numbers of staff need to be available to maintain high levels of care and to cope should an emergency arise, staff need to be deployed sensitively.

Effective communication between shifts, both in terms of 'handovers' and written messages, is also essential, and what information needs to be passed on must be decided upon. Staff in ward-type residential settings must also be consistent in enforcing rules and limits, and in how patients are approached. Drinkwater and Gudjonsson (1989) point out that in psychiatric settings, inconsistent treatment may intermittently reinforce disruptive and violent behaviour, because patients realize that they will achieve their objectives through such behaviour at least some of the time.

The availability of social and recreational activities for in-patients, and for planned and supportive contact between staff and patients is very important.

Information-gathering and its communication within any service is essential. Consider what information is to be collected, and how it is to be passed on. Besides specifying what information needs to be recorded to support the service's work, policies should also highlight the need to share this information with other agencies. Feedback should also be obtained from other agencies, so that the quality of decisions made can be audited and lessons learned.

In in-patient settings, care must be paid to staffing levels, skill-mix, and the deployment of staff. Patients should be treated in a consistent and fair manner, with expectations tailored to what can realistically be achieved. Flexibility is also required.

In community-based settings, how to trace staff whereabouts, communication, and contingency plans in the event of staff not making contact at specified times are paramount for safety.

Attention should be paid in all settings to everyday aspects of working practices, such as clothing, communication, and time-management.

Action points:

- quality and security of premises, and staff working practices influence safety;
- ask for a security review of your premises by Trust Security officers, or local Crime Prevention Officers.

In the community

While health-care workers in the community generally experience lower levels of physical violence, they are exposed to higher levels of non-physical violence (Beale *et al.* 1999). Because they are usually isolated in the community, they are at higher risk should an incident occur (Whittington 1997).

The sharing of information, both within and between teams, is of prime importance. This includes other factors such as the characteristics of carers or potentially dangerous pets, and general levels of crime in the area. A means of communication between team members and their base is also necessary.

Mobile telephones or short-wave radios are useful, but can be unreliable. Phoning a colleague before a worrying visit and leaving the phone on so that they can listen in may be reassuring; but why visit alone in these circumstances?

There are also problems associated with locating staff at work in the community. Staff should make their movements known to identified members of the team before leaving base. A time to ring back after appointments should be arranged so that, if contact is not made, the staff member's last location is known, and a contingency plan (perhaps worked out with the assistance of the local police) can be put into effect.

Action points:

- communicate with colleagues about risky situations;
- liaise with local police;
- a police walkabout may help orientate new community staff.

Risk can also be reduced by being sure of where one is visiting and how to get there. Blocks of flats or courts can be disorientating, so consider asking the patient or a carer to rendezvous in an easily identifiable location nearby. Council maps of difficult estates may be available. Vehicles should be parked as close as possible to the address, and parked ready to leave quickly. Avoid looking lost or disorientated. Do not become a target!

Possessions left in the car should be locked out of sight. Consider how conspicuously one should advertise one's status as a health-care worker. Identification should be carried, but more obvious signs (such as 'on call' stickers on cars, or bags or clothing bearing Trust logos) might attract thieves on the lookout for controlled drugs.

A personal alarm may be useful but must not give a false sense of security. When entering a patient's home, staff should be aware of exit routes, should they need to leave quickly.

Other precautions related to personal style and skill also apply wherever one works. Skilful time-management should take into account when one is at one's most efficient. Avoid allocating times when one is 'down' or tired to potentially risky appointments.

Allow sufficient time for appointments to avoid rushing them, to ensure that the person feels that he or she is being taken seriously, and treated appropriately. How much time is available, and how flexible this is, should be explicitly stated early in the meeting. Staff should always try to be punctual and, if possible, should inform the patient if they are delayed for any reason.

Clothing should permit free and rapid movement, and should not pose potential for harm. High heels, jewellery, and ties all present risks.

Home visits — managing aggressive pets

Pet dogs are a part of many households. They are protective and territorial, and can perceive raised tensions in the home, for example, at times of illness or domestic crisis. An unknown visitor may be perceived as an intruder, even by well-trained animals, though its owners may make light of the obvious signs of an aggressive reaction, for example, growling, raised hackles, and bared teeth. Always ask for dogs to be confined in another room before you enter the house. If regular calls to a patient with an aggressive dog are anticipated, an alternative may be to offer the dog a treat such as a 'Choc-drop' when visiting. This may make it less likely that future visits will be met with hostility, but check with the owner first. Some dog owners are very resentful of their dog receiving treats from strangers.

Box 7.1 Some do's and don'ts in the community

Don't

- ◆ Use an unreliable car.
- ◆ Wander about looking lost.
- ◆ Rely on second- or third-hand reports.
- ◆ Accept guidance from strangers.
- ◆ Be ashamed to ask for support.
- ◆ Rely on a personal alarm.
- ◆ Hang on to your bag if mugged.

Do

- ◆ Check the records beforehand.
- ◆ Know your patch.
- ◆ Dress with safety in mind.
- ◆ Take the dog.
- ◆ Avoid solo visits to risky situations.
- ◆ Beware intervening in rows between couples.
- ◆ Ask for a police escort, if necessary.
- ◆ Make sure colleagues know where you are.
- ◆ Make a swift exit if you feel unsafe.

Insurance

Insurance policies are now available that specifically cover injuries resulting from assault for doctors and other staff. Check the small print on any existing policies, as some injury policies exclude assault.

Better communication

In the waiting-room

Grievances and dissatisfaction can be reduced by:

◆ using a Suggestion Box in the waiting-room;

◆ actively keeping patients informed about likely waiting times and any delays;

◆ where delays are likely, using a 'Triage' system to give appropriate priority;

◆ establishing a Patient Participation Group;

◆ using a Practice Pamphlet to invite comments and complaints — these should be directed to a named team member, e.g. complaints partner or practice manager;

◆ ensuring that 'shop-front' staff, such as receptionists, receive appropriate training in interpersonal skills, and can ask health-care staff for advice as they need it;

◆ not expecting receptionists to carry out tasks for which they are not qualified, such as assessing a person's clinical condition.

On the phone

A telephone drill will establish which calls should take priority. Well-trained empathic telephonists minimize patients' frustration by taking basic details efficiently and deciding on each phone call's priority.

Phone-call recording systems are now available, and can be used to resolve later disagreement about the content of phone calls. These systems can make staff feel protected, as they know that unreasonable remarks are being recorded.

Example of a GP phone drill

1. **Contact doctor at once:** these are calls about sudden medical emergencies: where there is talk of difficulty in breathing, collapse, chest-pain, bleeding, meningitis, etc.

2. **Contact doctor at end of present consultation, having taken the number:** these are calls where a visit may be needed directly.

3. **Contact doctor at end of surgery:** these are calls for advice.

4. **Contact another team member, such as the practice nurse or social worker (immediately or later):** these are calls needing other team services.

5. **Contact receptionist for appointments, results of tests, or other enquiries:** these are administrative calls for appointments, results, and other enquiries.

6. **Personal calls:** family members: put through at once; friends and other enquiries: take details for doctor to call back.

Decision-making and decision-management

Carson (1996) argues that risk-management is a particular form of decision-making. Its quality depends as much upon on the extent and value of the information available to the decision-makers, as upon their skills. Good decision-management therefore depends upon managerial and organizational procedures, which support risk decision-making. Besides defining its own remit, a service must also recognize which decisions lie outside its remit and specify who is responsible for them.

Common causes of error (such as overlooking or discounting negative evidence) in risk decision-making should also be recognized, and structures implemented to reduce their influence (Carson 1994).

The extent to which decision-makers are supported by the availability of information upon which to base decisions, and feedback regarding the outcomes of decisions, and the extent to which the organizational context supports effective decision-making processes, have a direct effect on the quality of the decisions made.

Action point:

◆ risk-reduction is a management skill

Service co-ordination and system management

Control of risk is also affected by the extent to which different agencies are kept informed of developments and the extent to which their efforts are effectively co-ordinated. Multi-agency and multidisciplinary work is becoming the norm in modern health-care services, and it is essential that the different agencies and disciplines involved in providing a service share information. This has been found to be particularly pertinent to the management of the risk of violence, especially homicides committed by psychiatric patients (e.g. Richie *et al.* 1994). Lelliott *et al.* (1997) found that poor communication between agencies was a key theme in seven out of the ten published homicide inquiries in London between 1985 and 1996.

A basic problem is the failure to pass on information, both to other agencies involved in a patient's care and to the police. The key issue is the conflict between the obligation to respect confidentiality and the need for disclosure in the public interest. The Department of Health's guidance (1996a) is that mental health services should ensure that patients understand the multi-agency nature of the service and the implications that this has for sharing information.

The Department of Health (1996b) also states that information can be disclosed to those outside direct involvement in the patient's care in order to prevent serious crime or risk of violence on a 'need to know' basis.

Action point:

◆ sharing information across disciplines is not easy but it is essential.

Communication again: complaints procedures

Many complaints against health-care staff arise from failures of communication. Maintaining sound clinical standards is of course vital, but providing a good service implies more than this. Articulate patients who are dissatisfied may express themselves via an immediate verbal complaint or a subsequent written one. Less articulate people may not be able to use verbal or written complaints as an outlet, and may become increasingly frustrated, hence aggressive.

The consequences (which can be psychological, physical, and even legal) are always unpleasant. Dealing with dissatisfied patients at an early stage prevents later facing complaint procedures or angry patients.

Striving to deliver services efficiently and effectively at the clinical and personal levels can help prevent patients' dissatisfaction, whether in the form of a minor grumble, a formal complaint, or even an angry outburst.

If a patient complains verbally, he or she must be listened to carefully, and notes must be made of the details for later review. A reasonable complaint may be exaggerated, especially if patients feel that they are not being listened to. It is therefore important not to get drawn into arguments, however unreasonable the grievance may at first appear.

A written complaint needs a personal response, within an agreed timescale. Complaints must be taken seriously. Discuss complaints with colleagues, preferably in team meetings, so that procedures can be reviewed, in order to see whether there is any room for improvement.

Action point:

- managing complaints well saves trouble.

What to do if ...
You are criticized by a patient or relative about a mistake:

- Act promptly to put matters right. Apologize or explain what has happened. People who are worried about themselves (or about a friend or relative) are much less likely to tolerate perceived discourtesy.

A patient or relative complains about other members of staff:

- Anxious people often ask different staff the same question. Say: 'I will find out for you exactly what is happening. I will either come back and let you know myself, or one of my colleagues will. Is that all right?'

- Make it clear that you are in control of the situation and that you take the complaint seriously. Failure to explain delays or queues can be interpreted as discourtesy or as dismissing clients' perceptions of their problems.

Hospital policies

Department of Health guidelines resulting from the Hospital Complaints Act (1985) provide for a senior member of management to be responsible for dealing with patients' complaints.

Training for coping with violence can only be effective if it is embedded in a management structure that delegates the necessary authority to a group or committee for the prevention and management of violent behaviour. This committee will approve and recommend policies and procedures; will make recommendations to professional and educational training committees; will review all violent incidents; and will make recommendations to clinical teams. Examples of relevant committees are a Nursing Professional Advisory Committee, a Health and Safety Committee, and a Joint Staff Consultative Committee.

Policies will make it mandatory for all staff to respond in an emergency, but this response will vary with the setting and the staff available. Policies should also specify the physical-restraint techniques that are permissible, identify the staff who have training responsibilities, and state the kind and amount of initial and refresher training to be undertaken by staff. It is essential that this kind of policy structure protects staff who work in areas where violence and aggression are apt to occur.

Services that do not provide such training may be in breach of health and safety regulations. The Health and Safety at Work Act (1974) requires employers to ensure the health, safety, and welfare of their workers and others present in the workplace, so far as is reasonably practicable. This includes the provision of any necessary information, instruction, and training. An employer can be sued for breach of statutory duty if, for example, a staff member, patient, or visitor is hurt, if such training as could have reasonably been expected to have prevented the injury was not available. The Management of Health and Safety at Work Regulations (1992) state that employers must efficiently assess all significant workplace risks and respond to risk assessments by introducing preventative measures. If violence was found to present such a risk, these would include (among other measures) training in defusing and counteracting it. As we have discussed, violence in the health-care setting is a clearly foreseeable risk. Furthermore, besides putting themselves at risk, nurses who agree to practise without these safeguards also fail to comply with Section 10 of the UKCC Code of Professional Conduct, which deals with safe standards of practice.

Individual interventions

Staff need to know how to defuse potentially violent situations, and how to disengage themselves if they are actually assaulted. Staff in in-patient or residential settings may also need to be trained in safe and professionally acceptable methods of restraining assaultative patients.

De-escalation

Skilled communication with patients is central to all health-care work. The de-escalation of a potentially violent incident has traditionally been viewed as an instinctive or intuitive verbal and non-verbal ability, and there is little consensus in the literature regarding its practice. However, it has been argued that de-escalation can be developed as a set of practice skills (Paterson *et al.* 1997), taught and rehearsed in a structured way.

For de-escalation to be attempted, staff must be alert to warning signs of aggression. These are often missed or ignored in practice. Duff *et al.* (1996) note in their study of the management of violence in acute psychiatric units, that staff did not always observe obvious antecedents to violence.

Confusion, irritability, boisterousness, verbal and physical threats, and attacks on objects have been found to be significant predictors of imminent violence in psychiatric in-patients (Linaker and Busch-Iverson 1995). Such behaviours have been observed in patients up to three days before a violent incident (Whittington and Patterson 1996), but might be ignored in practice because many of these signs also occur in the absence of aggression. This is consistent with the results of Tanke and

Yesavage's (1985) comparison of assaultative patients who did or did not show cues of imminent violence, and non-assaultative patients. Low-cue patients were significantly more thought-disordered and withdrawn, and less hostile, suspicious, and active than high-cue patients, while more thought-disordered and more active than non-assaultative patients.

Once signs of imminent aggression have been noted, it may be possible to de-escalate the situation (assuming that it has not been possible to avoid potential triggers to an incident, nor to remove the target of aggression from the scene).

Non-verbal cues are involved as well as verbal communication. Patterns of non-verbal communication can vary between cultures as much as language and dialect. Some caution should therefore be exercised to avoid unwitting provocation where the cultural backgrounds of the staff member and potential aggressor differ.

In terms of non-verbal behaviour, the practitioner must be aware of both *postural* and *gestural* cues. Postural cues are largely unconscious indicators of attitudes or emotional state that may contradict the verbal channel of communication (often referred to as *non-verbal leakage*), while gestural cues are consciously controlled and purposive. In de-escalation, postural cues must be controlled while verbal attempts to reduce the patient's level of arousal are augmented by gestural cues. Attention must be paid to non-verbal cues of potential aggression on the part of the potential assailant.

The objectives of de-escalation are to prevent the potential assailant from becoming more aroused, to reduce their level of arousal, and to address the grievance that has provoked the situation, while ensuring a safe environment. In order to achieve these, attention has to be paid to specific aspects of communication. These include one's own verbal and non-verbal communication (including proxemics), non-verbal cues of imminent violence in the potential aggressor, and assertiveness.

Verbal behaviour

An angry person's level of arousal can be checked and reduced by verbal stratagems. The practitioner should identify him- or herself by name and role, and should address the person by name (ask for this if necessary). This serves to personalize the practitioner, to prevent the person from viewing him or her as just a representative of 'the System' with which they feel a grievance. It also pays attention to the person (thus implying that the grievance will be heard), and can also introduce a pause into the process. The practitioner should speak calmly and clearly, using short and simple sentences and without raising the voice. The angry person may also be reminded where they are and what situation they are in, if delusional interpretations of the situation or misidentification or confusion are thought to underlie their hostility.

The task here is to shift the interpretation of the situation from that of a confrontation between enemies to that of a normal social interaction. This can be achieved by acknowledging that the person feels aggrieved, and that the grievance can be addressed by negotiation. This can be enhanced by suggesting (not ordering!) that they sit down, and by offering drinks, cigarettes, etc., Besides punctuating the process of escalation, this further serves to generate an expectancy of reasonable, rational, non-violent action.

The practitioner should try to communicate that he or she is attending to the grievances by asking open questions, summarizing what has been said, and by using minimal prompts, such as reflective questions, to encourage further disclosure. Besides clarifying the grievance and facilitating its expression, this also encourages the use of thought rather than violence.

While the practitioner should speak and listen in a sympathetic and non-partisan manner, he or she should not make either threats or promises, and should tactfully clarify what help can realistically be provided, at least in the immediate term. Actual threats are inherently provocative. Both threats and promises have to be kept, which the practitioner may not be able to guarantee. Sarcasm or provocative remarks must be avoided. Non-threatening and face-saving alternatives to violence should be suggested. To allow further face-saving, other patients should be removed from the area.

It is essential to engage a potential aggressor because every bit of co-operation that is extracted increases control of the situation and therefore the chance that the matter can be resolved without violence.

Assertiveness versus aggression — a communication skill

Assertiveness is the skill of expressing one's own needs and wishes calmly and clearly while enabling the other person to present his or her own position, in order to find common ground for agreement. Asserting oneself in a difficult situation involves avoiding the behavioural extremes of aggression and passivity.

An aggressive response on the part of a health worker to an angry or complaining person increases the risk of further escalation through anger being met with anger. Passive people, however, may find hostile criticism particularly stressful, and feel victimized and resentful. Losing control of one's temper leads to the risks of over-reacting and triggering a violent episode. Yet a passive response to an angry patient may risk increasing his or her anger, as the response may be interpreted as a refusal to answer criticisms.

A health professional whose self-esteem is low, or who has learned that aggression generally forces compliance in others, will not have much incentive to learn assertiveness skills.

Assertiveness is an important part of communications skills for health-care staff, valuable not only when dealing with angry and complaining patients, but also when managing personnel — and negotiating with managers.

Non-verbal behaviour

The practitioner needs to be both aware of his or her non-verbal behaviour, as well as cues of increased arousal and possible aggression on the part of the potential aggressor. Avoid smiling at the person, as this may be misinterpreted as laughing at them. Eye contact should resemble that of normal conversation as much as possible, and should not be prolonged or staring, as this may be viewed as provocative (Mehrabian 1972); while the avoidance of eye contact may be viewed as submissive or fearful.

Posture should be calm and relaxed. Avoid clenching the fists, putting your hands on your hips, or crossing your arms, as these can be interpreted as aggressive. If the hands are open and in view, minimum threat is posed. Another important aspect of non-verbal behaviour is sensitivity and responsiveness to mood. Facing extreme anger with total calm in an attempt to model calm behaviour may be misinterpreted as indifference, which may actually precipitate further escalation in order to provoke the desired response.

If modelling calm behaviour does not pacify a patient who is angry and shouting loudly, it may be better to respond by matching the level of arousal (though *not* the angry emotional content) momentarily by raising one's voice to gain attention before gradually becoming quieter. This is a skilled intervention, which requires training and practice.

Non-verbal cues

These can give warning signals of increasing anxiety, tension, and anger. Few people are able to become violent without non-verbal warning signals. Signs of imminent aggression include:

- rapid breathing, pacing, fist clenching;
- restless, repetitive movements, e.g. jumping up and down, pacing;
- gesticulating, and violent gestures, e.g. pointing;
- loud speech and raised pitch of voice, chanting;
- facial flushing or pallor, flared nostrils, tightening of the lips over the teeth;
- dropping of the eyebrows and chin, lowering of the body;
- tension in the shoulders, and raising of the hands above the waist;
- the potential aggressor may also glance at possible targets to strike (target acquisition glances).

Action points:

- assertiveness and de-escalation skills can be learnt;
- recognize your own body-language response to angry signals;
- beware responding unconsciously to a hostile stance in a way that increases tension, before a word has been spoken;
- before seeing a patient who may be upset, make sure you are calm yourself;
- always be courteous to clients and patients whatever their behaviour;
- do not bring stressful baggage from a previous problem into the consultation.

Communication skills

When talking to angry people:

- pay close attention, and stand just outside their personal space, slightly out of arm's reach;
- try to stand on their non-dominant side (usually the side a wristwatch is worn or the hair parted);
- use a quiet, calm, but determined manner;
- use calm body language; relaxed posture, hands open, attentive expression;
- avoid staring eye contact;

- avoid pointing at or touching angry people, or entering their personal space;
- convey attentiveness; introduce yourself, say 'Good Morning'; use their names; attempt to identify and acknowledge concerns; appear relaxed and non-aggressive yourself;
- use neutral, non-directive techniques for eliciting information, e.g., 'Would you like to tell me how we can help you?'
- speak in a low, measured tone of voice, clearly audible but not loud;
- do not ignore your own feelings; be prepared to leave the encounter immediately if you feel unsafe or threatened;
- do not mirror their mood, or get drawn into an escalating spiral of aggression;
- if asking someone to leave health premises, e.g. because of intoxication, saying 'On your bike, Jimmy' with a smile may be better received than a pompous 'I must ask you to leave'.

What to do if . . .
A patient or one of his or her relatives is verbally aggressive towards you:

- say: 'I am sure that if you explain the problem to me I can find a way of helping you', to convey that you are in control, and that the problem can be resolved;
- keep an eye on whether the person is becoming more or less tense;
- offer the person a seat while he or she talks to you — he or she is less likely to be able to hit you while seated.

Proxemics

Proxemics refers to one's position in relation to other people and to other features of the environment (such as escape routes, potential weapons, etc.). Research on body-buffer zones (e.g. McGurk *et al.* 1981) suggests that habitually violent people have larger than normal areas of personal space. This implies that it is best to keep slightly further away from a potential aggressor than normal to minimize the risk of accidental provocation.

One's orientation towards the potential aggressor is also important. A directly-oppositional position (whether standing or seated) is extremely confrontational, and should be avoided. A forty-five degree orientation is less confrontational and allows more opportunity for natural breaks in eye contact. When standing, the body presents a smaller target area for attack. If weight is placed over the rear foot, one is less off-balance if pushed from the front, and it is easier to move quickly backwards, than if facing directly forward with both feet parallel.

The practitioner should try to position him- or herself near to a potential exit (or panic alarm), and should not attempt to block a potential assailant's exit.

There may be times when the potential assailant cannot be allowed to leave, for example, when he or she is a detained patient who is attempting to leave the ward. This should not be attempted without help, and training in restraint must be provided.

Action point:
- think about your stance, posture and position when seeing an angry patient.

Physical interventions — escape, restraint, medication

Assaults will sometimes occur despite the most conscientious attention to prevention and de-escalation. Training in physical self-protection techniques for use as a last resort has been available to staff in health-care settings (particularly mental health) for over a decade. Such programmes typically involve training in de-escalation skills and violence prevention, methods of safely disengaging from assault (termed 'breakaway techniques' in the UK), and methods for safely restraining a person who is assaultative or attempting deliberate self-harm (termed 'Control and Restraint', C & R in the UK).

Research into this training suggests that it can reduce the number of assaults and assault-related injuries, and reduce fear and anxiety in staff. It may improve their confidence in their ability to conduct restraints safely and professionally, and improve knowledge of and attitudes towards violence and its prevention and management (Beech 1999; Collins 1994; Infantino and Musingo 1985; Paterson *et al.* 1992). Such training also decreases the amount of fear and aggression shown towards patients and increases the value paid by trainees to non-violent outcomes (Phillips and Rudestam, 1995). Attempts made by untrained staff to restrain patients have been found to increase both the level of violence and the risk of injury (Dietz and Rada, 1982).

The DHSS Advisory Committee on Violence to Staff (1988) advises against training in self-defence for staff on the grounds that commonly taught techniques on these (martial arts-based) courses are inappropriate for clinical-care areas, and specifically recommends C&R training (presumably meaning the breakaway training component). However, if attempts to use breakaways are unsuccessful and one is in grave danger, more drastic courses of action may be acceptable. For more robust training, we recommend that readers check their local adult education colleges for self-defence courses, or ask the police for advice (the police organize self-defence training for the public in some areas). Such training should also include discussion of the law regarding self-defence (which can be quite complex and contradictory), and emphasize the need for post-incident reporting and care (McCaughey 1997).

Action points — breakaways:

- services should ensure that all staff who are in contact with patients receive training in breakaways, which is regularly updated;
- it may be wise to undertake additional self-defence training.

What to do if . . .

You are grabbed round the neck by an assailant:

- shout loudly for help (if possible) to startle them, and keep shouting;
- apply the appropriate breakaway technique and quickly leave the area to call for help;
- if you have not been trained, or if your attempted breakaway has been unsuccessful, try to bend their little fingers back to loosen their grip — if this does not work, it may be necessary to use more drastic measures (e.g. poking your fingers in the eyes) to escape.

You are approached by someone holding a weapon:

- Shout loudly for help and to surprise your assailant. Continue shouting if you can.

- Remain facing the person while backing away towards an exit or protection offered by furniture, etc.. Turn and run towards safety when possible.
- Continue talking to the person, to personalize yourself, to encourage the person to take a more realistic view, and to ask them to put the weapon down and move away from it.
- DO NOT attempt to disarm or fight off the assailant unless there is *absolutely* no other alternative.
- It may be possible to fend off the assailant using an improvised weapon (e.g. a chair) with a longer reach than the weapon you are facing, or to smother the weapon with a cushion, a blanket, or a coat.
- If the weapon involved is a gun or explosive device, do exactly as the person says. Avoid provoking them. Do not put yourself or others at risk.

You are physically attacked while out in the community:

- Keep shouting and yelling as loudly as possible for as long as possible.
- Try to attract attention from bystanders.
- If escape is not possible, defend yourself immediately, using any means that are proportionate to the level of threat presented. These may include breakaways or techniques learned in other self-defence training, such as kicking, gouging, scratching, biting, and using improvised weapons (e.g. car keys, or activating a rape alarm near the assailant's ears).
- Note: while a kick in the testicles is painful, it will not immediately disable a determined attacker.

Action points — restraint:

Restraint should only be carried out where other means of preventing or containing violence have failed or cannot feasibly be used. It should only be performed by specifically trained staff. There are several organizations offering training in restraint. Whichever system is adopted, it should have the following features:

- a co-ordinated response by team members, each of whom has specific responsibilities;
- one identified team member responsible for co-ordinating the procedure, and for communication during the procedure;
- appropriate to the age, size, and gender of the patient;
- not dependent upon the weight or size of the patient or staff involved;
- a hierarchy of physical responses;
- secure grips;
- minimal pain;
- maintain the patient's dignity;
- protection of the patient's head during any descent to the floor;
- use of controlled descents.

The following actions are not permissible in any form of restraint:

- slapping, kicking, or punching;

- obstructing the airway or neck compression;
- placing bodyweight on the chest or abdomen.

(Department of Health and the Welsh Office 1999; Royal College of Psychiatrists' Research Unit 1998.)

Emergency tranquillization

The aim of rapid tranquillization is to minimize risk to the patient or to others, and must only be carried out with great caution by specifically trained staff. Two categories of drugs are currently recommended:

1. Short-acting Benzodiazepines. Lorazepam 2–4mg orally, intramuscularly, or slowly intravenously is usually effective and safe. Risks include respiratory depression and loss of consciousness. Flumazenil is a specific antagonist.

2. Antipsychotics, e.g. Haloperidol are also safe and effective in experienced hands, and safer than Chlorpromazine. Risks include loss of consciousness, cardiovascular collapse, seizures, and extrapyramidal effects, as well as neuroleptic malignant syndrome.

It should be noted that Reilly *et al.* (2000) found substantially raised risk of dose-related QTc lengthening in patients receiving droperidol and thioridizine, therefore conferring an increased risk of drug-induced cardiac arrhythmia. Since 31 March 2001 the manufacturers have voluntarily withdrawn all preparations of droperidol because of these concerns about its safety.

Action points — emergency tranquillization:

- Debate and agree on this procedure with other staff on the spot before acting. Is it safe and appropriate?
- The lateral thigh may be the most accessible injection site.
- It may be necessary to inject through clothing.
- The patient should be able to respond to verbal messages during the procedure.
- Dosage should be titrated to effect. Use the lowest dose possible.
- The risks of over-sedation and interaction with alcohol or other drugs, as well as the effects of any underlying physical illness, on the patient must be considered in each case.
- Patients need constant monitoring (pulse, BP, respiration) in the recovery position after sedation of this kind. Resuscitation facilities and staff familiar with their use should be to hand.

(From: Royal College of Psychiarcists' Research Unit 1998.)

After an incident

Incident reporting

Write a report of any violent incident. This is useful as evidence needed later, since a contemporary record is acceptable in court. It also allows staff to do some mental processing of the events for themselves, to get some perspective, and perhaps to reassure themselves that they took an acceptable course of action.

Accurate assessments of violence risk and training needs in relation to violence in the workplace depend upon incidents being reported. An incident must be reported if it results in death or certain types of serious injury, or a stay in hospital of more than 24h or an absence from work of more than 3 consecutive days (Reporting of Injuries, Diseases and Dangerous Occurrences Regulations 1995). However, the need to report violent incidents is frequently ignored. The Health and Safety Executive report (1989) found that only 20% of violent incidents were actually reported. This can be attributed to various factors, for example (Stark and Kidd 1995):

- absence of available guidelines or operational policy, or lack of knowledge about them;
- no (or inadequate) incident recording form;
- time and effort required to complete the incident recording form;
- a perception that violence is 'part of the job', and therefore insufficiently unusual to report;
- concern that violent incidents represent professional failure;
- fear of litigation.

A recording system has several benefits. These include the assessment and monitoring of the scale of the problem, the identification of weak areas of performance, the gathering of concrete information upon which to base the management of risk posed by particular patients, and feedback on the effectiveness of interventions. Commitment to such a system must be fostered by not necessarily attaching blame for incidents recorded, and by convincing staff of the benefits of reporting. The data recorded can also indicate necessary system improvements, and can be used to inform the tailoring of training programmes. Incidents, therefore, need to be reported as soon as possible. General practice staff should report all such incidents to their health authority.

The document used should be easily understandable, and not too long or cumbersome. As a rule of thumb it should (Beale 1999):

- record hard factual information (e.g. who was involved, when and where the incident occurred, whether a weapon was used, what injuries were sustained);
- describe how the incident occurred and what the outcome was;
- allow staff to make suggestions or comments to management.

Action points:
- check that you have a user-friendly reporting procedure in place;
- use it.

Response to assault

With the patient
Where possible the service will have to review the incident with the patient concerned or their relatives, and the future management of the patient will also have to be considered.

In general practice

Removal of such patients from GPs lists has to be the rule. The patient's immediate family will need to be removed as well if there is any chance of encountering the person concerned on a home visit. GP computer records should be tagged so that the patient concerned cannot later quietly rejoin the list.

National initiatives currently proposed for violent patients include provision for access to general medical services in secure premises. Notify the health authority of all abusive incidents, violent or otherwise, to permit them to appreciate the scale of the problem, and allocate appropriate resources.

Prosecution of assailants

One important aspect of the organization's response to a violent incident is the issue of criminal prosecution. There is a need for the development of clear policies regarding prosecution, widely disseminated amongst patients and staff, and consistently and fairly adhered to. This issue has been particularly considered in relation to psychiatric settings.

A recent Health Service Circular obliges health authorities to make resources available to support GPs tackling violence, and to involve better use of the Criminal Justice System, as well as to make special secure facilities available for supplying general medical services to violent patients in the community.

Prosecution of assaultative patients is uncomfortable and confusing to staff because it is often seen as conflicting with the ethos of care, and with the practitioner's ethical and professional responsibilities, and as implying moral judgement. Prosecution may be also seen as motivated by a desire to punish or get rid of undesirable patients, or as scapegoating them instead of addressing failures of service quality and delivery that are associated with high rates of violence. Victims of assault may wish to withdraw from a distressing situation and minimize its importance, or may feel confused and irrationally guilty about their role in the incident.

The risks of bad publicity for the service, stigmatization of the patient through arrest and subsequent court appearance, discomfort about breaching confidentiality, and fears of compromising the therapeutic relationship and alienating the patient from services can also contribute to non-prosecution (Smith and Donovan 1990). These considerations must be balanced against the right to safety of both staff and patients — health-care workers' ethical and professional obligations do not require the passive acceptance of victimization.

There is also the misunderstanding that prosecuting assaultative psychiatric patients is a waste of time because the patient's mental state would make it unlikely that a case would come to trial. There are two issues here. First, the patient's symptoms may have caused the assault, or rendered the patient unaware of the nature or consequences of his or her actions, thereby negating the *mens rea* ('guilty mind' or criminal intent) component necessary for an offence. If this was found to be the case then it may be accepted as mitigation at the sentencing stage and the court may then order compulsory treatment under the Mental Health Act (with or without Home Office restrictions) rather than legal punishment. In this case, the seriousness of the assault has been acknowledged by the criminal justice system, and the patient has been referred on to more appropriate treatment.

The second issue is that the case may not come to court because the defendant's mental state at the time of the trial may compromise the fairness of the trial. Mental illness can obviously impair the defendant's inability to understand the charges, to instruct counsel, to distinguish between guilty and not guilty pleas, or to follow court proceedings. However, treatment can usually alleviate symptoms to the extent that the defendant is fit for trial, and even if this is not possible, then the court still has the option of detaining the defendant in hospital for treatment without a conviction being recorded.

While it may sometimes be unclear how responsible (and hence accountable) a person with a mental disorder is for his or her actions, some assaultative behaviour is clearly attributable to illness factors, and it is appropriate to address this clinically. However, non-clinical factors can also motivate violence independently of the presence of mental disorder. The decision to prosecute should therefore be made on a case-by-case basis after considering the patient's clinical condition, the probable outcome of the charges, and the impact of the process on both patients and staff (Miller and Maier 1987). It must never be left to the victim of an assault to decide these difficult issues.

Violence against health staff may in the past have been regarded in the same light as 'domestic' assaults, (i.e. a private matter). Neither form of violence is acceptable nowadays.

The police are obliged to take action after any crime comes to their notice. Depending on the seriousness of the incident and the likelihood of successful prosecution, they may issue a warning, formally caution an individual, or charge offenders. The victim may be asked if they wish to take part in proceedings, but does not have the responsibility, as is often believed, of 'pressing charges'.

In assault cases there has to be clear evidence of the offence. It is also necessary to prove that the offender meant to harm someone, or knew that his/her behaviour created a risk of harming someone.

Police action may have several benefits. It increases the likelihood that an incident is recorded in medical notes, and it may lead to more appropriate future treatment. It gives the firm message that violence will not be tolerated, and that the patient is responsible for his or her behaviour. *Ex gratia* payments to victims of violent crime made by the Criminal Injuries Compensation Board are conditional upon police involvement (Cembrowicz 1989).

As part of the cross-Government drive against violence to staff in the NHS (the NHS Zero Tolerance Zone), assaults against NHS staff are regarded as 'serious matters, worthy of prosecution'. The Code for Crown Prosecutors states that a prosecution is likely to be needed (in the public interest) if the offence was committed against a person serving the public (e.g. a nurse).

Action points:

- the NHS is a Zero Tolerance Zone;
- always involve the police after an assault;
- do not leave it to the victim to take action;
- make clear records at the time;
- psychiatric illness does not automatically excuse violence.

Care of victims

Following a violent incident, any physical injuries must receive treatment, and the emotional aftermath of the incident must also be addressed, as this can be as traumatic as the physical effects. Simply put, effective coping with the emotional aftermath of violence leads to a reduction in stress, increased job satisfaction, improved standards of care, and possibly improved retention of staff. Poor or maladaptive coping, on the other hand, leads to low staff morale and increased staff sickness and absenteeism rates (Chaloner 1995).

The employer's liability to cover psychological injury as well as physical injury has recently been established. The high level of risk of psychological injury that health-care workers face therefore makes the adequacy of employers' arrangements for both pre- and post-incident management of stress a key factor affecting judgements of liability and resultant damages in the event of injury and subsequent litigation (Paterson and Tringham 1999).

But current evidence shows that psychological debriefing does not prevent post traumatic stress disorder, nor reduce psychological morbidity, depression or anxiety. (Wessely, Rose, Bisson 2000). Perhaps rehearsal of an assault in an official setting can add to the trauma rather than help it to heal.

After the treatment of any physical injuries, the victim should be allowed a period of peace, quiet, and privacy to deal with the immediate emotional reaction. The victim should also be informed of their rights regarding welfare support, prosecution, and Criminal Injuries Compensation. A written summary should be provided and they should receive ongoing support — the victim should not be expected to cope with the frustrations of the bureaucratic process alone and unaided. It is good practice to offer any member of staff who is involved in, or witnesses, a violent incident the option of going home if they wish. Compulsory debriefing should not take place.

The national charity, Victim Support Scheme (VSS) offers skilled support to anyone injured as a result of a criminal act. It can also advise institutions on prevention and management of violent situations, as well as referring victims to more specialist counselling.

Action points — after a violent incident:

- write an account of what happened;
- offer staff involved the choice of going home at once;
- psychological trauma may be worse than physical injuries;
- never minimize another person's distress; ask 'How do you feel?' (not 'You're all right, aren't you?');
- check up on your colleagues in the days after an incident;
- injuries must be independently checked and recorded, e.g. by occupational health or an A&E department;
- ask for support from your professional organization;
- outside sources of support such as a local church, Victim Support Scheme, or women's support group may be helpful;
- look after yourself, your colleagues, and your staff.

Box 7.2 Some Do's and Don'ts when facing an angry patient

Do

- ◆ Protect your own safety first.
- ◆ Recognize your own mood and feelings.
- ◆ Introduce yourself by name.
- ◆ Use calming body language.
- ◆ Pay attention to your own intuition.
- ◆ Put yourself in the patient's shoes: they may be anxious or afraid, as well as angry.
- ◆ Apologize and explain if necessary.
- ◆ Assert yourself appropriately.
- ◆ Allow people to 'get things off their chest'.
- ◆ Be prepared to leave the room if you feel at risk.
- ◆ Be clear about your own limits.
- ◆ Know what you will do if someone steps over the line.
- ◆ Remove difficult customers from an audience.
- ◆ Ensure good lines of communication within the practice.
- ◆ Recognize the causes of complaint by patients, e.g. prolonged waiting-time without explanation, queues for registration, delays in the service.
- ◆ Identify clinical issues that may cause conflict, and agree on a practice policy, e.g. on the prescribing of tranquillizers or opiates for addicts, or on issuing sick notes. This makes it easier to say 'no'.

Don't

- ◆ Meet anger with anger.
- ◆ Invade personal space.
- ◆ Raise your voice, point, stare.
- ◆ Be drawn into an escalating situation.
- ◆ Lose your own temper.
- ◆ Ignore your own safety.
- ◆ Appear to lecture or preach to the patient.
- ◆ Feel that you have to win the argument.
- ◆ Make the patient feel trapped or cornered.
- ◆ Invade their personal space.

> **Box 7.3**
>
> Always
>   Aim to preserve your own dignity and that of your patient
>
> Never
>   Threaten any intervention unless you can carry it out immediately, effectively, and safely.

Conclusion

Assaults on doctors and nurses are common, and are caused by many different factors. These factors can mostly be addressed, both organizationally and individually, and at national or local level.

Planning beforehand, prevention, and training in specific interventions can reduce the likelihood that violence will occur, or increase the chance that the incident can be defused or contained safely.

Supportive action after an incident mitigates its damaging effects though compulsory debriefing must be avoided.

By tackling these issues, doctors, nurses, and their managers may be enabled to discharge their professional duties without unnecessary fear. The Zero Tolerance campaign states that aggression, violence, and threatening behaviour will not be tolerated by professionals working in the NHS. The Health Service's most precious asset is ourselves, its staff.

Some useful phone numbers/websites

(Also see Appendix).
RCN Work Injured Nurses Group (WING) 0181 681 4030
BMA Counselling Service 0645 200169
Unison 0171 3882366
The Suzy Lamplugh Trust 0181 3921839
Victim Support 0171 7359166
Criminal Injury Compensation Authority 0141 3312726
Department of Health *www.doh.gov.uk*
Home Office *www.homeoffice.gov.uk*

Further reading/resources

Management of imminent violence (1998)
Publications Dept, Royal College of Psychiatrists 17 Belgrave Square, London SW1X
    8 PG (*booksalesrcpsych.ac.uk*)
Tackling Violence towards GPs and their Staff The NHS (Choice of Medical
    Practitioner) Amendment Regulations 1999 HSC 2000/001
    (*http://www.doh.gov.uk/coinh.htm*)
Combating Violence in General Practice, guidance for GPs (available from BMA).

Violence at work; a guide to risk prevention for UNISON branches, stewards, and safety representatives (1999). Available from UNISON.

Personal safety at work: guidance for all employees. Available from The Suzy Lamplugh Trust.

Breakaway/restraint training: The National Control and Restraint (General Services) Association teaches and promotes an approach to breakaway and restraint techniques which are both effective and do not rely on pain compliance. Its website is at *http://homepages.enterprise.net/bonesy* Membership Secretary Gary Ennis (NCRGSA, PO Box 370, St. Albans, Herts.),

References

Acquilina, C. (1991). Violence by psychiatric in-patients. *Medicine, Science, and the Law*, **31**, 306–12.

Adams, J., and Whittington, R. (1995). Verbal aggression to psychiatric staff: traumatic stressor or part of the job? *Psychiatric Care*, **2**, 171–4.

Anderson, E. (1997). Violence and the inner-city street code. In *Violence and childhood in the inner city*, (ed. J. McCord) Cambridge University Press, Cambridge.

Anonymous (1995). GPs are haunted by the spectre of violence. *British Medical Journal News Review* (January).

Ball-Rokeach, S. (1973). Values and violence: a test of the subculture of violence thesis. *American Sociological Review*, **38**, 736–49.

Bandura, A. (1983). Psychological mechanisms in aggression. In *Aggression: theoretical and experimental reviews*, Vol. 1 (ed. R.G. Geen and E.I. Donnerstein) Academic Press, New York.

Beale, D. (1999). Monitoring violent incidents. In *Work-related violence: assessment and intervention* (ed. P. Leather, C. Brady, C. Lawrence, D. Beale, and T. Cox), pp.69–86. Routledge, London.

Beale, D., Leather, P., Cox, T., and Fletcher, B. (1999). Managing violence and aggression towards NHS staff working in the community. *Nursing Times Research*, **4** (2), 87–99.

Beck, A.T. (1976). *Cognitive therapy and the emotional disorders*. International Universities Press, New York.

Beech, B. (1999). Sign of the times? A 3-day unit of instruction on 'aggression and violence in health settings for all students during pre-registration nurse training'. *Nurse Education Today*, **19**, 610–6.

Bernstein, H.A. (1981). Survey of threats and assaults directed towards psychotherapists. *American Journal of Psychotherapy*, **35**, 243–5.

Binder, R.L., and McNeil, (1994). Staff assault and the frequency of staff assault on doctors and nurses. *Bulletin of the American Academy of Science and the Law*, **22**, 545–50.

Blom-Cooper, L., Halley, H., and Murphey, E. (1995). *The falling shadow: one patient's mental health care 1978–1993*. Gerald Duckworth & Co., London.

Bottoms, A.E., and Wiles, P. (1997). Environmental criminology. In *The Oxford handbook of criminology* (ed. M.R. Maguire, R. Morgan, and R. Reiner) Clarendon Press, Oxford.

Brickman, A.S., McManus, M., Grapentine, W.L., and Alessi, N.E. (1984). Neuropsychological assessment of seriously delinquent adolescents. *Journal of the American Academy of Child Psychiatry*, **23**, 453–7.

Bryant, E., Scott, M.L., Golden, C.J., and Tori, C.D. (1984). Neuropsychological deficits, learning disability, and violent behaviour. *Journal of Consulting & Clinical Psychology*, **52**, 323–4.

Carmel, H., and Hunter, M. (1989). Staff injuries from inpatient violence. *Hospital & Community Psychiatry*, **40**, 41–6.

Carson, D. (1994). Dangerous people: through a broader conception to 'risk' and 'danger' to better decisions. *Expert Evidence*, **3**, 51–69.

Carson, D. (1996). Developing models of risk to aid co-operation between law and psychiatry. *Criminal Behaviour and Mental Health*, **6**, 6–10.

Cembrowicz, S. (1989). Dealing with 'difficult' patients: what goes wrong. *The Practitioner*, **233**, 486–9.

Cembrowicz, S.P., and Shepherd, J.P. (1992). Violence in the Accident and Emergency department. *Medicine, Science and the Law*, **32**, 118–22.

Cembrowicz, S., Ford, P.G.T., Winn, J.C., Goodman, M., and Dyer, C. (1984). Assault on a GP. *British Medical Journal*, **294**, 616–8.

Chaloner, C. (1995). Strategies for coping with violent incidents: the psychological consequences of exposure to violence. *Psychiatric Care*, **2**, 162–6.

Cohn, N.R. (1961). *The pursuit of the millennium* (2nd edn). Harper & Row, New York.

Collins, J. (1994). Nurses' attitudes towards aggressive behaviour, following attendance at 'The Prevention and Management of Aggressive Behaviour Programme'. *Journal of Advanced Nursing*, **20**, 117–31.

Convey, J. (1986). A record of violence. *Nursing Times*, **82**(46), 36–8.

Cooper, A.J., and Mendoca, J.D. (1990). A prospective study of patient assaults on nurses in a provincial psychiatric hospital in Canada. *Acta Psychiatrica Scandanavica*, **84**, 163–6.

Cottle, M., Kuipers, E., Murphy, G., and Oakes, P. (1995). Expressed emotion, attributions and coping in staff who have been victims of violent incidents. *Mental Handicap Research*, **8**, 168–83.

Davies, W. (1988). How not to get hit. *The Psychologist*, **1**, 175–6.

Davies, W. (1989). The prevention of assault on professional helpers. In *Clinical approaches to violence* (ed. K. Howells and C.R. Hollin) John Wiley & Sons, London.

Davies, W., and Burgess, P.W. (1988). Prison officers' experience as a predictor of risk of attack: an analysis within the British prison system. *Medicine, Science, and the Law*, **28**, 135–8.

Davies, M., and Schlich, T. (1999). Determining whether senior and specialist registrars choose or reject a career in general adult psychiatry. *Psychiatric Bulletin*, **23**, 607–9.

Delgado, J.M.R. (1971). *The physical control of the mind: towards a psychocivilised society*. Harper & Row, New York.

Department of Health (1996a). *The protection and use of patient information*. HSG (96)18, LASSL(96)5.

Department of Health (1996b). *Security in clinical information systems*.

Department of Health and Social Security (1988). *Violence to staff*. Report of the DHSS Advisory Committee on Violence to Staff. HMSO, London.

Department of Health and the Welsh Office (1999). *Mental Health Act 1983 Code of Practice*. HMSO, London.

Depp, F.C. (1982). Assaults in a public mental hospital. In *Assaults within psychiatric facilities* (ed. J.R. Lion and W.H. Reid), pp. 21–46. Grune & Stratton, New York.

Dietz, P.E., and Rada, R.T. (1982). Interpersonal violence in forensic facilities. In *Assaults within psychiatric facilities* (ed. J.R. Lion and W.H. Reid), pp.47–60. Grune & Stratton, New York.

Drinkwater, J., and Gudjonsson, G. (1989). The nature of violence in psychiatric hospitals. In *Clinical approaches to violence* (edn K. Howells and C.R. Hollin), pp.311–28). Wiley, Chichester.

Duff, L., Gray, R., and Bristow, F. (1996). The use of control and restraint techniques in acute psychiatric units. *Psychiatric Care*, **3**, 230–4.

Erlanger, H. (1974). The empirical status of the subculture of violence thesis. *Social Problems*, **22**, 280–92.

Estroff, S.E., and Zimmer, C. (1994). Social networks, social support, and violence among persons with severe, persistent mental illness. In *Violence & mental disorder: developments in risk assessment*. In (ed. J. Monahan and H.J. Steadman) Chicago University Press, Chicago.

Falshaw, L., Browne, K.D., and Hollin, C.R. (1996). Victim to offender: a review. *Aggression and Violent Behaviour*, **1**, 389–404.

Farrington, D.P. (1978). The family backgrounds of aggressive youths. In *Aggression and antisocial disorder in children* (ed. M. Berger and D. Schaffer) Pergamon Press, London.

Fenton, G.W. (1984). Epilepsy, mental abnormality, and criminal behaviour. *Mentally abnormal offenders* In (ed. M. Craft and A. Craft) Ballière-Tyndall, Eastbourne.

Fesbach, S., and Price, J. (1984). The development of cognitive competencies and the control of aggression. *Aggressive Behaviour*, **10**, 185–200.

Friis, S., and Helldin, L. (1994). The contribution made by the clinical setting to violence among psychiatric patients. *Criminal Behaviour and Mental Health*, **4**, 341–52.

Golding, A. (1996). Violence and public health. *Journal of the Royal Society of Medicine*, **89**, 501–5.

Gournay, K., Ward, M., Thornicroft, G., and Wright, S. (1998). Crisis in the capital: in-patient care in inner London. *Mental Health Practice*, **1**, (5), 10–8.

Graham, H.D., and Gurr, T.R. (1979). *Violence in America* (2nd edn). Sage, Beverley Hills.

Gunn, J., and Bonn, J. (1971). Criminality and violence in epileptic prisoners. *British Journal of Psychiatry*, **118**, 337–43.

Gunn, J., and Fenton, G. (1971). Epilepsy, automatism, and crime. *The Lancet*, **1**, 1173–6.

Harris, A. (1989). Violence in general practice. *British Medical Journal*, **298**, 263–4.

Health Services Advisory Committee (1987). *Violence to staff in the health services*. HMSO, London.

Health and Safety Executive (1989). *Violence to staff*. (IND (G) 189 M100). HMSO, London.

Hiday, V.A. (1995). The social context of mental illness and violence. *Journal of Health and Social Behaviour*, **36**, 122–37.

Hobbs, F.D.R. (1991). Violence in general practice: a survey of general practitioners' views. *British Medical Journal*, **302**, 329–32.

Hodgkinson, P., McIvor, L. and Phillips, M. (1985). Patient assaults on staff in a psychiatric hospital: a two-year retrospective study. *Medicine, Science, and the Law*, **25**, 288–94.

Home Office (1998). *Criminal statistics England and Wales 1997*. HMSO, London.

Hope, T. (1998). Community crime prevention. In *Reducing offending: an assessment of research evidence on ways of dealing with offending behaviour*. (ed. P. Goldblatt and C. Lewis) Home Office. Home Office Research Study 187. Home Office, London.

Huesmann, L.R., Eron, L.D., Lefkowitz, M.M., and Walder, L.O. (1984). Stability of aggression over time and generations. *Developmental Psychology*, **20**, 1120–34.

Infantino, J.A., and Musingo, S.-Y. (1985). Assaults and injuries among staff with and without training in aggression control techniques. *Hospital & Community Psychiatry*, **36**, 1312–4.

James, D.V., Fineberg, N.A., Shah, A.K., and Priest, R.G. (1990). An increase in violence in an acute psychiatric ward. *British Journal of Psychiatry*, **156**, 846–52.

Jamieson, K.G. (1971). Prevention of head injury. In *Head injuries*. Proceedings of an international symposium. Churchill Livingstone, Edinburgh.

Katz, P., and Kirkland, F.R. (1990). Violence and social structure on mental hospital wards. *Psychiatry*, **53**, 262–77.

Kidd, B., and Stark, C.R. (1992). Violence and junior doctors working in psychiatry. *Psychiatric Bulletin*, **16**, 144–5.

Lamplugh, D. (1988). *Beating aggression: a practical guide for working women.* Weidenfeld and Nicholson, London.

Lancee, W.J., Gallop, R.G., McCay, E., and Toner, B. (1997). The relationship between nurses' limit-setting styles and anger in psychiatric in-patients. *Psychiatric Services*, **46**, 609–13.

Lanza, M.L., Kayne, H.L., Hicks, C., and Milner, J. (1991). Nursing staff characteristics related to patient assault. *Issues in Mental Health Nursing*, **12**, 253–65.

Lanza, M.L., Kayne, H.L., Hicks, C., and Milner, J. (1994). Environmental factors related to patient assault. *Issues in Mental Health Nursing*, **15**, 319–35.

Larkin, E., Muntagh, S., and Jones, S. (1985). A preliminary study of violent incidents in a special hospital (Rampton). *British Journal of Psychiatry*, **153**, 226–31.

Lelliott, P., Audini, B., Johnson, S., and Guite, H. (1997). London in the context of mental health policy. In *London's mental health: the report to the King's Fund London Commission.* (ed. S. Johnson, R. Ramsay, G. Thornicroft, L. Brooks, P. Lelliott, E. Peck, *et al.*) King's Fund Publishing, London.

Linaker, O.M., and Busch-Iversen, H. (1995). Predictors of immanent violence in psychiatric in-patients. *Acta Psychiatrica Scandanavica*, **92**, 250–4.

Mark, V.H., and Ervin, F.R. (1970). *Violence and the brain.* Harper & Row, New York.

Marsh, P. (1985). Patterns of aggression — not unnaturally. In *Current issues in clinical psychology* (ed. E. Karas Vol. 2), Plenum, London.

McCaughey, M. (1997). *Real knockouts: the physical feminism of women's self-defence.* New York University Press, New York.

McGurk, B.J., Davies, J.D., and Graham, J. (1981). Assaultive behaviour, personality and personal space. *Aggressive Behaviour*, **7**, 317–24.

McNeil, D.E., and Binder, R.L. (1989). Relationship between preadmission threats and later violent behaviour by acute psychiatric in-patients. *Hospital & Community Psychiatry*, **40**, 605–8.

Megargee, E.I. (1982). Psychological determinants and correlates of criminal violence. In *Criminal violence* (ed. M.E. Wolfgang and N.A. Weiner). Sage, Beverly Hills, CA.

Mehrabian, A. (1972). *Non-verbal communication.* Aldine–Atherton, Chicago.

Miller, L. (1992). Neuropsychology, personality, and substance abuse in the head injury case: clinical and forensic issues. *International Journal of Law & Psychiatry*, **43**, 303–16.

Miller, R.D., and Maier, G.J. (1987). Factors affecting the decision to prosecute mental patients for criminal behaviour. *Hospital & Community Psychiatry*, **38**, 50–5.

Mirlees-Black, C., Mayhew, P., and Percy, A. (1996). *The 1996 British Crime Survey: England and Wales.* London: Government Statistical Service.

Morrison, E.F. (1990). Violent psychiatric in-patients in a public hospital. *Scholarly Inquiry for Nursing Practice: An International Journal*, **4**, 65–82.

Nachson, I. (1988). Hemisphere function in violent offenders. In *Biological contributions to crime causation* (ed. T.E. Moffitt and S.A. Mednick), Martinus Nijhoff, Dordrecht, Holland.

Noble, P., and Rodger, S. (1989). Violence by psychiatric in-patients. *British Journal of Psychiatry*, **155**, 384–90.

Novaco, R.W., and Welsh, W. (1989). Anger disturbances: cognitive mediation and clinical prescriptions. In *Clinical approaches to violence* (ed. K. Howells and C.R. Hollin). John Wiley, London.

Novaco, R.W. (1994). Anger as a risk factor for violence among the mentally disordered. In Violence and mental disorder: developments in risk assessment. (ed. J. Monahan & H.J. Steadman). pp. 21–57. Chicago: University of Chicago Press.

Olweus, D. (1980). The consistency issue in personality psychology revisited: with special reference to aggression. *British Journal of Social & Clinical Psychology*, **19**, 377–90.

Paterson, B., and Tringham, C. (1999). Legal and ethical issues in the management of violence. In *Aggression and violence: approaches to effective management* (ed. J. Turnbull and B. Paterson). Macmillan, Basingstoke.

Paterson, B., Turnbull, J., and Aitken, I. (1992). An evaluation of a training course in the short-term management of violence. *Nurse Education Today*, **12**, 368–75.

Paterson, B., Leadbetter, D., and McComish, A. (1997). De-escalation in the management of aggression and violence. *Nursing Times*, **93**, (36), 59–61.

Paterson, B., McComish, A.G., and Bradley, P. (1999a). Violence at work. *Nursing Standard*, **13**, (21), 43–6.

Paterson, B., Leadbetter, D., and Bowie, V. (1999b). Supporting nursing staff exposed to violence at work. *International Journal of Nursing Studies*, **36**, 479–86.

Pearson, P. (1998). *When she was bad: how women get away with murder.* Virago, London.

Phillips, D., and Rudestam, K.E. (1995). Effect of non-violent self-defence training on male psychiatric staff members' aggression and fear. *Psychiatric Services*, **46**, 164–8.

Powell, G., Caan, W., and Crowe, M. (1994). What events precede violent incidents in psychiatric hospitals? *British Journal of Psychiatry*, **165**, 107–12.

Prins, H. (1993). *Report of the committee of inquiry into the death of Orville Blackwood and a review of the deaths of two other Afro-Caribbean patients.* SHSA, London.

Ray, C.L., and Subich, L.M. (1998). Staff assaults and injuries at a psychiatric hospital as a function of three attitudinal variables. *Issues in Mental Health Nursing*, **19**, 277–89.

Reilley J.G., Ayis, S.A., Ferrier, I.N., Jones, S.J., and Thomas, S.H.L. (2000). QTc-interval abnormalities and psychotropic drug therapy in psychiatric patients. The Lancet, 355 1048–1052.

Richie, H., Dick, D., and Lingham, R. (1994). *The report of the inquiry into the care and treatment of Christopher Clunis.* HMSO, London.

Robins, L. (1978). Study predictors of adult antisocial behaviour: replications from longitudinal studies. *Psychological Medicine*, **8**, 611–22.

Royal College of Psychiatrists' Research Unit (1998). *Management of imminent violence: clinical practice guidelines to support mental health services.* Royal College of Psychiatrists, London.

Ryan, J., and Poster, E. (1993). Workplace violence. *Nursing Times*, **89**, (48), 38–41.

Sampson, R.J., Raudenbush, S.W., and Earles, F. (1997). Neighbourhoods and violent crime: a multilevel study of collective efficacy. *Science*, **277**, 918–24.

Shepherd, J.P., and Farrington, D.P. (1993). Assault as a public health problem: a discussion paper. *Journal of the Royal Society of Medicine*, **86**, 89–92.

Siann, G. (1985). *Accounting for aggression: perspectives on aggression and violence.* Allen & Unwin, London.

Smith, J., and Donovan, M. (1990). The prosecution of psychiatric patients. *Journal of Forensic Psychiatry*, **1**, 379–83.

Stark, C., and Kidd, B. (1995). The role of the organisation. In *Management of violence and aggression in health care* (ed. B. Kidd and C. Stark, pp.123–39. Gaskell, London.

Tanke, E.D., and Yesavage, J.A. (1985). Characteristics of patients who do and do not provide visible cues of potential violence. *American Journal of Psychiatry*, **142**, 1409–13.

Tuchman, B. (1978). *A distant mirror: the calamitous 14th century*. Ballantine, New York.

Turnbull, J. (1999). Violence to staff: who is at risk? In *Aggression & violence. Approaches to effective management* (ed. J. Turnbull and B. Paterson), pp.8–30. Macmillan, London.

Walmsley, R. (1986). *Personal violence*. Home Office Research and Planning Report; Home Office Study no. 89. HMSO, London.

Wessely, S., Rose, S., and Bisson, J. (2000). Brief psychological interventions ("debriefing") for trauma related symptoms and prevention of post traumatic stress disorder (Cochrane Review) in: *The Cochrane Library*, 4, 2000. Oxford: Update Software.)

White, M., Kasl, S.V., Zahner, G.E.P., and Will, J.C. (1987). Perceived crime in the neighbourhood and mental health of women and children. *Environment and Behaviour*, **19**, 588–613.

Whittington, R. (1997). Violence to nurses: prevalence and risk factors. *Nursing Standard*, **12**,(5), 49–54.

Whittington, R., and Patterson, P. (1996). Verbal and non-verbal behaviour immediately prior to aggression by mentally disordered people: enhancing the assessment of risk. *Journal of Psychosocial and Mental Health Nursing*, **3**, 47–54.

Whittington, R., and Wykes, T. (1992) Staff strain and social support in a psychiatric hospital following assault by a patient. *Journal of Advanced Nursing*, **17**, 480–6.

Whittington, R., and Wykes, T. (1994a). An observational study of associations between nurse behaviour and violence in psychiatric hospitals. *Journal of Psychiatric and Mental Health Nursing*, **1**, 85–92.

Whittington, R., and Wykes, T. (1994b). Violence to staff in psychiatric hospitals: are certain staff prone to being assaulted? *Journal of Advanced Nursing*, **19**, 219–25.

Whittington, R., and Wykes, T. (1996). Aversive stimulation by staff and violence by psychiatric patients. *British Journal of Clinical Psychology*, **35**, 11–20.

Whittington, R., Shuttleworth, S., and Hill, L. (1996). Violence to staff in a general hospital setting. *Journal of Advanced Nursing*, **24**, 326–33.

Widom, C.S. (1989). The cycle of violence. *Science*, **24**, 160–6.

Wolfgang, M.E., and Ferracutti, F. (1967). *The subculture of violence*. Tavistock, London.

Yeudall, L.T., and Fromm-Auch, D. (1979). Neuropsychological impairments in various psychopathological populations. In *Hemisphere asymmetries of function and psychopathology* (ed. J. Gruzelier and P. Flor-Henry). Elsevier/North Holland, New York.

Yeudall, L.T., Fromm-Auch, D., and Davies, P. (1982). Neuropsychological impairment of persistent delinquency. *Journal of Nervous & Mental Diseases*, **170**, 257–65.

Chapter 8

The effects of assault on health-care professionals

Gillian Mezey

St George's Hospital Medical School London SW17

Health professionals work with members of the public at all times of the day and night, a factor that makes them vulnerable to violent assault and victimization. Attacks on health-care professionals may be committed by other staff, patients, or members of the public. They may be a consequence of the assailant's mental disorder or altered level of arousal due to drug or alcohol intoxication. They may be committed with or without intent or prior planning on the part of the assailant. The definition of violence includes relatively minor acts, such as verbal abuse, intimidation, harassment, and threats, which cause damage because of their potential to escalate and impact on staff morale and confidence, as well as more serious physical or sexual assaults. In the most extreme cases, it may result in serious injury or even the death of the health professional.

Most victims of violence agree that the emotional impact of their experiences far exceeds the impact of the physical injury (Conn and Lion 1983; Wykes and Whittington 1994) and for that reason this chapter will focus only on the psychological effects of assault.

Prevalence

Table 8.1 provides figures for major injuries and minor injuries requiring over 3 days off work as a result of violence, grouping them by profession. Assaults on staff who work in the health service are common and would appear to be on the increase (Haller and Deluty 1988; Health Services Advisory Commission 1987; Noble and Rodgers 1989). The Health and Safety at Work Act 1974 gave Health Authorities a statutory duty to provide a safe working environment for their employees. However, a report by the Health Services Advisory Commission found that one in ten employees had suffered minor injuries as a result of being assaulted by a patient (HSAC 1987). In 1996 a national audit report on health and safety estimated that health-care workers may be three times more at risk of assault than other workers (National Audit Office 1996). In 1997, Unison found that around one in five family doctors had been assaulted in the course of their work and reported, 'violence can poison the lives of GPs and their practice staff' (Unison 1997). Another study found that 63% of the 1093 GPs who responded had suffered some form of aggression in the previous year (Hobbs

Table 8.1 Major injuries and minor injuries requiring over 3 days off as a result of violence by certain professions

	major injury (%)	minor injury (%)	Total number of injuries
Ambulance staff	11	89	62
Bus/coach driver	10	90	263
Care assistants	9	91	358
Doctors	31	69	13
Medical support	6	94	82
Nurses and asst. nurses	10	90	692
Police	13	87	378
Prison officers	14	86	162
Social support	15	85	205
Teachers	14	86	130
Other public sector	25	75	163

The Economic & Social Research Council (ESRC) Violence Research Programme (1998) *Taking Stock: What do we know about violence?* p. 23.

1994). Most of the incidents reported had taken place in the surgery; 3% involved actual injury. About one-third (37%) of the assaults were by male patients and a quarter (25%) by male relatives of patients. Mental illness was only noted as a factor in 15% of incidents. Anxiety (29%) was the most common reason quoted, closely followed by drugs or alcohol (27%) (D'Urso and Hobbes, 1989).

The actual level of victimization is likely to be much higher, due to the marked reluctance of health professionals to report such incidents (Lanza 1985). Health workers at most risk include: ambulance staff, nurses (particularly those in training grades), Accident and Emergency workers, and mental health professionals (HSAC 1987; Mackay 1994). Risk factors include lack of training, working in isolation, low staff levels, and inadequate security. Within psychiatric settings, assaults on staff are particularly associated with little therapeutic activity (Ekblom 1970) and trivial disputes over food, space, or personal possessions, which have particular significance for individuals who are confined within a restricted space (Pearson *et al.* 1986).

The effects of assault on the victim

General: making sense of violence

Although there are a number of studies of violence in the workplace, less is known about the effects of assault on the victim. Health-care professionals who are assaulted at work have, in general, a similar range of responses to other victims of workplace-related violence and should have a similar entitlement to treatment. The workplace, like the home, is generally regarded as a safe place; the experience of violence challenges certain basic assumptions the individual may hold about their environ-ment and the people they work with. However, there may be particular issues for health professionals who are assaulted, which impact on their recovery.

A general response to misfortune is to attempt to 'make sense' of the experience, in terms of what is already known and understood about the world and immediate envi-ronment. Janoff-Bulman (1985) has argued that three core assumptions are violated as a result of being threatened or assaulted: that the world is benevolent; that events in the world are meaningful; that the self is positive and worthy. Victims of violence can no longer take these assumptions for granted. They are confronted with a world that is unsafe and unpredictable, where events are random and meaningless, and the self is vulnerable and weak. A further theoretical basis for understanding the responses of victims of assault is the 'Just World Hypothesis', which argues that, in a just world, people get what they deserve and deserve what they get (Lerner and Mathews 1967). Essentially this means that, if someone is hit, it is either because of the sort of person they are, or because they did something to deserve it. This theory tends to divert the responsibility for violence away from the perpetrator and towards the victim; it denies the often arbitrary nature of the violence and the selection of the victim, and is there-fore likely to increase the victim's tendency to blame themselves.

The tendency of health professionals who are assaulted at work to feel responsible for what has happened may be exacerbated by the response of their colleagues or managers. An unsympathetic, critical, or unsupportive response is bound to reinforce feelings of failure, anger, guilt, and self-blame. One study that examined the attitudes of non-assaulted employees to their assaulted colleagues, found evidence of extremely negative attitudes towards, and scapegoating of, the victims (Lanza 1987). There is considerable under-reporting of such incidents for reasons that include: the effort required, the fact that such violence becomes regarded as part of the backdrop of working life, and the view that being assaulted by a patient represents performance failure (Lanza 1985).

The experience of victimization is difficult to reconcile with the sorts of experiences people hope for when they enter the 'helping profession'. Many health professionals feel humiliated and taken advantage of, and feel that their professionalism has been attacked and undermined. They may even believe that becoming a carer should confer on them an immunity to other people's aggression. Most health workers perceive themselves as altruistic people, and to respond to such altruism with aggression seems undeserved and unfair.

The impact of violence on the individual and the organization can be profound, although many researchers have remarked on the tendency of health workers to deny and minimize the severity and impact of their assaults (Lanza 1983, 1984; Madden et al. 1976). This attitude has been particularly described amongst psychiatric nurses (Shouksmith and Wallis 1988), who perhaps need to convey an image of themselves as psychologically well-adjusted. It may be important to minimize the effects of the violence simply to allow the worker to continue to function within that environment. Becoming a victim entails dependency and relinquishing a degree of control and autonomy. It means moving from the role of carer to cared for — a transition that some health professionals find very difficult.

Psychological effects

The effects of an assault vary, depending on: the seriousness of the incident (in particular perception of life threat and injuries sustained); the victim's previous personality, including previous victimization; and the response of their colleagues, social network, and the organization in which they work. Occasionally, even apparently trivial assaults may trigger emotions associated with past episodes of violence, or cause unresolved personal conflicts to surface and produce a severe and chronic reaction (Lanza 1983).

Being physically assaulted can result in emotional, behavioural, and cognitive changes. The experience often alters the victim's relationship with their colleagues, as well as with their patients (Ryan and Poster 1989). In a study of 60 social workers who had been assaulted, only three of them claimed to have suffered no emotional response; 10% reported that it had had a permanent effect on their confidence, an additional 18% reported a temporary effect (Rowet 1986).

Common responses include depression, general and phobic anxiety, self-doubt, apprehension, and fear (see Tables 8.2 and 8.3). Anger was reported as the most common emotional response in a study of nursing staff in the United States (Ryan and Poster 1989). In the weeks following an assault at work, increased fatigue, irritability, anxiety, headaches, and increased alcohol and cigarette consumption were symptoms commonly reported by assaulted nursing staff (Whittington and Wykes 1989, 1992). Persisting anger may be self-directed as guilt and self-blame or directed towards others — the boss, the institution, or colleagues — for having failed to protect them. The assaulted worker commonly describes associated somatic symptoms, including dry mouth, tightness in the chest, palpitations, sweating, and restlessness. They may self-medicate with alcohol and drugs (including nicotine) in an attempt to manage their hyper-arousal and anxiety; this can then become a problem in itself.

Being assaulted at work often produces a loss of trust, which can spill over into relationships with partners, children, and friends outside the workplace. Many individuals describe disrupted concentration following an assault; their thoughts are frequently interrupted by ruminations about the assault, 'Why did it happen?' 'Why me?' — constantly ruminating over the event in an attempt to make sense of what has happened.

Recovery following an assault at work can be prolonged: the study by Ryan and Poster (1989) found that at least one-fifth of respondents were still experiencing

Table 8.2 Psychological responses following assault

- Anxiety
- Depressed mood
- Fears and phobias
- Guilt and self-blame
- Anger and irritability
- Cognitive effects
- Psychosomatic responses

Table 8.3 Behavioural responses following assault

- Substance-misuse (drugs, alcohol, cigarettes)
- Absenteeism from work
- Avoidance of patient contact
- Loss of interest and involvement in work
- Avoidance of reminders of assault
- Social withdrawal
- Relationship failure

severe psychological and emotional effects one year after an assault. If post-traumatic stress disorder develops, then the condition is likely to become chronic, without specific treatment (Kessler 2000).

Compensation following an assault at work is rare; what most health workers primarily desire is an apology from the perpetrator, expressions of care and concern from colleagues and management, and acknowledgement of their distress. Where the perpetrator is a patient and, particularly where criminal prosecution is not proceeded with, the victim of the assault may feel resentment that their assailant has been 'allowed to get away with it'. Within psychiatric settings, assaulted staff often express the view that the patient is, in fact, simply feigning mental illness in order to avoid responsibility. The prosecution of psychiatric patients is extremely rare, partly because of the police reluctance to press charges where the patient is known to be suffering from mental disorder and is already in psychiatric treatment (Hoge and Gutheil 1987).

Specific psychiatric conditions

Burnout syndrome

Burnout syndrome (Freudenberger 1974) can be the end-point of chronic stress at work and involves disillusionment, impaired work performance, psychosomatic complaints, absenteeism, and eventually departure from the work place. Burnout reflects a dissonance between the individual's internal expectations of the job and their contribution, and the external demands placed on them. Although there are many potential sources of stress experienced by health professionals, the experience of assault may contribute to a sense of being devalued and not appreciated, thus leading to the development of 'burnout'.

Acute stress disorder and post-traumatic stress disorder

Post-traumatic stress disorder is a recognized psychiatric condition, which may develop following serious violent assault (APA 1994) (Table 8.4). The disorder includes physiological, behavioural, and cognitive responses and has two major components: re-experiencing symptoms and avoidance symptoms related to the traumatic event. Re-experiencing symptoms include nightmares, flashbacks, and a feeling that the event is recurring. These re-experiencing symptoms are accompanied by physiological

Table 8.4 Post-traumatic stress disorder (APA 1994)

A. The person has been exposed to a traumatic event in which both of the following were present:

   (1)   the person experienced, witnessed, or was confronted with an event or events that involved actual or threatened death or serious injury, or a threat to the physical integrity of self or others;

   (2)   the person's response involved intense fear, helplessness, or horror.

B. The traumatic event is persistently re-experienced in one (or more) of the following ways:

   (1)   recurrent and intrusive distressing recollections of the event, including images, thoughts or perceptions;

   (2)   recurrent distressing dreams of the event;

   (3)   acting or feeling as if the traumatic event were recurring (includes a sense of reliving the experience, illusions, hallucinations, and dissociative flashback episodes, including those that occur on awakening or when intoxicated);

   (4)   intense psychological distress at exposure to internal or external cues that symbolize or resemble an aspect of the traumatic event;

   (5)   physiological reactivity on exposure to internal or external cues that symbolize or resemble an aspect of the traumatic event.

C. Persistent avoidance of stimuli associated with the trauma and numbing of general responsiveness (not present before the trauma), as indicated by three (or more) of the following:

   (1)   efforts to avoid activities, places, or people that arouse recollections of the trauma;

   (2)   inability to recall an important aspect of the trauma;

   (3)   efforts to avoid thoughts, feelings, or conversations associated with the trauma:

   (4)   markedly diminished interest or participation in significant activities;

   (5)   feelings of detachment or estrangement from others;

   (6)   restricted range of affect (e.g. unable to have loving feelings):

   (7)   sense of foreshortened future (e.g. does not expect to have a career, marriage, children, or normal lifespan).

D. Persistent symptoms of increased arousal (not present before the trauma), as indicated by two (or more) of the following:

   (1)   difficulty falling or staying asleep;

   (2)   irritability or outbursts of anger:

   (3)   difficulty concentrating:

   (4)   hyper-vigilance;

   (5)   exaggerated startle response.

E. Duration of the disturbance (symptoms in Criteria B, C, and D) is more than 1 month.

F. The disturbance causes clinically significant distress or impairment in social, occupational, or other important areas of functioning.

   Specify as:
   Acute: if duration of symptoms is less than 3 months.
   Chronic: if duration of symptoms is 3 months or more.
   With delayed onset: if onset of symptoms is at least 6 months after the stressor.

hyper-arousal including increased startle response, irritability, and intensification of distress when exposed to reminders of the trauma (which may mean patients, the ward, or the hospital, for health workers who are assaulted at work). Alternating with the re-experiencing symptoms is avoidance of trauma-related situations, which are liable to trigger or intensify distress, and a general constriction of emotional responsiveness. The condition cannot be diagnosed until the symptoms have been present for at least four weeks and, after three months the condition is described as chronic. Post-traumatic stress disorder is associated with high levels of distress and impairment in the individual's social, interpersonal, and occupational functioning.

Post-traumatic avoidance may be particularly difficult to pick up and yet may profoundly affect professionals' capacity to function effectively: they may avoid confrontation with distressing reminders by taking extended sick leave; they are likely to avoid contact with the perpetrator of the assault, which can be a problem if this involves a current patient; they may request transfer to another ward or leave altogether. Although the avoidance produces some short-term gain, in terms in minimizing the current anxiety and apprehension, it can also make it more difficult, with prolonged periods of absence, to confront the feared situation, leading to further loss of confidence and self-esteem. Post-traumatic stress disorder is a serious condition that is likely to become chronic in the absence of specialist treatment (Kessler 2000). Eventually, without counselling or specific treatment, the individual may just decide to leave altogether, a decision that carries costs, not only for the individual concerned, but for the organisation, which has to recruit and retrain new staff to replace them.

The risk to health professionals of being assaulted needs to be recognized within all settings, and appropriate measures introduced in the workplace to minimize the risk of violent victimization. For those staff who are assaulted, it is important that the emotional and psychological effects are recognized and responded to appropriately to prevent long-term damage to the individual.

References

American Psychiatric Association (1994). *Diagnostic criteria from DSMIV*. APA, Washington.

Conn, L., and Lion, J. (1983). Assaults in a University Hospital. In *Assaults within psychiatric facilities* (ed. J. Lion and W. Reid. W. B. Saunders, Philadelphia.

D'Urso, P., and Hobbs, F.D.R. (1989). Aggression and the general practitioner. *British Medical Journal*, **298**, 97–8.

Ekblom, B. (1970). *Acts of violence by patients in mental hospitals*. Svenska Bokforlaget, Uppsala, Sweden.

Freudenberger, H.J. (1974). Staff burn out. *Journal of Social Issues*, **30**, 159–65.

Haller, R.M., and Deluty, R.H. (1988). Assaults on staff by psychiatric inpatients. *British Journal of Psychiatry*, **152**, 174–9.

Health Services Advisory Committee (1987). *Violence to staff in the health services*. HMSO, London.

Hobbs, R. (1994). Aggression towards general practitioners. In *Violence in health-care professionals* (ed. Til-Wykes) pp. 73–87. Chapman and Hall, London.

Hoge S.K., and Gutheil, T.G. (1987). The prosecution of psychiatric patients for assaults on staff. A preliminary empirical study. *Hospital and Community Psychiatry*, **38**,(1), 44–49.

Janoff-Bulman, R. (1985). The aftermath of victimisation: rebuilding shattered assumptions. In *Trauma and its wake* Vol. 1, (ed. C.R. Figley), pp. 15–35. Brunner–Mazel, New York.

Kessler, R.C. (2000). Post-traumatic stress disorder: the burden to the individual and to society. *Journal of Clinical Psychiatry*, **61**, 4–12.

Lanza, M.L. (1983). The reactions of nursing staff to physical assault by a patient. *Hospital and Community Psychiatry*, **34**, 44–7.

Lanza, M.L. (1984). A follow-up study of nurses' reactions to physical assault. *Hospital and Community Psychiatry*, **35**,(5), 492–4.

Lanza, M.L. (1985). How nurses react to patient assaults. *Journal of Psychological Nursing*, **23**,(6), 6–10.

Lanza, M.L. (1987). The relationship of assault to blame placement for assault. *American Psychiatric Nursing*, **1**(a), 269–79.

Lerner, M.J., and Mathews, G. (1967). Reactions to suffering of others under conditions of indirect responsibility. *Journal of Personality and Social Psychology*, **5**, (3), 319–25.

MacKay, C. (1994). Violence to health-care professionals: a health and safety perspective. In *Violence and health-care professionals* (ed. Til-Wykes) pp. 9–22. Chapman and Hall, London.

Madden, D.J., Lion, J.R., and Penna, M.W. (1976). Assaults on psychiatrists by patients. *American Journal of Psychiatry*, **133**, (4),422–5.

National Audit Office (1996). *Report by the controller and auditor on general health and safety in the NHS*. Hospital Trusts in England. HMSO, London.

Noble, P., and Rodger, S. (1989). Violence of psychiatric inpatients. *British Journal of Psychiatry*, **155**, 384–90.

Pearson, M., Wilmot, E., and Padi, M. (1986). A study of violent behaviour among inpatients in a psychiatric hospital. *British Journal of Psychiatry*, **149**, 232–5.

Rowett, C. (1986). Violence in social work. *Institute of Criminology*. Occasional Paper, Cambridge University.

Ryan, J., and Poster, E. (1989). The assaulted nurse: short-term and long-term responses. *Archives of Psychiatric Nursing*, **3**, 323–31.

Shouksmith, G., and Wallis, D. (1988). Stress amongst hospital nurses. In *Stress and organisational problems in hospitals: implications for management.* (ed. D. Wallis and C.J. de Wolf) Croom Helm, London.

Stanko, E. (1988). *Taking stock: what do we know about violence?* ESRC Violence Research Programme, Middlesex.

Unison Primary Health Office (1997). *Violence in GPs' surgeries — results of Unison's survey.* Unison, London.

Whittington, R., and Wykes, T. (1989). Invisible injury. *Nursing Times*, **42**, 30–2.

Whittington, R., and Wykes, T. (1992). Staff strain and social support in a psychiatric hospital following assault by a patient. *Journal of Advanced Nursing*, **17**, 480–6.

Wykes, T., and Whittington, R. (1994). Reactions to assault, In *Violence and health-care professionals* (ed. Til Wykes). Chapman and Hall, London.

Chapter 9

The care of victims

Jonathan I. Bisson

Victims of violence may experience a variety of emotional and psychiatric reactions to their traumatic experience. Often these represent a post-traumatic stress response, which will spontaneously resolve, but some individuals will develop specific psychiatric disorders requiring treatment. The psychological and psychiatric care of victims of violence should not be considered in isolation from other forms of care. As discussed elsewhere in this book, victims of violence may receive care from a variety of different agencies including the police, victim support, general practitioners, and social services. It is likely that many victims will benefit most from a well co-ordinated package of care involving different agencies.

Psychological complications of violence

Perhaps the most widely reported psychiatric disorder following violence at present is post-traumatic stress disorder (PTSD) but it is important to consider other common psychological reactions to violence including substance-misuse, anxiety, and depression. These conditions may occur as co-diagnoses with PTSD but may also be precipitated by violence and be present without coexisting PTSD.

Post-traumatic stress disorder

PTSD is precipitated by a major traumatic event and was first described in 1980 (APA 1980). Its definition has been refined over the years and is included in the tenth edition of the *International classification of diseases* (ICD-10) (WHO 1992) and the fourth edition of the *Diagnostic and statistical manual of mental disorders* (DSMIV) (APA 1994). Characteristic features include distressing re-experiencing of the event, avoidance, numbing of general responsiveness, and hyper-arousal. (see Chapter 8).

Depression

A depressive episode is characterized by lowered mood, loss of interest and enjoyment, and reduced energy. Other common symptoms include reduced self-esteem and self-confidence, ideas of guilt or unworthiness, pessimistic views of the future, ideas of self-harm and suicide, disturbed sleep, and disturbed appetite.

Anxiety

Typical anxiety symptoms include apprehension, restlessness, tension headaches, palpitations, overbreathing, sweating, abdominal discomfort, shakes, and dry mouth.

Phobic anxiety disorder is probably the commonest form of anxiety disorder following an episode of violence. In this condition the individual's anxiety is predominantly evoked by specific situations that are not currently dangerous (e.g. places that remind the individual of the trauma).

Disorders of substance-use

Disorders of substance-use include acute intoxication, harmful use, and dependence syndrome, which is characterized by a sense of compulsion to take the substance, difficulties in controlling substance-taking behaviour, physiological withdrawal, tolerance, primacy of substance use over other activities, and persisting use despite clear evidence of its harmful consequences. Alcohol is the commonest substance misused but illegal substances, such as cannabis and amphetamine, are also regularly misused.

Adjustment disorders

Adjustment disorders are commonly diagnosed following traumatic events and are states of subjective distress and emotional disturbance following a stressor. Symptoms vary but often comprise a mixture of anxiety, depressive and PTSD symptoms without satisfying the full criteria for these or another major psychiatric disorder.

Enduring personality change

ICD-10 (WHO 1992) also recognized that some individuals experience a change in personality following major trauma and introduced the diagnosis 'enduring personality change after catastrophic experience', which may be preceded by PTSD but cannot be diagnosed at the same time as PTSD. The criteria include a permanent significant personality change that can be traced back to the catastrophic experience and results in inflexible and maladaptive behaviour not present before the pathogenic experience.

Prevalence of psychological reactions after violence

Post-traumatic stress disorder

There have been no good epidemiological studies of the prevalence of PTSD amongst the general community in the UK. In the USA there have been several. The findings of the Epidemiologic Catchment Area Survey were the first to be published. Helzer *et al.* (1987) reported a 1% lifetime prevalence rate for PTSD amongst 2493 individuals interviewed in St Louis with the Diagnostic Interview Schedule (DIS). Davidson *et al.* (1991) reported a 1.3% lifetime prevalence and 0.44% current prevalence of PTSD also using the DIS in 2985 individuals in North Carolina. Breslau *et al.* (1991) used the DIS with a population of 1007 American adults aged between 21 and 30. Almost 40% had been exposed to a major traumatic event; the lifetime prevalence rate for PTSD was 9%. The biggest study to date is the National Comorbidity Survey (Kessler *et al.* 1995), which interviewed a representative sample of 5877 Americans aged between 15 and 54 years old: 60.7% of males and 51.2% of females reported having been involved in a significant traumatic event. The lifetime prevalence of PTSD was 10.4% in females and 5.0% in males.

Research has suggested that exposure to higher impact trauma (e.g. rape) is associated with much higher rates of PTSD than exposure to lower impact trauma (e.g. physical assault). In Breslau *et al.*'s (1991) study, 11.6% of those who had suffered a sudden injury or serious accident and 22.6% of those physically assaulted developed PTSD compared to 80% of women who reported rape. Kessler *et al.* (1995) found a lifetime prevalence of PTSD following serious accident of 20.7% in men and 23.6% in women. For physical attack, the rates were 12.4% in men and 30.8% in women; and for rape, 65% in men and 45.9% in women.

Prevalence of other psychological sequelae following traumatic events

In over 50% of cases when PTSD is diagnosed, another major psychiatric disorder can additionally be made. The commonest co-diagnoses include major depressive disorder, panic disorder, other anxiety disorder, and substance-abuse/dependence. It is therefore essential to consider the coexistence of other disorders when PTSD is present. The National Vietnam Veterans Readjustment Study (Kulka *et al.* 1990) found that of those suffering from PTSD at the time of the study, 50% could be diagnosed as suffering from one of the above disorders in addition. Further evaluation of the subjects revealed a 99% lifetime co-morbidity. Kessler *et al.* (1995) found co-morbidity to be present in 88.3% of males and in 79% of females diagnosed as suffering from PTSD. The PTSD was felt to be the main diagnosis in approximately 40% of males and 50% of females.

The natural course of post-traumatic stress disorder symptoms

There are few good prospective studies to determine the natural course of PTSD symptoms but those that have been conducted suggest that there is a gradual reduction in symptoms over time. Rothbaum and Foa (1992) have conducted prospective studies of rape victims and victims of non-sexual criminal assault. Sixty-four rape victims were interviewed within two weeks of their trauma, weekly to 12 weeks and then at 6 and 9 months. Unfortunately there was a high dropout rate with only 24 individuals completing the 9-month follow-up. At initial interview, 94% met the PTSD symptom criteria, at 1 month this had reduced to 65%, was 47% at 3 months, 42% at 6 months, and 47% at 9 months. A similar but more marked reduction in PTSD symptoms was found in the 51 assault victims they studied: 65% satisfied the PTSD symptom criteria at 1 week, 37% at 1 month, 15% at 3 months, and 12% at 6 months when, unfortunately, only 26 remained in the study. At 9 months none of the 15 interviewed met the criteria for PTSD.

Kessler *et al.* (1995), in their retrospective study of 5877 individuals, found that PTSD symptoms were reported to have reduced most rapidly in the first 12 months and then reduced more slowly, but over a third of individuals continued to suffer from PTSD 6 years after diagnosis, irrespective of whether or not treatment had been received.

Predictors of psychological sequelae

The studies described above and other studies have found several factors that appeared to be associated with PTSD following a traumatic event, in addition to the severity of the trauma. These include behavioural difficulties before the age of 15 (Helzer *et al.* 1987), family history of psychiatric disorder (Breslau *et al.* 1991; (Davidson *et al.* 1991), reduced social support (Davidson *et al.* 1991), pre-trauma anxiety or depression (Breslau *et al.* 1991; McFarlane 1988; Resnick *et al.* 1992), neuroticism (Breslau *et al.* 1991), female sex (Kessler *et al.* 1995), previous trauma (McFarlane 1988), early symptoms of PTSD (Brewin *et al.* 1998) and early symptoms of depression (Freedman *et al.* 1999). Victims of assault have also been found to fare worse than victims of road-traffic accidents (Shepherd *et al.* 1990). In a study of victims of traumatic facial injury (Bisson *et al.* 1997), we found that psychological outcome at 6 weeks after the traumatic injury was well predicted by early symptoms of PTSD but equally well predicted by asking junior dentists, with no psychological training, to predict outcomes on a 0–5 scale.

Interventions

Given the natural history of psychological sequelae in assault victims, with a rapid reduction in levels of distress over time, it seems reasonable to predict that most individuals will not require formal intervention. However, there has been considerable debate on this point with some individuals arguing for routine intervention for everyone (e.g. Dyregrov 1989) and others arguing for evidence-based interventions for those with psychological symptoms (e.g. Bisson 1997).

Early intervention

One-off interventions

Wessely *et al.* (1999) performed a systematic review of randomized controlled trials (RCTs) of single-episode early interventions compared to no intervention. Six studies were included, three of which used psychological debriefing (PD): a technique that involves detailed consideration of the traumatic event and the normalization of psychological reactions. In the psychological debriefing studies, a total of 299 subjects were randomized and 233 subjects completed follow-up. In the other three studies involving techniques similar to debriefing, a total of 163 subjects were randomized and 142 subjects completed follow-up. Overall, the quality of the studies was found to be poor: only one study scored greater than 50% on a quality ratings scale devised for studies of psychiatric interventions. The single-episode early psychological interventions had no effect on subsequent rates of development of PTSD, despite being well-received by a majority of participants.

Three studies have specifically considered the benefit of individual psychological debriefing in victims of violence and are considered in more detail below.

Rose *et al.* (1999)

Rose et al. considered 118 male and 39 female victims of violent crime who had an average age of 35 years (SD = 13). Participants were randomly allocated to either assessment only, education about post-traumatic stress symptoms, or psychological debriefing followed by education. There were no significant differences in symptoms of PTSD or depression between the three groups, although, as predicted by previous research, symptoms reduced in all groups over time. The mean Impact of Event Scale (a well-validated questionnaire measure of PTSD symptoms) score for the assessment-only group reduced from 28.0 (SD = 19.3) at baseline to 15.9 (SD = 19.4) at 11-month follow-up, compared with the education group, which reduced from 24.2 (SD = 19.0) to 14.7 (SD = 19.5) and the debriefing plus education group, which reduced from 28.5 (SD = 18.4) to 15.9 (SD = 16.0).

Dolan et al. (1999)

Dolan et al. reported a study of 100 patients who had presented to an Accident and Emergency department following a road-traffic accident, assault, or other traumatic injury. Patients were randomly allocated to receive a single session PD, 7–11 days post-trauma or to receive no intervention. Analyses of co-variance with severity of injury as co-variate revealed no differences in symptoms of PTSD, anxiety, and depression between intervention and control groups at 1-month and 6-month follow-up.

Stevens and Adshead (cited in Hobbs and Adshead, 1996)

Stevens and Adshead described a study of individuals who had presented to an Accident and Emergency department following acute physical trauma: 44 males and 19 females were recruited, and 21 were lost to follow-up. Those in the intervention group received a standardized interview within 24 h of attendance, which reviewed the experience and their emotions. Although not adhering to a specific PD technique, it contained several components of PD. Individuals were reassessed 1 week, 1 month, and 3 months post-attendance.

There was no significant difference between those patients who were counselled and those who were not, in terms of PTSD, depression, and anxiety symptoms — except for those showing high initial anxiety and depression symptoms, who did better if in the counselled group. Two-thirds said that they found the intervention useful and one-third stated that they did not. Reasons given by this latter group for finding the counselling unhelpful were that they felt it had been offered too early, or that personally they felt they had not needed it. A major flaw in this study was the fact that those individuals who displayed significant emotional responses during the counselling session were excluded from follow-up. This may have caused significant bias probably resulting in the intervention appearing more effective than it was.

Other early interventions

As a result of concerns about the lack of effectiveness of one-off early interventions, more complex early interventions have been developed. This area has been less well-researched to date but appears to be a natural progression from one-off interventions.

Foa et al. (1995) investigated the effectiveness of a four-session cognitive behavioural intervention in rape survivors shortly after the rape. Individuals were invited to attend four sessions of a group-intervention programme in which individuals were provided with education regarding traumatic stress, encouraged to expose themselves to fear-provoking cues, and provided with some cognitive strategies. This was not an RCT, but a group of women who presented to the same centre a year earlier were used as controls. The intervention group did significantly better in terms of reduction of symptoms of PTSD.

There have also been three randomized controlled trials of brief early interventions. Brom *et al.* (1993) compared three to six sessions of an intervention, which compared educational and cognitive-behavioural techniques with no treatment among 151 survivors of road-traffic accidents at least 1 month after their trauma. There were no differences in outcome between the intervention group and the control group.

Bryant *et al.* (1998) considered a more formalized cognitive-behavioural intervention for survivors of road-traffic accidents (RTA). In an attempt to focus the intervention on those individuals at highest risk of developing PTSD phenomena, they included only those individuals who satisfied the criteria for a diagnosis of acute stress disorder (ASD) at 2 weeks following the trauma. This condition requires an individual to suffer from distressing re-experiencing phenomena, avoidance phenomena, and hyper-arousal phenomena as is typical in PTSD but, in addition, individuals must have dissociative phenomena such as derealization, depersonalization, or psychogenic amnesia. Harvey and Bryant's (1998) prospective study of ASD suggested that 80% of RTA victims with ASD have PTSD at 6 months and without treatment a similar number do so at 2 years.

Twenty-four individuals were included in the RCT. The intervention was of five 1½ h sessions in which individuals received prolonged exposure, education, and cognitive restructuring. The control group received supportive psychotherapy for the same length of time. This involved focusing on here and now difficulties with attempts to avoid discussion of the trauma and represented a placebo control condition. The group who received the cognitive-behavioural intervention fared significantly better at treatment and follow-up. The authors concluded that the intervention appeared useful but required replication. In a recent presentation, Bryant discussed the results of a larger trial using the same methodology in a larger group of RTA victims with ASD with similarly positive results (Bryant 1999).

The other recently completed study was by the Cardiff Violence Group and reported at the same meeting (Bisson *et al.* 1999). This study included 53 victims of violence amongst 152 acute physical injury sufferers presenting to the Emergency Department in Cardiff. Individuals were randomly allocated to a four-session cognitive-behavioural intervention or to no treatment. The main finding in this study was that symptoms of PTSD decreased significantly more in the intervention group than in the control group at 13-month follow-up. Avoidance symptoms of PTSD had decreased significantly more at 3 months. There were no other significant differences between the groups at 3 months, although anxiety and depression symptoms (as measured by the HADS) and PTSD symptoms (as measured by the CAPS) decreased more in the intervention group than the control group. Time had a marked effect. Symptoms in both groups decreased significantly over the 13 months on all measures.

Conclusions

The results of published RCTs of individual PD raise serious questions about the future usefulness of PD and the wisdom of advocating one-off interventions post-trauma. Apart from the inappropriate use of resources that would result through routine use of an intervention that was not effective, other potential adverse effects, such as service providers being secondarily traumatized through being exposed to the ventilation of powerful emotions by the victims of the trauma (e.g. Raphael 1986), passive participation (Flannery 1991), and delay in referral for treatment of psychiatric disorder (McFarlane 1989), could be avoided.

Given the current state of knowledge, neither one-off group or individual PD can be advocated as being able to prevent the subsequent development of PTSD following a traumatic event. However, there may be benefits to aspects of PD, particularly when employed as part of a comprehensive management programme.

In my opinion, given the evidence at present, our limited resources should be primarily used to provide more complex, evidence-based treatments for individuals who develop significant psychological difficulties following traumatic events. There is no evidence to support the preventive value of debriefing delivered in a single session but there is a strong argument for providing acute psychological first aid and forming a treatment alliance as early as practical following a traumatic event. Early contact may provide a method of addressing the major problem of the general reluctance of people with PTSD to accept treatment.

Later interventions

If an individual does develop a psychiatric disorder following a traumatic event, it would seem appropriate to offer more formal evidence-based treatment at an early stage. The form of treatment offered will depend on the expertise available locally. As previously discussed, PTSD is one of several psychiatric disorders that can be precipitated by violence. It is essential to treat the underlying condition and although approaches may be similar, difficulties will be missed and left unaddressed unless victims are thoroughly individually assessed, their needs determined, and specific management plans formulated and followed.

Post-traumatic stress disorder

Psychological treatments

Sherman (1998) conducted a meta-analysis of controlled trials of psychological treatments for PTSD. Eleven studies included a form of exposure therapy, three a form of cognitive therapy (including stress inoculation therapy), and three eye-movement desensitization and reprocessing. Other therapies identified included relaxation, supportive counselling, psychodynamic psychotherapy, and hypnotherapy.

Sherman's (1998) combined sample represented 690 participants from 17 studies. Approximately 50% of participants were Vietnam or Israeli combat veterans; 180 were female rape/assault victims; the remainder had experienced other traumatic events including violent crime, traumatic bereavement, and road-traffic accidents.

Sherman used a composite of PTSD symptoms, anxiety, and depression measures to calculate post-treatment effect sizes but analysing effect size for the individual symptoms made no real difference to outcome. All the trials revealed a positive outcome for therapy against no therapy with effect sizes immediately after treatment ranging from 0.03 to 8.4. The overall effect was significant, d = 0.54, r = 0.26 (95% C.I. = 0.39 to 0.68). Twelve studies provided follow-up between 3 months and 1 year. The effect sizes ranged from −0.25 to 1.69, with an overall effect of d = 0.53, r = 0.25 (95% C.I. = 0.37 to 0.69). This means that around 70% of control scores would be below the average experimental score.

Cognitive behavioural therapy

No meta-analyses have solely considered cognitive-behavioural therapy, although 14 of the 17 studies considered by Sherman (1998) were of cognitive-behavioural therapy. There have been a number of RCTs of varying quality. They have all described a positive effect of the exposure therapy. Amongst the best methodologically was that of Foa *et al.* (1991) who performed a RCT in 55 female victims of sexual assault, including rape. The interventions considered were prolonged exposure (PE), stress-inoculation training (SIT), supportive counselling (SC) (unconditional support from the therapists and 'here and now' problem-solving), and a waiting-list group. The treatments took place over nine sessions of 90 min occurring bi-weekly; 55 individuals were randomized; 45 completed the study. Immediately after treatment, Sherman (1998) calculated the effect size to be; 0.92 (95% C.I. = 0.57 to 1.27) for SIT; 0.33 (−0.03 to 0.69) for PE; and 0.14 (−0.21 to 0.49) for SC. At 3-month follow-up, the effect sizes were; 1.1 (0.66 to 1.5) for SIT; 1.67 (1.2 to 2.1) for PE; and 0.55 (0.17 to 0.94) for SC. At follow-up, 55% of the PE and SIT groups, and 45% of the supportive counselling group, no longer fulfilled the criteria for PTSD.

Eye movement desensitization and reprocessing (EMDR)

EMDR was first reported by Shapiro in 1989. The patient is asked to focus on the traumatic event, a negative cognition associated with it, and the associated emotions. The patient is then asked to follow the therapist's finger as it moves from side to side. There is no proven theoretical basis for EMDR, although several hypotheses have been postulated, and the necessity for eye movements has been challenged by some studies (e.g. Pitman *et al.* 1996).

There have been no well-designed systematic reviews or meta-analyses to date, although there are at least nine RCTs of EMDR in PTSD of variable and overall poor quality. The majority show EMDR to be effective at reducing symptoms of PTSD and of similar effectiveness to other active treatments such as cognitive-behavioural therapy (Bisson 1999).

Other psychological approaches

A variety of other psychological treatments have been advocated for use in the treatment of PTSD but to date have not been subjected to as rigorous evaluation as CBT and EMDR. One RCT of 112 PTSD sufferers from a variety of traumatic events found 18 sessions of psychodynamic psychotherapy to be as effective as exposure therapy and hypnotherapy, and better than waiting-list control (Brom *et al.* 1989). Trauma symptoms reduced from 79.2 (SD = 21.8) to 56.2 (SD = 24.1) in the desensitization group, 85.0 (SD = 16.9) to 65.4 (SD = 29.4) in the hypnotherapy group, 81.6 (SD = 25.2) to 57.0 (SD = 21.1) in the psychodynamic group, and 73.2 (SD = 18.2) to 66.4 (SD = 24.3) in the waiting-list group. These improvements were maintained at follow-up. Zlotnick *et al.* (1997) randomized 48 female survivors of childhood sexual abuse to a 15 week affect-management group or to a wait-list control. All patients additionally received individual psychotherapy and pharmacotherapy for at least 1 month before the study and for the duration of the study. The 16 individuals who completed the affect-management group showed a reduction of PTSD symptoms on the Davidson scale from a mean of 66.88 (SD = 22.00) to 45.76 (SD = 34.12). The wait-list control group showed a reduction from 74.69 (SD = 25.83) to 73.06 (SD = 29.86). Psychological treatments that have not yet been subjected to RCTs include drama therapy and music therapy.

Pharmacological treatments

There has been one published systematic review of placebo-controlled drug trials for PTSD to date (Penava *et al.* 1997). Six studies were identified with a total of 242 participants. The PTSD effect size across all trials was 0.41. The strongest effect size was 0.77 for the specific serotonin reuptake inhibitor fluoxetine ($n = 64$ in one trial). The monoamine oxidase inhibitor phenelzine had an effect size of 0.39 ($n = 63$ in two studies), tricyclic antidepressants 0.32 ($n = 149$ in three studies) and alprazolam, a benzodiazepine, 0.25 ($n = 16$ in one study). Differences in effect size were found between the tricyclics with amitriptyline (0.37, $n = 62$ in one study) faring better than imipramine (0.26, $n = 60$ in one study). In addition to helping reduce PTSD symptoms, the drugs were also found to reduce associated symptoms of depression and anxiety. Drugs that were more serotonin-specific were more effective, although the small number of studies and differing populations severely limits the conclusions that can be drawn regarding differential effects of the different medications. One selective serotonin reuptake inhibitor (sertraline) has now been licensed for the treatment of PTSD and other antidepressants are likely to follow.

With the somewhat limited and methodologically compromised information currently available, the treatments that have the best evidence-base for use are exposure therapy, cognitive therapy, EMDR, and antidepressant medication. It would seem reasonable to offer PTSD sufferers a choice of any of these given the current research, if they are available. Other treatments or combinations of treatment (e.g. medication and psychological treatment) may help and are widely used but have not been adequately researched to date.

Depression

The treatment of depression is much better researched than PTSD and there have been many RCTs and systematic reviews that have identified effective treatments. Like PTSD, both pharmacological and psychological treatments have been shown to be effective in depression. The choice of treatment for mild and moderate severity depression lies between medication and psychotherapy. Antidepressants have evolved over the years and it would be usual and totally appropriate to be started on an antidepressant, either a tricyclic such as dothiepin or the newer lofepramine or a specific serotonin re-uptake inhibitor such as fluoxetine or sertraline. Other antidepressants include the monoamine oxidase inhibitors such as phenelzine and moclobemide and the serotonin and noradrenaline re-uptake inhibitor venlafaxine. There is good evidence for the effectiveness of all these antidepressants in the treatment of depression. Joffe *et al.* (1996) performed a systematic review and estimated the average effect size to be 0.5 for antidepressant drug over placebo, meaning that 69% of those taking an antidepressant fared better than the outcome of the average person taking a placebo.

Cognitive-behavioural therapies, and particularly cognitive therapy, have been the most researched psychological treatments. If there are good cognitive therapists available, then there appears to be little to choose between this or an antidepressant in terms of effectiveness. Gloaguen *et al.* (1998) performed a meta-analysis of cognitive therapy in depression and found an effect size of 0.82 for cognitive therapy over placebo, meaning that 79% of those who received cognitive therapy fared better than the outcome of the average person who received a placebo. Interestingly, some research has suggested that in severe depression a combination of antidepressant medication and cognitive therapy or interpersonal therapy is better than either on their own (Thase *et al.* 1997).

If standard treatments for depression do not work, other management strategies can be beneficial in treatment resistant depression. Standard treatment algorithms have been developed (e.g. The Bethlem and Maudsley NHS Trust Prescribing Guidelines 1999) and include increasing the dose of antidepressant, changing antidepressant, and augmenting medication treatments such as lithium carbonate. Electro-convulsive therapy has been shown to be effective in severe depression, particularly if accompanied by psychotic features. Other psychological treatments that have been widely advocated but lack robust research support include psychodynamic treatments.

Anxiety disorders

Again the treatment approaches that have been shown to be beneficial are pharmacological and psychological (Gale and Oakley-Browne 1999). Antidepressants have anxiety-reducing properties and several are licensed specifically for the treatment of anxiety disorders in addition to depression. Another group of anxiety-relieving drugs are the benzodiazepines, such as diazepam and temazepam. These are undoubtedly effective at relieving symptoms of anxiety but have fallen into something of a state of disrepute due to their addictive potential and the problems caused by this. However, if used cautiously they can have a role in the short-term treatment of individuals with anxiety disorders. Cognitive-behavioural therapies have been found to have similar effect sizes (around 0.7) to pharmacological approaches in meta-analyses (Gale and Oakley-Browne 1999).

A proposed model of care

Despite the need for further research in this area, there is sufficient evidence available to propose a model of care for victims of violence. As stated previously, this model should be incorporated into the care offered by other organizations.

1. *Education.* It seems appropriate to offer individuals some form of education when they first present following a violent act. This is most likely to be in written form and contain general advice about issues following violence. Specific mention should be made of psychological aspects including the normal post-stress response and the availability of effective help should the psychological reaction not settle or cause marked distress.

2. *Detection of high-risk groups.* Given the evidence that some individuals are at higher risk than others of developing difficulties, it would seem appropriate to try to detect these individuals. With basic training, Emergency Department staff, the police, Victim Support, and other individuals in contact with victims of violence could detect those individuals at highest risk and direct them to appropriate services. Specific questionnaire measures, such as the Impact of Event Scale (Horowitz *et al.* 1979), are available and could be used to screen for psychological distress.

3. *Brief cognitive-behavioural intervention.* Individuals with symptoms of post-traumatic stress disorder, which are continuing a month after the incident, could be offered a brief cognitive-behavioural intervention, such as the one used by ourselves (description in the Appendix 1). This is evidence-based and has been shown to reduce symptoms of post-traumatic stress.

4. *Treat specific psychiatric disorder.* If an individual develops a psychiatric disorder such as PTSD, depression, or phobic anxiety then it is appropriate to offer an evidence-based treatment at an early stage. All individuals involved in the aftercare of victims of violence should be familiar with the common psychiatric disorders that can develop and know how to put such individuals into contact with appropriate services.

Concluding remarks

There has been a marked increase in the amount of interest and research in the area of PTSD over the last two decades. This has resulted in a developing knowledge of how best to cater for victims of trauma, including victims of violence. Effective evidence-based interventions and treatments are now available, although there remains considerable work to be done to determine the best possible ways to intervene.

Appendix: description of Cardiff intervention

This is a four-session intervention and contains several elements used in standard cognitive-behavioural therapy. In all the sessions, progress, levels of functioning, and homework compliance are reviewed. Clients are asked regularly to rate their levels of distress during the sessions using a subjective 0–10 distress rating scale.

Session one

The therapist discusses the incident and psychological symptoms with the individual. Individuals are educated regarding the normal stress response to an act of violence and physical injury, if present, reassured that a significant proportion of people experience similar symptoms following violence, and receive an explanation of the rationale behind the intervention. They are then encouraged to describe the traumatic incident in detail, in the first person present tense, including thoughts, feelings, sights, smells, noises, emotions, and physical reactions. The therapist records the sequence of events on paper and the participant is asked to read it at least once a day as homework.

Session two

The client is asked to read the text aloud so that it can be recorded onto an audiotape. Homework involves listening to the audiotape of this recording for at least half-an-hour every day. The therapist also attempts to identify, discuss, and challenge any cognitive distortions, such as unrealistic beliefs about being responsible for their injury.

Session three

The client listens to the taped account and discussion, then focuses on areas where habituation is not taking place and a number of approaches are suggested to overcome any avoidance as follows. Image Habituation Training (IHT) (Vaughan and Tarrier 1992) is used where the client is being troubled by specific distressing intrusive images. A graded *in vivo* exposure programme is devised if the client is avoiding real-life situations, e.g. car travel. Homework tasks comprise listening to the tape daily, using IHT where necessary, and the achievement of any agreed exposure goals.

Session four

The client again listens to the tape and discussion focuses on problems and successes over the course of therapy. The client is given a written summary that outlines successes, areas for attention, potential problem areas and how to cope with these, and any other relevant details.

References

American Psychiatric Association (1980). *Diagnostic and statistical manual of mental disorders* (3rd edn). APA, Washington DC.

American Psychiatric Association (1994). *Diagnostic and statistical manual of mental disorders* (4th edn). APA, Washington DC.

Bisson, J.I. (1997). Is post-traumatic stress disorder preventable? *Journal of Mental Health*, 6, 109–11.

Bisson, J.I. (1999). Post-traumatic stress disorder. *Clinical Evidence*, 2, 373–7.

Bisson, J.I., Shepherd, J.P., and Dhutia, M. (1997). Psychological sequelae of facial trauma. *Journal of Trauma, Injury, Infection and Critical Care*, 43, 496–500.

Bisson, J.I., Shepherd, J.P., Joy, D., and Probert, R. (1999). Randomised controlled trial of a four session intervention post-trauma. *Abstracts of 15th Meeting International Society of Traumatic Stress Studies*, p. 63. Miami.

Breslau, N., Davis, G.C., Andreski, M.A., and Peterson, E. (1991). Traumatic events and post-traumatic stress disorder in an urban population of young adults. *Archives of General Psychiatry*, 48, 216–22.

Brewin, C.R., Andrews, B., Rose, S., and Kirk, M. (1998). Acute stress disorder and post-traumatic stress disorder in victims of violent crime. *American Journal of Psychiatry*, **156**, 360–66.

Brom D., Kleber R.J., and Defares P.B. (1989). Brief psychotherapy of posttraumatic stress disorders. *Journal of Consulting and Clinical Psychology*, **57**, 607–12.

Brom, D., Kleber, R.J., and Hofman, M.C. (1993). Victims of traffic accidents: Incidence and prevention of post-traumatic stress disorder. *Journal of Clinical Psychology*, **49**, 131–40.

Bryant, R.A. (1999). Treating acute stress disorder: cognitive-behaviour therapy and hypnosis. *Abstracts of 15th Meeting International Society of Traumatic Stress Studies*, p. 36. Miami.

Bryant, R.A., Harvey, A.G., Dang, S.T., Sackville, T., and Basten, C. (1998). Treatment of acute stress disorder: a comparison of cognitive-behavioral therapy and supportive counselling. *Journal of Consulting and Clinical Psychology*, **66**, 862–6.

Davidson, J.R., Hughes, D., Blazer, D.G., and George, L.K. (1991). Post-traumatic stress disorder in the community. *Psychological Medicine*, **21**, 713–21.

Dolan, L., Bowyer, P.S., and Freeman, C. (1999). Post-trauma debriefing at home: is it effective? *European Society for Traumatic Stress Studies, 6th Conference Abstracts*, pp.29–30. Istanbul.

Dyregrov, A. (1989). Caring for helpers in disaster situations: psychological debriefing. *Disaster Management*, **2**, 25–30.

Flannery, R.B., Fulton, P., Tausch, J., and DeLoffi, A.Y. (1991). A program to help staff cope with psychological sequelae of assaults by patients. *Hospital and Community Psychiatry*, **42**, 935–8.

Foa, E.B., Rothbaum, B.O., Riggs, D.S., and Murdock, T.M. (1991). Treatment of Posttraumatic stress disorder in rape victims: a comparison between cognitive-behavioural procedures and counselling. *Journal of Consulting and Clinical Psychology*, **59**, 715–23.

Foa, E.B., Hearst-Ikeda, D., and Perry, K.J. (1995). Evaluation of a brief cognitive-behavioural program for the prevention of chronic PTSD in recent assault victims. *Journal of Consulting and Clinical Psychology*, **63**, 948–55.

Freedman, S.A., Brandes, D., Peri, T., and Shalev, A. (1999). Predictors of chronic post-traumatic stress disorder. *British Journal of Psychiatry*, **174**, 353–9.

Gale, C.K., and Oakley-Browne, M. (1999). Anxiety Disorder. *Clinical Evidence*, **2**, 347–53.

Gloaguen, V., Cottraux, J., Cucherat, M., *et al.* (1998). A meta-analysis of the effects of cognitive therapy in depressed patients. *Journal of Affective Disorders*, **49**, 59–72.

Harvey, A.G., and Bryant, R.A. (1998). The relationship between acute stress disorder and post-traumatic stress disorder: a prospective evaluation of motor vehicle accident survivors. *Journal of Consulting and Clinical Psychology*, **66**, 507–12.

Helzer, J.E., Robins, L.N., and McEvoy, L. (1987). Post-traumatic stress disorder in the general population: findings of the epidemiologic catchment area survey. *New England Journal of Medicine*, **317**, 1630–4.

Hobbs, M., and Adshead, G. (1996). Preventive psychological intervention for road crash survivors. In *The aftermath of road accidents: psychological, social and legal perspectives* (ed. M. Mitchell), pp.159–71. Routledge, London.

Horowitz, M., Wilner, N., and Alvarez, W. (1979). Impact of event scale: a measure of subjective stress. *Psychosomatic Medicine*, **41**, 209–18.

Joffe, R., Sokolov, S., and Streiner, D. (1996). Antidepressant treatment of depression: a meta-analysis. *Canadian Journal of Psychiatry*, **41**, 613–6.

Kessler, R.C., Sonnega, A., Bromet, E., Hughes, M., and Nelson, C.B. (1995). Post-traumatic stress disorder in the national comorbidity survey. *Archives of General Psychiatry*, **52**, 1048–60.

Kulka, R.A., Schlenger, W.E., Fairbank, J.A., Hough, R.L., Jordan, B.K., Marmar, C. *et al.* (1990). *Trauma and the Vietnam war generation: report of findings from the national Vietnam veterans readjustment study.* Brunner Mazel, New York.

McFarlane, A.C. (1988). The longitudinal course of post-traumatic morbidity: the range of outcomes and their predictors. *Journal of Nervous and Mental Disease,* **176**, 30–9.

McFarlane, A.C. (1989). The prevention and management of the psychiatric morbidity of natural disasters: an Australian experience. *Stress Medicine,* **5**, 29–30.

Penava, S.J., Otto, M.W., Pollack, M.H., and Rosenbaum, J.F. (1997) Current status of pharmacotherapy for PTSD; an effect size analysis of controlled studies. *Depression and Anxiety,* **4**, 240–2.

Pitman, R.K., Orr, S.P., Altman, B., Longpre, R.E., Poire, R.E., and Macklin, M.L. (1991). Emotional processing during eye movement desensitization and reprocessing therapy of Vietnam veterans with chronic posttraumatic stress disorder. *Comprehensive Psychiatry,* **37**, 419–29.

Raphael, B. (1986). *When disaster strikes: a handbook for caring professions.* Hutchinson, London.

Resnick, H.S., Kilpatrick, D.G., Best, C.L., and Kramer, T.L. (1992). Vulnerability-stress factors in development of post-traumatic stress disorder. *Journal of Nervous and Mental Disease,* **180**, 424–30.

Rose, S., Brewin, C.R., Andrews, B., and Kirk, M. (1999). A randomised controlled trial of individual psychological debriefing for victims of violent crime. *Psychological Medicine,* **29**, 793–9.

Rothbaum, B.O., and Foa, E.B. (1992). Subtypes of post-traumatic stress disorder and duration of symptoms. In *Post-traumatic stress disorder: DSMIV and beyond* (ed. J.R. Davidson and E.B. Foa), pp.23–35. American Psychiatric Press, Washington DC.

Shapiro, F. (1989). Eye movement desensitisation: a new treatment for post-traumatic stress disorder. *Journal of Behaviour Therapy and Experimental Psychiatry,* **20**, 211–7.

Shepherd, J.P., Qureshi, R., Preston, M.S., and Levers, B.G. (1990). Psychological distress after assaults and accidents. *British Medical Journal* **301**, 849–50.

Sherman, J.J. (1998). Effects of psychotherapeutic treatments for PTSD: a meta-analysis of controlled clinical trials. *Journal of Traumatic Stress,* **11**, 413–36.

Taylor, D., McConnell, D., McConnell, H., Abel, K., and Kerwin, R. (1999). *The Bethlem & Maudsley prescribing guidelines,* (5th edn). Martin Dunitz, London.

Thase, M.E., Greenhouse, J.B., Frank, E., *et al.* (1997). Treatment of major depression with psychotherapy or psychotherapy-pharmacotherapy combinations. *Archives of General Psychiatry,* **54**, 1009–1015.

Wessely, S., Rose S., and Bisson J. (1999). *A systematic review of brief psychological interventions ('debriefing') for the treatment of immediate trauma related symptoms and the prevention of post-traumatic stress disorder.* The Cochrane Library, published on CD-ROM Update Software Inc, CA, USA and Oxford, UK.

World Health Organisation (1992). *The ICD-10 classification of mental and behavioural disorders: clinical descriptions and diagnostic guidelines.* WHO, Geneva.

Zlotnick, C., Shea, T., Rosen, K., Simpson, E., Mulrenin, K., Begin, A. *et al.* (1997). An affect-management group for women with posttraumatic stress disorder and histories of childhood sexual abuse. *Journal of Traumatic Stress,* **10**, 425–36.

Chapter 10

Compensation for personal injuries caused by crime in Great Britain

David Miers

Introduction

Violence at work

This chapter is concerned with the possibility of a health-care worker who becomes the victim of an act of violence at work obtaining compensation for any injuries thereby sustained. The definition of violence at work used by the British Crime Survey (BCS) in a recent survey (Budd 1999, p. 2), is: 'All assaults or threats which occurred while the victim was working and were perpetrated by members of the public'. This therefore excludes assaults and threats committed by co-workers, but clearly includes patients, the patient's friends or relatives, or persons who are visiting the place of work (which could include a patient's private home or a nursing home and the like). The compensation possibilities that will be described in this chapter apply equally to those injured on or off duty: a nurse who is indecently assaulted while walking home from the theatre is in the same position, so far as these possibilities are concerned, as one assaulted by a patient, but we are not particularly concerned in this chapter with offences committed against health-care workers otherwise than when they are in the course of their employment. For our purposes, too, the distinction between co-workers and members of the public is of little practical importance. The nurse would have the same compensation possibilities were the offender to be another nurse. This latter event would of course raise disciplinary issues for the health authority as the victim's and the offender's employer; but these are not germane to this discussion.

The Home Office definition speaks of 'assaults' and 'threats'. Assaults include two of the most frequently occurring offences against the person: common assault and wounding, together with robbery and snatch theft, being property offences, which involve some violence being used against the victim in their commission.[1] Threats may include both verbal threats and non-verbal intimidation (which might also have a racial or sexual element),[2] typically to the victim's personal safety, but may also include

---

[1] In law, there is no such offence as 'snatch theft'. Theft is not usually accompanied by the use or threat of violence but, where it is, it may be treated by the police as a crime of violence (i.e. robbery).

[2] See Sections 29–32 of the Crime and Disorder Act 1998.

threats relating to the victim's property. Like theft, burglary is a crime against property, and the shock that victims suffer upon discovering that they have been burgled may be no different in its impact upon their well-being than that suffered in consequence of a direct personal assault. It is, however, important to maintain the distinction between property offences and personal victimization, for, as we shall see, the best compensation possibility for victims of crime, the Criminal Injuries Compensation Scheme, excludes trauma arising as a result of property loss or damage.

Before focusing more closely on the health-care worker's particular risk of becoming a victim of violence at work, it is useful to take an overview of the everyday risk of personal victimization. Despite the headlines, crimes of violence against the person are not that common. In 1998, of 4.5 million offences known to the police, 7% (353 200) consisted of offences of violence against the person (256 100), sexual offences (34 100) and robbery (63 000).[3] To these figures, which are based on its traditional recording methods, the Home Office added in 1998 the numbers of recorded offences of common assault and assault on a constable. Hospital staff will be very familiar with the sequelae of these offences, which are numerous (272 000), and which range from, for example, spitting at a constable to actual physical injury. The British Crime Survey has estimated that the total number of notifiable offences falling into the traditional group, i.e. including those that are not reported, is 10.2 million. (Home Office 2000, table 2A). Of these, the estimated number of offences of wounding is 714 000 and of robbery 897 000; taken together, these represent 16% of the total. This much higher proportion is inflated primarily by the 75% under-reporting of robbery; in the case of wounding, the proportion of non-reported offences (7%) is only slightly higher than those which are (5%). Because many of the reasons why offences are not reported (unknown offender, previous violent encounters between the victim and the offender, absence of any other person occupying a policing role, the victim's unwillingness to involve the police, or the sense that there is little point in doing so) do not apply with the same force where the offence occurs, say, in a hospital, we might expect a yet closer correspondence between reported and unreported offences of violence at work.[4]

That said, violence at work is relatively rare. 'The 1998 BCS estimates that 2.8% of working adults were victims of at least one violent incident at work in 1997 . . . [650 000 individuals]. Overall, the risks of physical assault while working are lower than the risks away from work' (Budd 1999, p.10). Measured against the average risk for all occupational groups within the survey (1.2%), nurses (5%), care workers (2.8%) and other health professionals (1.4%) are members of a broadly defined high-risk occupation. The category 'nurses', who are more than four times at risk than the national average, includes auxiliary nurses; 'care worker' covers such as workers in residential establishments, hospital and ward assistants, ambulance staff, and hospital porters. One important variable is shift work, in particular night duty: more than half of the assaults and a third of the threats occurred after 6.00 p.m.

---

[3] Home Office 2000, table 2.21. The figures in the text have been rounded.
[4] Budd (1999, p.37) reports that 'violence at work is relatively well reported compared to non-work violence; with some 55 per cent of assaults and 37 per cent of the threats coming to the attention of the police'.

The majority of offences against the person result in no serious injury to the victim (Hough and Mayhew 1983). In the case of violence at work, Budd (1999, pp. 33–4) reports that 'just under a half (46%) of all assaults at work resulted in some type of injury to the victim, though for most the injury was relatively minor .... Almost one in ten of those assaulted at work, and 1% of those threatened, saw a doctor as a result of the incident. However, less than 1% of victims of violence at work required an overnight stay in hospital as a result of the incident'. With the usual caveats about sampling errors and over-generalization, of the 1.2 million incidents of violence at work estimated by the BCS for 1997, 50 000 resulted in victims requiring medical attention, and 5000 in an overnight admission. For many, violence at work is just 'part of the job' (Budd 1999, p.40); nevertheless, the impact upon their sense of well-being and of confidence can be, even for victims of minor assaults, at the very least temporarily disabling (Maguire and Corbett 1987). On this matter, Budd (1999, p. 34) reports that nearly 75% of those who had been the victims of violence at work said that they were emotionally affected by the event. However, so far as compensation is concerned, the key issue is the depth of that emotional response; shock, fear, and distress, however acutely they may be felt at the time, will not be compensable as a head of damage in its own right, unless it meets what the law regards as a medically recognizable condition. The severity of the injury is a central dimension of the compensation arrangements that are described in this chapter.

The standard legal position

Employers have a duty to provide their employees with a safe system of work,[5] and thus where a health-care worker on duty is injured by a patient, it is in theory possible to succeed in a civil action in negligence against a hospital management or a health authority. It would have to be proved that the patient was known to the management or authority to have violent propensities, and that, in the circumstances, they had failed to take reasonable care to contain them, and that the worker's injury was closely related to that neglect. There might be liability, for example, where a female nurse is instructed to treat a male patient whose violent propensities are known to the management of the hospital in which he is being compulsory detained under the Mental Health Act 1983, the ward sister having failed first to check that any prescribed drug regime had been complied with. It would certainly be otherwise if a nurse working elsewhere in the hospital were injured following the patient's escape from the constraints normally imposed upon such a person. However, in the analogous context of the prison service, the courts have been reluctant to impose liability upon the management unless it had, in effect, accepted the prisoner's potential for violence and had instituted procedures (which proved fallible) explicitly designed to contain it.[6] Such

---

[5] The Health and Safety Executive (1998) has produced useful notes on employers' responsibilities concerning the effects of crime in the workplace.

[6] Important recent decisions include *Reeves v. Commissioner of Police for the Metropolis* [1999] 3 All E.R. 897 (liability of a police authority for the suicide of a prisoner known to have suicidal tendencies and in respect of whom the police had taken steps to minimize any risk of suicide while he was in police custody), *Costello v. Chief Constable of Northumbria* [1999] 1

civil action holds out little hope to injured nurses; it would certainly not extend to drunk and violent patients brought into an Accident and Emergency department.

The same can be said of instances in which health-care workers are attacked by strangers in hostels or other residences managed by the hospital trust or health authority and in which the worker resides, even for a short time. Even where a series of offences, e.g. indecent assaults, have been apparently committed by one man breaking into ground-floor bedrooms, no liability would be imposed upon those managing the hostel or residence for failing to prevent further assaults, unless they had, perhaps, unreasonably failed to repair a broken door or window.[7]

When a crime of violence is committed, we do not normally think of the civil obligation that the offender now owes the victim; yet every criminal offence against the person (and against property) is also a civil wrong (called a tort). Accordingly, where he or she is injured by a patient, a health-care worker should initially think of the possibility of a civil action. This will be an action for assault and battery, which, depending on the severity of the injury, will be heard in the County Court or the High Court. Provided that there are credible witnesses to give evidence of the assault (and there will need to be such witnesses if criminal proceedings are to succeed) and that the patient has sufficient funds (which, if the injury is minor, may well be the case), there is every reason to consider this possibility. Civil actions against offenders are rare, largely because victims believe, probably correctly, that their offenders, often being young or unemployed, are unlikely to have much money.

In general, victims leave to the police, and hence to the Crown Prosecution Service (CPS), any proceedings that should be taken. Where the offence is not committed by a patient and the offender's identity is otherwise unknown, there can clearly be no question either of civil action or of criminal proceedings. Even if the offender is apprehended and prosecuted to conviction, there is no guarantee that he or she will have sufficient funds to warrant a subsequent civil action. These considerations are relevant to the choice between what constitutes the two most realistic possibilities for health-care workers to obtain compensation for injuries arising from their becoming the victim of an offence involving personal violence. The first is that,

....

All E.R. 550 (liability of police authority for injuries sustained by a police officer at the hands of a violent prisoner in circumstances in which a second officer had been given responsibility for the first officer's safety), and *Kent v. Griffiths* [2000] 2 All E.R. 474 (liability of an ambulance service to answer a 999 call within a reasonable time). For an earlier analysis of the liability of health authorities for the criminal acts of psychiatric patients, see Miers (1996), and cases since that review: *Clunis v. Camden London Borough* [1998] 3 All E.R. 180, *Barrett v. Enfield London Borough* [1999] 3 All E.R. 193, *Palmer v. Tees Health Authority* (1999) 45 B.M.L.R. 88.

[7] Even where the offender was known to the police for his repeated victimization of the victim he ultimately murdered, the Court of Appeal held, on an application to strike the action out, that it would not be just and reasonable to impose civil liability on the police authority: *Osman v. Ferguson* [1994] 4 All E.R. 444. The European Court of Human Rights has ruled that this decision contravened Article 6(1) of the European Convention on Human Rights (right to institute civil proceedings); *Osman v. United Kingdom* [1999] *Criminal Law Rev.* 82.

following the conviction of the offender, the court makes a compensation order in the worker's favour, payable by the offender via a Magistrates' Court. Clearly, this possibility is dependent on the offender's being convicted, and upon his or her having some funds with which he or she can pay the order. Where the offender is not prosecuted (possibly because his or her identity was never known) or, if convicted, is without sufficient funds, the second possibility is an award made by the Criminal Injuries Compensation Authority (CICA), to which it is necessary to make an application. Each possibility has its advantages and disadvantages, which will be detailed in the next two sections.

Compensation orders

Injuries covered

The law governing compensation orders is to be found in Sections 130–4 of the Powers of Criminal Courts (Sentencing) Act 2000, replacing legislation first enacted in 1973 and subsequently amended in 1982 and 1988. In essence, Section 130 permits a Crown Court or a Magistrates' Court to impose an order upon an offender convicted before it, requiring him to pay compensation to anyone who has sustained any personal injury, loss, or damage as a result of the offence or of one taken into consideration. Some of the advantages of the compensation order can be seen here.

First, although this chapter is principally concerned with compensation for injuries arising from personal violence, a compensation order can be made in respect not only of personal injury, but also of the loss of or damage to property. Suppose a health-care worker is robbed on the way home. Upon conviction the offender can be ordered to pay for the theft of a wallet or handbag (assuming they are not returned), for the repair of clothing or personal accoutrements torn or broken in the attack, as well as for such personal injuries as cuts or bruises sustained by the victim. Second, while the court may order the offender to pay compensation for personal injury arising from the offence, the offence itself does not have to be a crime of violence. Suppose the worker returns home to find that he or she has been burgled. There is well-substantiated research that shows that burglary victims frequently suffer shock (Maguire 1982). This arises from a combination of feelings, of having one's privacy invaded (some female victims speak of a feeling akin to being sexually compromised), of anger, of depression, and of a heightened fear of crime. There is no doubt that the court could include in the order a sum by way of compensation for this trauma.

So far as crimes of violence against the person are concerned, a compensation order can be made in respect both of physical injuries and of mental injuries, such as might arise from a straightforward case of an offence of wounding or assault occasioning actual bodily harm (Sections 20 and 47 of the Offences against the Person Act 1861, respectively). Such an event is not unusual in an A&E department on a Friday or Saturday night: cuts, scarring, broken noses and jaws, shock, and distress may result. There may be some difficulty where the offender is mentally ill, as this could preclude a conviction if he or she didn't know what he or she was doing; and where the offender is elderly (and possibly suffering from some form of dementia),[8] the CPS may consider a prosecution inappropriate. If the injury is serious, an application to the CICA may succeed (see below). It is, however, no impediment to a conviction for these offences that the offender was voluntarily intoxicated, whether through drink or drugs. The courts take a robust view of self-induced intoxication; they treat this as reckless conduct, and it is no defence to a charge involving an offence that can be committed recklessly, that the perpetrator was so intoxicated that he or she didn't know what he or she was doing.

Compensation can also be ordered in respect of convictions for sexual offences, whether, as is typically the case in rape, they result in physical injury, or, as in indecent exposure or assault, they result primarily in shock. In any of these cases, an order may be made in favour of a victim who suffers physical or mental injury or both.[9] A 'peeping tom' does not by definition commit a criminal offence; however, if it is his intention, for example, to frighten a nurse by peering through her bedroom window while she is undressing, he may be guilty of an offence under Section 47 of the Offences against the Person Act 1861, if as a consequence the nurse suffers clinically recognizable mental harm.[10] It is also possible that a 'peeping tom' could commit an offence under Section 5(1) of the Public Order Act 1986 (threatening, abusive or insulting words, or behaviour), in which case a compensation order could be made against him on conviction. A person who 'stalks' a nurse, makes silent phone calls,[11] or otherwise harasses her (this includes alarming or causing the victim distress) commits an offence under Sections 1–2 of the Protection from Harassment Act 1997. An actual or apprehended breach of Section 1 may be the subject of a claim in civil proceedings by the person who is or may be the victim of the course of conduct in question, and damages may be awarded for (among other things) any anxiety caused by the harassment and any resulting financial loss. A conviction for such an offence will likewise open the possibility that the court may order the offender to compensate the victim: while the standard of proof is lower in civil than in criminal proceedings, the victim may prefer that the burden of proof is carried by the state (the CPS). Of course, even

---

[8] See Budd (1999, p.19), reporting a care assistant's comments: 'I work in a home for elders and I am often hit by the residents who have Alzheimer's disease. They get angry because they are helpless and lash out at the staff.'

[9] For example, a compensation order of £500 was made against a man (aged 42) convicted of indecently assaulting a 16-year-old girl at a party. He had been drinking heavily, propositioned and cornered her, and then repeatedly licked her face after she had refused to kiss him (*The Times*, 5 November 1999).

[10] *R v. Chan-Fook* [1994] 1 W.L.R. 689. In *Smith v. Chief Superintendent, Woking Police Station* [1983] 76 Cr. App. Rep. 234, the court held that a man who stood in the garden of a private house looking through the window at the victim with the intention of frightening her, committed an assault notwithstanding that there were no spoken threats. He had put her in fear because she was uncertain what he would do next, and whether that would involve violence against her.

[11] The House of Lords has held that silent phone calls can, if their impact on the victim is sufficiently severe, constitute an offence under Section 18 of the 1861 Act (causing grievous bodily harm with intent); *R v Ireland and Burstow* [1997] 4 All E.R. 225.

where there is a conviction, the victim can refuse the offer, even if the offender is well able to pay. Clearly, this may well be the case in such circumstances as sexual harassment and other sexual offences, where the last thing the victim wishes is to be reminded of the offender's unwanted presence in her life.

So far we have assumed that the health-care worker who has suffered the personal injury specified by Section 130 of the 2000 Act is the same person as the victim of the offence for which the offender is convicted. Of course, in most cases it will be, but it need not be: the worker who suffers shock as a consequence of being a witness to an offence against another, or, perhaps, who comes upon another person who is lying unconscious having been the victim of a crime, is also covered by this section. A paramedic who attends upon the victims of a terrorist bomb explosion, for example, is in theory covered, though it is no doubt unlikely that an order would be made in such a case, the offender being sent to prison for many years. Nevertheless, there is an important point here to which we shall return.

Compensation orders can also be made in respect of an offence that is taken into consideration by the court when sentencing the offender. This process is a common occurrence with minor property offences; it enables the police to treat the offences as 'cleared up', and in practice it means that the offender will not be convicted and sentenced for all of them. Thus, it may be possible for a victim of theft, of taking a vehicle without consent, or of criminal damage, to obtain compensation even though no conviction is returned. In the case of personal injury, however, this is unlikely, as a court would not, as a general rule, be prepared to take offences of violence against the person into consideration upon sentence.

There are, however, a number of limitations on the scope of compensation orders. They are not payable where the offender has been cautioned. Cautioning is a standard response to first-time offenders committing property offences; it is thus unlikely to affect, one way or the other, health-care workers who are the victims of crimes of violence. Injuries arising from road-traffic offences are, with one small exception, excluded. Neither can compensation be ordered in respect of loss of dependency, that is the loss of income of the deceased, occasioned by homicide. The exception here is for what is called bereavement. Suppose a murdered worker had been married; a compensation order may be made in favour of his or her spouse. The only other case allowed by law will, in the nature of health-care employment practices, not apply, since it relates to a case where the deceased was under 18. Where the bereavement award is payable, it is for a sum not exceeding the maximum laid down in the Fatal Accidents Act 1976, currently £7500.

Assessing the offender's means

All that has been said so far is, of course, dependent on the offender having sufficient funds to pay compensation. Before it makes an order, the court must comply with its statutory duty to take the offender's means into account. If the offender indicates a willingness to pay compensation, a court will usually take that at its face value, though it must satisfy itself about the sources from which these funds will be drawn. The problem for the court is that if it makes an order with which the offender cannot comply, the offender is likely to return to crime so as to meet it. If there is a capital asset, a car perhaps, there is no objection to the court making an order on the basis that the offender will have to sell it, provided that it can place reasonably clear value upon it. Nor is there any objection to an order's being made against an offender on income support. The Home Office has in the past indicated that, in such circumstances, payment of £5.00 a week may be proper; this does, of course, have serious implications for the total amount that the offender may be able to pay. An unwillingness to pay should not deter the court from making an order if it is obvious that the offender has some financial resources.

A Crown Court judge can make a compensation order for any amount at all; but in the Magistrates' Courts, where the vast majority of orders are made, Section 131(1) of the 2000 Act imposes a maximum of £5000 for any one offence (this is in line with the limit on magistrates' powers to fine offenders). Within either this statutory limit or the limit imposed in practice by the amount the offender is able to pay, the order is payable as a lump sum or in instalments, usually over not more than 3 years. As we will see, the number of victims who recover under compensation orders is low, as is the amount that they recover.

Assessing the amount of compensation

On the assumption that there are some funds, the next step is for the court to determine how much the offender ought to pay the victim. This depends first on how extensive are those resources, and second on the severity of the injuries sustained. Clearly, if the offender is on income support and the victim was blinded in one eye (an injury that would attract £18 000–22 000 general damages in a civil action, or £20 000 under the Criminal Injury Compensation Scheme's tariff provisions), the order will come nowhere close to compensating the victim. Indeed, in a case where there is a great discrepancy between what the offender can afford and the severity of the injuries, the court may well not make any order. Here we see the principal obstacle to a health-care worker's obtaining full compensation from the offender for the injuries sustained. If the injuries are minor, full compensation may be made, albeit in instalments; but if their value exceeds what the court thinks it proper for the offender to pay, the victim will only receive some of the 'ideal' value of the injuries. Of course it remains open to the worker to sue the offender. A civil court does not have to take the defendant's means into account when making its order, which could of course result in bankruptcy; but given an offender with little resources, the health-worker may not think it worth the trouble. As we shall see, if the injuries are severe and uncompensated by the offender, the worker may well succeed in an application to the CICA; but there are some limitations there.

Like the assessment of damages in a civil action, the evaluation by a criminal court of a victim's injury in respect of which it is considering making a compensation order comprises two elements: one sum to reflect general damages, i.e. to include what is called pain and suffering and loss of amenities; and the second to reflect special damages, i.e. to include material losses, such as loss of income and expenses.

General damages

In 1988 a set of guidelines was published indicating the figure that would be appropriate for given personal injuries, being the ones most commonly appearing before magistrates. These were updated in 1993, and it would be appropriate to regard them all as being index-linked since then. The figures are based on the likely effects of an injury of the specified kind being sustained by a person of between 20 and 35 years of age, of average health, and with no particular susceptibilities. The guidelines recommend that the age and the sex of the victim be treated as factors that may materially affect the assessment. Particular mention is made of the impact of the offence on an elderly or disabled victim, and on the effect of scarring; a scar that can be seen when the victim is fully clothed, especially if it is on the face, should normally be treated as more serious than one that is concealed. Generally speaking, a court will regard as more serious scarring on a woman than a man.

The figures given in Table 10.1 reflect what the law calls 'pain and suffering', i.e., the normal physical and mental distress associated with the particular injury. They also include the normal 'loss of amenity' that such injury causes, for example, being unable to pursue a hobby or to engage in a sport. Where there is a particular sensitivity that aggravates the injury, or where, for example, the worker is a county standard squash player now unable to compete in a national competition, it may be possible to persuade the court to increase the amount payable; but as always, this will be subject to what the court considers the offender can be properly ordered to pay. Moreover, magistrates are unwilling to become involved in more complicated assessments of the loss to the victim. If an offender is on trial at the Crown Court, a Circuit or High Court judge will be better placed to assess general damages in such a case; but in general, if the injury requires anything other than a simple assessment (especially if the prognosis is unclear), the court will be reluctant to make an order.

Special damages

'Special damages' covers all those material losses that flow from the injury, for example, loss of earnings, the cost of dental treatment such as the repair or replacement of dentures, hearing-aids, and spectacles, and expenses incurred in travelling to and from the worker's GP or to an out-patients' department. Health-care workers who have a contract of employment with a health authority or trust will usually not lose any earnings, as they will continue to be paid; on the other hand, a bank or agency nurse is usually not paid unless working. It is therefore very important that such a worker keeps a clear and accurate record of the number of days lost as a consequence of the injury.[12] Some health-care workers who live at home also look after their elderly parents; if the consequence of the injury is that someone else has to be engaged to care for the house and/or parents, this expense too is covered by the heading 'special damages'. As ever, whether an order is made to cover this expense will depend on the offender's resources.

Whatever the material loss for which the victim is seeking compensation, the court will in every case require evidence of the loss, and may ask for receipts, pay slips, bills,

---

[12] Budd (1999, pp.35–6) notes that 'victims of violent incidents while working rarely took time off work as a result of the incident, only 4 per cent did so . . . [those who did] usually had a day off, though in a few cases one or two weeks were taken and in one case the victim was off work for about two months'.

Table 10.1 Pain and suffering guidelines in Magistrates' Courts (Home Office 1988, 1993)

Type of injury		Suggested award (£)
Graze	Depending on size	up to 50
Bruise	Depending on size	up to 75
Black eye		100
Cut (no permanent scarring)	Depending on size and whether stitched	75–500
Sprain	Depending on loss of mobility	100–1000
Loss of a non-front tooth	Depending on cosmetic effect and age of victim	250–500
Other minor injury	Causing reasonable absence from work (2–3 weeks)	550–850
Loss of front tooth		1000
Facial scar	(However small) resulting in permanent disfigurement	750+
Facial scar	A vicious slash wound from ear to the corner of the mouth or under the chin	6000–9000+
Jaw	Fractured (wired)	2750
Nose	Undisplaced fracture of the nasal bone	750
Nose	Displaced fracture of the nasal bone requiring manipulation under general anaesthetic	1000
Nose	Not causing fracture but displaced septum requiring a sub-mucous resection	1750
Wrist	Simple fracture with complete recovery in a few weeks	1750–2500
Wrist	Displaced fracture (limb in plaster for some 6 weeks; full recovery 6–12 months)	2500+
Finger	Fractured little finger, assuming full recovery after a few weeks	750
Leg or arm	Simple fracture of tibia, fibula, ulna or radius with full recovery in three months	2500
Laparotomy	Stomach scar 6–8 in long (resulting from exploratory operation)	3500

and other documentary evidence of payments made or owed by the worker as a result of the injury. A victim is strongly advised to make sure that these details are kept safely. Even if there is limited success in obtaining a compensation order, these details will be needed should a claim be made to the CICA.

What you need to do

Unlike the CICA, there is no official application procedure that you need to follow for the court to consider whether it should order your offender to pay you compensation. Remember that the court is not obliged to make an order in your favour. However, the court is under a statutory duty to give reason why it hasn't made an order in a case in which it has power to do so. If you have appeared as a prosecution witness in your offender's trial, and during your evidence you told the court about the injuries that were inflicted on you, the court would be acting unlawfully if it did not then give a reason why it has not, upon conviction, ordered the offender to compensate you. If the reason it gives is that it has considered the offender's means to be insufficient, then you have no ground for complaint. Likewise if it makes an order for a smaller sum than the full value of your injuries; but if it makes no order and says nothing at all, then you should seek legal advice.

Another reason that the court could properly give for not making an order in your case is that it had insufficient evidence upon which to establish to its satisfaction the kind of injury you sustained and its impact upon you: your evidence that the offender ran up to you and hit you with a broken bottle may be quite sufficient to convict of an offence of wounding, but it will not be sufficient to determine what amount of compensation you should be paid, even given that the offender is apparently well off. Even though you may be the chief prosecution witness, you have no right to speak to the court about your injuries except in answer to the questions put to you; you cannot address the court in your own right about your loss of earnings or medical expenses. Neither do you have any right to speak up at the sentencing stage, which is the time when the court will be considering the question of compensation. How then, is the court going to know about your injuries and the impact they have had on you?

The answer is to make sure that when you report the offence to the police (or if someone else reports on your behalf) that the police fill in, or let you fill in, a 'Compensation Schedule'. If you are asked to attach copies of receipts and bills, always make sure you keep your own copy. All police forces have been instructed by the Home Office to give assistance to victims of crime, and to use this Schedule, which asks for details of any injury, loss, or damage, as a means by which the court will be informed of your circumstances. The Schedule is attached to the case papers forwarded to the CPS, who should in turn notify the magistrates or the trial judge of its contents. If the police to whom you speak do not know about the Schedule, refer to the Home Office circulars.[13]

An alternative is to get in touch with the national organization, Victim Support (for address and telephone number see Appendix I), which is a charity specifically established

---

[13] In May 2000 the Home Secretary announced a new 'Victim Personal Statement' scheme to be introduced nationwide in order to give victims of crime a greater say in the criminal justice system. Victims and their families will be able to give a personal statement on how a crime has affected them. This will be seen and taken into account by the police, the Crown Prosecution Service (in deciding whether to prosecute) and the courts (in deciding on sentence). The scheme is intended to be introduced early in 2001. It will be available to any individual victim of crime and others including relatives and partners in homicide cases, and parents of children who are victims.

to help victims of crime. Besides exploring compensation possibilities, it operates a volunteer-counselling service. Victim Support has some 380 branches, listed in local telephone directories. You may well find that, if your injury is serious, the local branch will get in touch with you (each one is routinely informed by the police of offences of personal violence, given of course, that the police have recorded the offence).

Success rates

While, in theory, compensation orders offer a quick and simple means by which a victim of a crime of violence can obtain compensation from the offender, their use is irregular. During the mid-1990s there was a marked decrease in the number of orders made by comparison with the earlier years of the decade: from 19 000 in 1994 to 13 300 in 1997 (violence against the person, sexual offences and robbery, Magistrates and Crown Court proceedings; Home Office 2000, table 7.22). In 1998 (the last available year published in the Criminal Statistics) a total of 13 900 orders were made in respect of these three offence categories: 11 300 by magistrates and 2900 by the Crown Court. In the case of indictable offences of violence against the person, 10 700 orders were made by magistrates (against 44% of all offenders sentenced for this type of offence) and 2500 were made by the Crown Court (19% of offenders). There were 600 orders made by magistrates on conviction for robbery (against 48% of offenders) and 100 at the Crown Court (3% of offenders). For sexual offences, 300 orders were made following summary conviction (against 24% of offenders), and less than 100 were made by the Crown Court (1% of offenders)

There are no clear reasons why the number of orders made in 1997 fell so dramatically by comparison with the preceding years. What is beyond dispute is that no amount of Schedules, guidelines, or statutory duties will make any difference if your offender is of limited means. In 1997, the average amount ordered to be paid by magistrates in the case of violence against the person was £218, and in the case of sexual offences, £159. In the Crown Court, these amounts were £484 and £396, respectively. By comparison, the highest average figure in the Magistrates' Court for any one offence was £322 (fraud and forgery) and the average for all indictable offences was £208; in the Crown Court these averages were £3090 (fraud and forgery) and £961, respectively. The figures for personal injury are, therefore, very low; even if the average figure in a magistrates' court (£218) was an amount payable only in respect of pain and suffering, it is an amount commensurate with virtually the lowest figure on the Home Office's recommended tariff, payable in respect of a black eye or sprain (£100) or a minor cut (£75–£200). As it is unlikely that all 13 900 victims in whose favour orders were made in 1997 sustained only such minor injury, the primary reason for these low figures is almost certainly that in most cases the court considered that this was all the offender could afford, irrespective of the tariff value of the injury.

It is, however, of interest to note that the average figures for offences of violence (£218 and £484 in the Crown Court) are broadly in line with the compensation levels that the BCS victims gave when they were asked the question: 'Apart from any financial losses what would you say would be a reasonable sum to compensate you for the upset and inconvenience you and/or your household suffered?'. The average value that victims placed on their experience was £147; in the specific instance of assault, £285.

These figures are well within the actual levels reported in the Criminal Statistics for 1998 and thus suggest that health workers should actively follow up the exhortation that the Lord Chancellor made to the magistracy in October 1999, that they should take stern action against offenders convicted of offences against NHS employees.[14]

Two studies conducted some years ago showed that around 80% of offenders eventually comply with the orders made against them. Payment by instalments may well take over a year (that is, of course, after the delay in bringing the offender to trial, which may be a few weeks in the Magistrates' Courts, but months in the Crown Court). Despite these considerations, a health-care worker who suffers a fairly minor injury, caused by an offender with means, stands a good chance of becoming the beneficiary of a compensation order. If the injuries are severe, it is very unlikely to reflect their 'value' according to law. In this case, the only recourse is to apply to the CICA.

The criminal injuries compensation scheme

Injuries covered

The Criminal Injuries Compensation Authority (CICA) administers a Scheme established under the Criminal Injuries Compensation Act 1995 by which victims of crimes of violence may be compensated for the injuries they sustained, and, where they die in consequence, by which their dependants can be compensated. This Scheme, which had existed in a non-statutory form since 1964, applies throughout England, Wales, and Scotland and is funded by the government; there is therefore no question of the making of the award or of the payment of the compensation being dependent on the offender's resources.[15] Clearly, this is a very substantial advantage by comparison with compensation orders. So far as its scope is concerned, the Scheme differs from compensation orders in two main ways.

First, the Criminal Injuries Compensation Scheme only applies to personal injuries. With one exception to be mentioned later, no compensation can be awarded for any loss of, or damage to, property, or for injury arising from the commission of an

---

[14] Part of the NHS Zero Tolerance Policy is to encourage prosecutions of those who attack staff (Burke 1999; Editorial 1999). Sections 67–68 of the Crime and Disorder Act 1998 introduce reparation orders as a further measure that may be imposed on young offenders. Such orders have been available in respect of adult offenders since 1973, but are infrequently used. Under the 1998 Act, a reparation order may be made upon conviction in respect of anyone affected by the offence, which thus may include someone other than the immediate victim. A reparation order cannot be used for the purpose of effecting direct monetary compensation (though a compensation order could be made in addition), but could include, for example, a young person undertaking remedial work at the hospital where the offence was committed.

[15] Note that in Northern Ireland there are separate statutory provisions concerning the compensation of victims of crimes of violence. These provisions are similar to those in Great Britain, but there are important dissimilarities that are a response to the particular political circumstances obtaining there. A useful recent overview is to be found in Bloomfield et al. (1999).

offence against property. A health-care worker who is robbed can be compensated for the physical and mental injury that is caused, but not for the loss of or damage to possessions. There can, however, be no compensation for the shock of discovering that one has been burgled, no matter how great the burglary or the shock, because burglary is a crime against property. The kinds of injury that constitute 95% of the claims that the CICA receives arise from offences such as assault occasioning actual bodily harm, wounding, and causing grievous bodily harm under Sections 47, 20, and 18, respectively of the Offences against the Person Act 1861. Depending on the severity of the injury, and whether it was recklessly or intentionally inflicted, this part of the Scheme covers, for example, nurses and porters injured by offenders under the influence of alcohol or drugs, robberies, or other violent assaults. The Scheme will also cover the offences of rape, indecent assault, and harassment under the Protection from Harassment Act 1997 discussed earlier. Threats of harm will, as in those cases where the only consequence of an assault is mental injury, come within the Scheme only where the victim is able to demonstrate that the injury is, at the very least, medically verified.[16] Serious trauma or psychiatric disturbance will almost always fall within the Scheme.

There are four other circumstances in which a health-care worker may sustain an injury which are covered by this Scheme.

1.   The worker could sustain injuries arising from an offence of arson; for example, while attending at the scene a person who has been burnt or overcome by fumes in an arson attack on a building, the worker is him or herself injured by the collapse of a part of the building, or is overcome by fumes.

2.   Injuries caused by an offence of poisoning are within the Scheme.

3.   It is possible that a member of the nursing or medical teams on duty in an A&E department could become involved in trying to restrain a patient, perhaps by going to a colleague's assistance, and in so doing, sustain an injury. Injuries arising from such efforts by the victim to enforce the law, perhaps by giving help to a policeman, are compensable under the Scheme. Suppose a nurse tries to sedate the violent offender whom a policeman is endeavouring to restrain, and is injured by a weapon held in the offender's flailing hands. The nurse who could show that the offender intentionally or recklessly inflicted the injury would clearly come within the scope of the Scheme's main provision, namely, that injury was caused by the commission of a crime of violence. If, however, the injury was sustained accidently (being now sedated, the offender falls against the nurse) or as a result of the offender's negligence (now wishing to give himself up, he throws the weapon to one side, where it strikes the nurse), he or she would not be the victim of a crime of violence. However, the nurse

---

[16] The following reports: 'I was working in casualty and I tried to take a dressing off a man's arm, he tried to grab me and threatened to push my teeth down my throat' and 'A patient didn't like our systems in the practice and threatened to hit me if I didn't examine his child and used foul language to me and my receptionist' (Budd 1999; p.19) would not, though no doubt common enough experiences, appear on the face of them to be sufficiently serious to come within the Scheme's ambit.

who was taking an exceptional risk in helping the policeman will come within the Scheme. What is an 'exceptional' risk will depend upon the circumstances, but where a private citizen assists in the restraint of an armed offender, the risk would probably be so regarded.

4. In all three of these possibilities, the injury sustained could, like standard offences of personal violence, be physical or mental in its impact on the worker. Where the only injury that the health worker suffers is mental injury, the Scheme restricts compensation to those cases where the victim 'was put in reasonable fear of immediate harm to his own person'. A nurse or ambulance driver who sustains mental, but no physical, injury as a result of being involved, say, in treating the victims of a siege in which hostages have been taken and shot, will be within the Scheme if, as is likely on these facts, they were themselves put in fear. But such mental injury alone will not be compensable where the worker deals with the aftermath of the siege, the offender by now having committed suicide or been disabled by the police. The same result will follow in the terrorist scenario used earlier. Paramedics who attend at the aftermath of a terrorist bombing and who suffer mental injury only will fall outside the Scheme unless it could be shown that at the time of so attending, they were themselves in fear of physical injury; for example, that there might be a second explosive device in the vicinity.

The second main difference between the terms of the Scheme and a compensation order is that there is no requirement for an award of compensation under the Scheme that there be a conviction against the offender (though this will help), or even that the offender be identified. This is obviously of great importance where the worker is attacked by someone who is not a patient. It is also of importance where the worker is attacked by a patient against whom, because of his or her mental condition, criminal proceedings are unlikely to be taken or to succeed. Indeed, the nurse or care worker may, in these circumstances, 'feel that the offender was not entirely responsible for their actions and therefore not view the incident as one within the remit of a crime survey. This will result in an underestimation of incidents against health care workers' (Budd 1999, p.19). It will also result in the worker being unable to pursue a claim under the Scheme, if it is not reported as a crime, even if the offender is, in effect, beyond prosecution.

Although, in the usual case, there need be no identification of the offender, it is vital that the health-care worker should, without delay, report the incident giving rise to the injury to the police. Where the offence takes place while the worker is on duty, it is quite likely that it will be reported to the police by the hospital management. In the Home Office survey, this was the reason victims gave most frequently for not reporting the matter to the police themselves (Budd 1999, p.38). This is quite understandable, but unless there are very good reasons why the victim did not make a report (e.g. because the offence was disabling), this will not do for the purpose of obtaining compensation from the CICA. The Scheme is explicit: *the worker him- or herself must report the incident to the police.*[17]

---

[17] Some 30% of the nil award claims fail because the victim did not report the incident to the police or thereafter co-operate with them, the medical authorities, or the Authority itself (National Audit Office 2000, para. 2.19).

As has been indicated, the Scheme also applies to cases in which the worker is killed in the assault; the various points made above apply equally here, with appropriate adjustments. The Scheme does not apply to injuries or fatalities arising from traffic accidents, unless the accident was a result of a deliberate attempt to hit the victim.

Eligibility for compensation

At the expense of repetition (but it is important) the first requirement is that the health-care worker him- or herself reports the incident to the police without delay. Thereafter the worker must co-operate with them in their enquiries. If the police wish to hold an identification parade, he or she must attend; fear of reprisal will not be an acceptable excuse. It is not necessary to press charges, but if the Crown Prosecution Service do, the worker must be willing, if called upon, to give evidence at the trial. The worker must also co-operate with the CICA after making the claim for compensation; withholding evidence of injury, for example, for fear of embarrassment, will not be acceptable.

The claim for compensation must be made within two years of the incident. It is sometimes the case that many years pass before an injury's full effects become evident; the CICA has a discretion to allow claims made out of time, but the circumstances of the claim will be closely scrutinized.

Third, there is a minimum financial threshold in the Scheme: the injury has to be 'worth' £1000. As we shall see in more detail below, the compensation that is payable under the Scheme falls broadly into two categories. The first is a 'tariff' award, being a fixed sum related to the nature of the injury sustained. The second is a calculated award, related to loss of earnings or the provision of special care or provision for severely injured victims. The tariff will only be activated where the injury sustained meets one of the minimum £1000-injury descriptions. The kind of injuries that are worth exactly this amount are given in Table 10.2, which gives all of the current £1000

Table 10.2 Injuries to the head worth £1000 (the minimum CICA financial threshold)

Head: ear: fractured mastoid
Head: ear: temporary partial deafness — lasting 6 to 13 weeks
Head: ear: tinnitus (ringing noise in ear — lasting 6 to 13 weeks
Head: eye: blurred or double visions — lasting 6 to 13 weeks
Head: facial: multiple fractures to face
Head: nose: undisplaced fracture of nasal bones
Head: teeth: fractured/chipped tooth/teeth requiring treatment
Head: teeth: chipped front tooth requiring crown
Head: teeth: fractured tooth requiring crown
Head: teeth: damage to tooth/teeth requiring root-canal treatment
Head: teeth: loss of one tooth other than front
Head: teeth: slackening of teeth requiring dental treatment

injuries to the head. They are cited in full as an illustration both of their medical descriptions and of the manner in which the tariff is set out. There are altogether 310 tariff injuries, of which 27 are stated at the £1000 minimum. A tariff system operating in this way naturally poses difficulties where a victim sustains multiple injuries, none of which alone meets the minimum amount. The Scheme recognizes this as follows.

> Minor multiple injuries will only qualify for compensation where the applicant has sustained at least three separate injuries of the type illustrated below, at least one of which must still have had significant residual effects six weeks after the incident. The injuries must have necessitated at least two visits to or by a medical practitioner within that six week period. Examples of qualifying injuries are:
>
> (a)   grazing, cuts, lacerations (no permanent scarring)
>
> (b)   severe and widespread bruising
>
> (c)   severe soft tissue injury
>
> (d)   black eye(s)
>
> (e)   bloody nose
>
> (f)   hair pulled from scalp
>
> (g)   loss of fingernail.

This is an important provision, given that many common assaults result only in minor injuries of this kind; this will be true, in particular, of the thousands of common assaults now recorded in the Criminal Statistics. The Home Office research found that of those 46% of assaults that did result in some type of injury, 'bruising or black eyes were most common, with 40% of incidents resulting in such injuries. Scratches and cuts were each reported in about a tenth of incidents, and broken bones in 1%' (Budd 1999, p.33). As the Scheme makes clear, the victim will have had to sustain a combination of such injuries if an award is to be made. It will be noted that the qualifying injuries are all physical injuries. It is thus not open to workers to argue that they should be compensated where they have sustained two of the illustrated injuries, together with mental injury in the form of anxiety or loss of confidence.[18] This is so in part because the tariff includes an element of compensation for the degree of shock that an applicant in normal circumstances would experience as a result of an incident

---

[18] These are two of the forms of psychological symptoms of nervous shock given in Note 2 to the tariff:
shock or 'nervous shock' may be taken to include conditions attributed to post-traumatic stress disorder, depression, and similar generic terms covering:
(a) such psychological symptoms as anxiety, tension, insomnia, irritability, loss of confidence, agoraphobia and pre-occupation with thoughts of guilt or self-harm; and
(b) related physical symptoms such as alopecia, asthma, exczema, enuresis and psoriasis. Disability in this context will include impaired work (or school) performance, significant adverse effects on social relationships and sexual dysfunction.

resulting in injury. And threats alone, unless they amount, in the tariff description, to 'Shock: Disabling, but temporary mental anxiety, medically verified', will not be compensable.

The final condition of eligibility concerns the victim's own behaviour. The Scheme provides that the CICA may disqualify from compensation a claimant who has a conviction for a serious offence, but as such a history would in any event preclude someone from becoming a health-care worker in the first place, this can be set aside. However, the Scheme also provides that the CICA may disqualify a claimant from compensation because of his or her conduct before, during, or after the events giving rise to the claim, or because of his or her unlawful conduct. If the worker provoked the assault, or was intoxicated (whether through drink or illicit drugs), and certainly if he or she struck the first blow, the CICA could well refuse any or all of the claim. Again, one must assume that such conduct would not arise where the health worker was on duty.

Assessing the amount of compensation

Like compensation orders, a CICA award includes both general damages and special damages. However, under the arrangements introduced from 1 April 1996 (which apply to all injuries arising after that date), these assume a different guise to their counterparts in common law, on which the replaced non-statutory scheme was based. In short, where the victim survives the criminal injury, the new Scheme provides that compensation payable under an award will be:

1 a standard amount of compensation determined by reference to the nature of the injury (the tariff);

2 where the applicant has lost earnings or earning capacity for longer than 28 weeks as a direct consequence of the injury (other than an injury leading to his death), an additional amount in respect of such loss of earnings; and

3 where the applicant has lost earnings or earning capacity for longer than 28 weeks as a direct consequence of the injury (other than an injury leading to his death) or, if not normally employed, is incapacitated to a similar extent, an additional amount in respect of any special expenses, backdated to the date of injury.

In the case of fatal injuries, there are, similarly, three kinds of compensation: the standard amount, an additional amount for loss of dependency, and an additional amount for loss of a parent's services. Before turning to consider these categories in more detail, we should note first that, unlike the old Scheme (and the position at common law), the new Scheme imposes a total maximum amount payable in respect of the same injury of £500 000. This applies both to personal and to fatal injury applications. The Scheme also introduces further tariff limits where the victim suffers multiple injuries. In that event the victim will receive the full tariff award for the most serious injury, followed by 10% and then 5% of the tariff level for the second and third highest rated injuries. We deal first with the tariff award (the 'standard amount of compensation'), and then with the categories of additional amounts.

The tariff

The 1995 Act requires the tariff to show, in respect of each description of injury, the standard amount of compensation payable in respect of that description of injury. There are, as noted above, currently 310 such descriptions ranging in value over 25 levels of award from £1000 to £250 000, the maximum payable for any single injury. The examples given in Table 10.2 were all valued at £1000. The examples set out in Table 10.3 are, in each case, the complete set of descriptors for the category in question. They have been picked at random, to give a further indication of the manner in which the tariff is has been constructed.

It will be apparent that a victim's inclusion in any one of these descriptions will depend on the medical evaluation of the injury and its prognosis. This is of course no different from the position at common law, but in the case of the tariff the medical practitioner's evaluation assumes a categorical role, given that there is no scope within the Scheme for any modification of an award, once the victim's injury has been allocated to one of the descriptions. Many of the descriptions do make distinctions between injuries according to their impact on the victim (for example, whether the victim has made a full or a partial recovery from an injury to a limb, or whether an injury to the hand involves the thumb or the index finger: there are 65 different descriptions of injuries to the 'upper limbs'), but they do not permit many of the

Table 10.3 Examples of tariff descriptions of injury (brain, neck, shock)

Description of injury	Levels	Standard amount (£)
Brain damage: moderate impairment of social/intellectual functions	15	15 000
Brain damage: serious impairment of social/intellectual functions	20	40 000
Brain damage: permanent — extremely serious (no effective control of functions)	25	250 000
Neck: scarring: minor disfigurement	3	1 500
Neck: scarring: significant disfigurement	7	3 000
Neck: scarring: serious disfigurement	9	4 000
Shock		
Disabling, but temporary mental anxiety, medically verified	1	1 000
Disabling mental disorder, confirmed by psychiatric diagnosis:		
lasting up to 28 weeks	6	2 500
lasting over 28 weeks to one year	9	4 000
lasting over one year but not permanent	12	7 500
Permanently disabling mental disorder, confirmed by psychiatric prognosis:	17	20 000

standard factors applicable at common law (and which may figure in the making of a compensation order) to be taken into account. For example, 'significant disfigurement' caused by scarring of the neck will attract an award of £3000 whether the victim is young or old, male or female.

The Secretary of State has the power to add to, or to remove from, the tariff any description of injury, to increase or reduce the amount shown as the standard amount of compensation for any given injury, or to alter the tariff in such other way as he/she considers appropriate. In its consultation exercise conducted in 1999, the Home Office has indicated that a number of changes — both by way of addition to and deletion from — the current list will be made. These changes arise as a result of the first full year's work by the CICA. The changes include awards in respect of sexually transmitted diseases arising from sexual offences (Home Office, 1999; para. 33).

The position with regard to the death of the victim is too complex to be pursued here; in any event, homicide at a place of work is a rare occurrence. It is sufficient to note that where the victim died as a result of the criminal injury, a tariff award of £10 000 is payable where there is only one qualifying claimant, and where there is more than one, £5000 each. A 'qualifying claimant' means the victim's spouse or former spouse, parent or child (of any age), and a person who, though not formally married to the victim, had at the date of death being living with the victim as husband and wife for at least two years. The Scheme does not, at present, cater for homosexual partnerships, of whichever gender.[19]

Additional payments

There are two kinds of additional payment available under the Scheme where the victim survives the criminal injury. By the terms under which they become payable, they will only apply to more serious and to disabling injuries. As we have seen, the most serious case identified by the Home Office survey resulted in 2 months absence from work, considerably less than the 28-week minimum. The main rules for the payment of additional compensation for loss of earnings are that the injury must have been the direct cause of the applicant's loss of earnings or of earning capacity, and that the loss must have lasted for 28 full weeks. That period will normally run from the date of injury. Any payment made under this provision will commence from the 29th week. The 28-week period was chosen because it coincides with the period of time for which statutory sick pay is payable.

The rules governing the calculation of loss of earnings and earning capacity are complex. In essence, as the CICA puts it in its Guide to earnings and expenses (1996, para. 13):

> the calculation is based on a comparison of your earnings or other income before and after the injury. If there is a loss to you as a direct result of the injury, we take that figure and deduct from it any financial benefits you have received which also result from the injury.

---

[19] It may be noted that the single payment is more than the equivalent payable in a fatal accident action: £7500. The exact categories of 'qualifying claimant' are more detailed than I have described. See Miers 1997; para. 8.5.1.2.

In the standard case of an applicant in regular employment there will generally be little difficulty in calculating loss of earnings by reference to wage or salary slips. If the worker has a contract of employment, he or she is unlikely to lose any earnings, at least in the short term. Agency and bank nurses should make sure they keep an account of how much income they have lost while unable to work. Note that any social security benefits you receive will be taken into account when calculating your loss. There is also a maximum amount that can be awarded under this heading: it shall not exceed one-and-a-half times the gross average industrial earnings, as published by the Department for Education and Employment.

The second kind of additional compensation relates to loss or damage to certain kinds of property, costs associated with National Health Service and private health treatment, and costs associated with the applicant's long-term care. To qualify under any one of these headings, applicants must satisfy the 28-week time condition; that is, that at the date of the application they have either sustained or are likely to sustain 28 weeks' loss of earnings or of earning capacity, or, in the case of someone retired from work, has been or is likely to be incapacitated for more than 28 weeks. If the condition is met, compensation is payable for such expenses from the date of the injury, not just from the 29th week.

1 Compensation may be payable for loss of or damage to property or equipment belonging to the applicant which was relied on as a physical aid, where the loss or damage was a direct consequence of the injury. This includes such items as spectacles, dentures, hearing aids, and artificial limbs.

2 Private medical expenses are payable, but only where a claims officer considers that, in all the circumstances, both the private treatment and its cost are reasonable.

3 Compensation may be payable for long-term care. This can include special equipment, adaptations to accommodation or care, whether in a residential establishment or at home, where these are not provided or available free of charge from the National Health Service, local authorities or any other agency.

Where the victim dies as a result of the injury, there are, similarly, two kinds of additional compensation. The first may be payable to a qualifying claimant, where a claims officer is satisfied that the claimant was financially dependent on the deceased. Unlike additional compensation in cases where the victim survives the injury, the period of loss begins from the date of the deceased's death and continues for such a period as a claims officer may determine. Like other aspects of the Scheme, this can be a complex calculation. It begins with the assessment of the total net annual loss to the qualifying claimant. In a case where the deceased was the principal source of income, this will involve a determination of the victim's earnings and earnings prospects at the date of death. Where the deceased provided a secondary income, or was primarily responsible for looking after their domestic arrangements, including any children of the marriage, the claims officer will have to calculate the value of those latter services, in addition to the loss of the income. As in the case where the victim survives, the Scheme also requires that any income received by the applicant by way of pensions or social security benefits resulting from the death be taken into account. If there was no dependency, then no compensation is payable.

The second category concerns the loss of parental services. This is a novel legal provision, and one that is not conditional upon the claimant demonstrating financial dependence on the deceased. It extends to qualifying claimants under 18 years of age at the time of the parent's death, in cases where the claimant was dependent on the victim — mother or father — for parental services. The additional compensation comprises a payment for loss of that parent's services at an annual rate of level 5 of the Tariff (currently £2000), and such other payments as a claims officer considers reasonable to meet other resultant losses.

What you need to do

To obtain an application form write to:

Criminal Injuries Compensation Authority
Tay House
300 Bath Street
GLASGOW G2 4JR.

It is also possible that your local police station may have forms. If you have trouble filling them in, ask for help from your local branch of Victim Support, or write to them in London if there is no branch near you (see Appendix I for details).

Before you send your completed form, make a copy. Your claim will be dealt with initially by letter. The CICA's 'claims officer' dealing with your application will seek to verify what you have said by writing to the police, your employer, and those who have given you medical treatment. They may also write to you for clarification of matters raised by your claim. Do not be tempted to exaggerate your injuries; give as succinct and accurate an account of their impact as you can. You will in due course receive a letter giving the CICA's determination of your claim. You may accept it; but you also have the right to question it. There are two steps that you can take, in the following order. First, you may ask the CICA to conduct a 'review' of its decision in your case. This review is carried out by another, more senior, claims officer than the one who made the initial decision. If you are dissatisfied with that reviewed decision, you may appeal to the Criminal Injuries Compensation Appeal Panel. This body is wholly separate from the CICA. It decides some appeals solely on documentary evidence; in more serious cases there is an oral hearing. In this case, it may help if you can elicit the support of your union or professional body, or a solicitor (but not one who asks for a cut from any compensation you should be awarded!).

When the CICA first tells you its initial decision, it will send you details about reviews and appeals. Be careful! If you question a low award, you suspend any entitlement you would otherwise have to it; in other words, if on appeal the CICA thinks its original 'low' award was too high, it is free to reduce it further, and you will have no remedy. This Appeals Panel has a similar power. Consult a lawyer if you wish to question the CICA's decision.

Success rates

The CICA receives around 80 000 claims for compensation a year; just over a half are successful. Of those that are rejected, a third do not present injuries that qualify for the minimum award. It aims to issue its first decision in 90% of cases within 12 months of receipt of the claim. In 1998–99, it achieved a 82% success rate; a typical claim takes 11.7 months to reach a first decision (National Audit Office 2000, para. 4.3). You may well have to wait for some months, therefore, before you are told of the CICA's initial decision. The delay will be longer if your injury is medically complicated, or the prognosis unclear. There is provision within the Scheme to revisit a compensated injury, should your condition later deteriorate; but it is best to wait until you have a firm prognosis before applying.

Summary

1   If the injury you have sustained is fairly minor (as most are) — bruising; cuts requiring a few stitches; a broken tooth; wrist, neck, or shoulder sprain; or a small scar — and your offender is to be prosecuted for an offence that caused it, try for a compensation order.

2   If you do, make sure you fill in or get the police to fill in a Compensation Schedule. Keep a record of any costs, including loss of earnings, that you have incurred as a result of the injury. Keep copies.

3   Make a note of the name of the police officer who deals with your claim, and of his/her station phone number.

4   If you are not called as a prosecution witness, pester your local Crown Prosecution Service (make a note of their telephone number) to tell you the date of the trial. If your offender is convicted and is remanded for sentencing, pester the CPS to tell you when the sentencing hearing will be. That is when the question of compensation will arise.

5   Do not have great expectations of large sums by way of compensation. The average figure ordered by magistrates in 1997 for offences of wounding and occasioning actual bodily harm was £205. If your offender really is penniless, you probably will not get anything.

6   If your injury is complex, or its prognosis unclear, it is likely that the court will not make an order.

7   If the injury you have sustained involves at least scarring, a broken arm, leg, rib, jaw, or nose, or the loss of more than one tooth, you should certainly make a claim to the Criminal Injuries Compensation Authority.

8   If you do, you MUST *personally* report the incident to the police without delay.

9   Write to the Criminal Injuries Compensation Authority in Glasgow for a claim form. Keep a copy of the completed form that you return. Keep a record of any costs, including loss of earnings, that you have incurred as a result of the injury (but remember that there is no compensation for the first 28 weeks' loss of earnings). Also keep a note of any sick pay or other payments you receive in consequence of the injury.

10 Any compensation you receive from the offender by way of a compensation order will be deducted from the award. When the CICA notifies you of the award, you

are required to confirm that you will in turn pay over any such moneys you may receive.

11 The CICA will not reimburse any expenses that you incur in making your claim, whether or not it is successful.

12 Take legal advice before questioning the CICA's initial determination.

13 You will see that there are two groups of victims who are likely to fall between these two remedies:

(a) those victims whose offenders were convicted but against whom a compensation order was not made, or was made in an amount less than the value of the injuries they sustained, if those injuries are worth less than £1000; and

(b) those victims whose offenders were not convicted and whose injuries are worth less than £1000.

There is no practical hope for compensation in either case. The irony is that if a victim's offender is neither convicted nor worth pursuing through either the criminal or the civil courts, the health-care worker's best chance of compensation is if she or he is caused more harm than the minimum loss specified by the tariff Scheme.

14 If you need some practical help, get in touch with your local branch of Victim Support.

References

Bloomfield, K., Gibson, M., and Greer, D. (1999). *Report of the review of criminal injuries compensation in Northern Ireland.* A report to the Secretary of State for Northern Ireland.

Budd, T. (1999). *Violence at work: findings from the British crime survey.* Home Office Information and Publications Group, Research, Development and Statistics.

Burke, K. (1999). Staff demand protection after violent attack in A&E. *Nursing Standard,* **13**, (50), 4, (1 September 1999).

Criminal Injuries Compensation Authority (1996). *Guide to earnings and expenses.*

Criminal Injuries Compensation Authority (1999). *Third report: accounts for the year ended 31 March 1999.* House of Commons Paper HC 353 (March 2000).

Criminal Injuries Compensation Appeals Panel (1999). *Third report: accounts for the year ended 31 March 1999.* (March 2000). Cm 460 HMSO, London.

Editorial (1999). Violence: a worldwide epidemic. *Nursing Standard,* **13**, (52), 31, (15 September 1999).

Health and Safety Executive (1998). *Violence and aggression to staff in health services: guidance on assessment and management.*

Home Office (1988). *Guidelines on compensation in the criminal courts.* HO Circular No.85/1988.

Home Office (1993). *Compensation in the criminal courts.* HO Circular No.53/1993.

Home Office (1998). *Keeping victims informed of developments in their case.* HO Circular No.55/1998.

Home Office (1999a). *Victims of crime.* HO Communication Directorate 6/99.

Home Office (1999b). *Compensation for victims of violent crime: possible changes to the criminal injuries compensation scheme.*

Home Office (2000). *Criminal statistics, England and Wales 1998.* Cm 4649. HMSO, London.

Hough, M., and Mayhew, P. (1983). *The British Crime Survey.* Home Office Research Study 76. HMSO, London.

Maguire, M. (1982). *Burglary in a dwelling.* Heinemann, London.

Maguire, M., and Corbett, C. (1987). *The effects of crime and the work of Victim Support schemes.* Gower, Aldershot.

Miers, D. (1996). Liability for injuries caused by violent patients. *Journal of Personal Injury Litigation,* 314–323.

Miers, D. (1997). *State compensation for criminal injuries.* Blackstone Press, London.

National Audit Office (2000). *Compensating victims of violent crime.* House of Commons Paper HC 398 (14 April 2000).

Chapter 11

The future: the contribution of Accident and Emergency departments to community violence prevention

Jonathan Shepherd

Accident and Emergency departments (AEDs) interface not only with medical services but also with local communities. They have extensive opportunities to work with local public services, of which police services are most important in maintaining law and order and preventing violence. In the context of violence as an important health issue, this chapter summarizes work that demonstrates the substantial extent to which violence, including violence that results in AED treatment, is not reported to the police; states why reporting is important; lists the obstacles to reporting; and identifies strategies and practical ideas about how these might be overcome to the benefit both of communities and of victims. It is concerned primarily with violence in which adults are injured. In setting out directions for future research, it identifies the need for evaluations of interventions that focus on both injury outcomes and process outcomes so that the benefits of AED-police collaboration can be maximized.

Importance of violence as a health issue

The importance of violence as a health issue is now well-established. It is an important cause of death, and physical and psychological morbidity (Joy *et al.* 2000; Rivara *et al.* 1993; Shepherd and Farrington 1993). Even in countries like the UK, which have strict weapon control, violence affects health substantially, particularly in terms of the facial deformity caused by blunt trauma (Bisson *et al.* 1997; Shepherd 1990a). Leaving aside the injuries that violence produces, fear of crime can have a paralysing effect on communities and reduce quality of life for individual citizens. In turn, violence has been recognized as a public health problem, partly in the hope that, 'It would be better to reduce violence through the positive aim of promoting health rather than through the negative aims of retribution, deterrence and incapacitation' (Moore 1995; Shepherd and Farrington 1993). However, on their own, health, community safety, or criminal justice solutions to violence are not enough. There is now a consensus internationally that the key to community violence prevention is inter-agency co-ordination at the local level (Graham *et al.* 1998).

Health-criminal justice collaboration is important — not only at the operational level, but at the policy level as well. One of the most interesting recent developments in medicine is scrutiny of the impact of criminal laws by epidemiologists. It has been shown, for example, that accidental shooting deaths of children can be reduced by laws requiring gun-owners to keep firearms locked away (Cummings *et al.* 1997). An evaluation of state laws that restrict handgun purchase by persons with criminal records, has demonstrated decreases in violent offending by would-be purchasers who were denied handgun purchase (Wright *et al.* 1999). Targeted police work has been found to prevent alcohol-related violence in Australia by increasing deterrence (Homel *et al.* 1997). Studies like these suggest that law enforcement can produce changes in behaviour.

This health perspective of the criminal justice system is of great strategic importance. It provides a robust way of finding out whether criminal justice systems and criminal laws prevent violence, and has been influential in improving criminal justice responses to handgun violence, alcohol-impaired driving, domestic violence, and child abuse. Although it might be assumed that criminal laws are built on good evidence of effectiveness, few have been quantitatively evaluated using methods commonplace in medicine. The reasons for this include more reliance on qualitative approaches in legal and social sciences, and reliance on incomplete and unreliable police crime statistics as measures of violent offending (Shepherd *et al.* 1989).

Low police reporting rates for violence

Another important reason to develop health-criminal justice partnerships is that AEDs detect far more assaults in the community than are recorded by the police (Clarkson *et al.* 1994; Shepherd *et al.* 1989). Cross-referencing AED and police data concerning community violence has not been done systematically on a national basis, but studies in regional centres in the UK have shown that overall, only about 25–50% of offences that led to AED treatment appeared in police records (Clarkson *et al.* 1994; Shepherd *et al.* 1989). This proportion is consistent with the findings of biennial British Crime Surveys, which compare householders' accounts of crime with police records (Mirrlees-Black *et al.* 1998). In a UK study, assaults on men and assaults in bars, night-clubs and in the street, which resulted in AED treatment, were less likely to be recorded by the police than assaults on women and assaults in other locations (Shepherd *et al.* 1989). Differential rates of recording were also found according to time of day and day of week: this has obvious implications for the organization of community policing and law enforcement (Shepherd *et al.* 1989). In the US, low rates of police recording/investigation of intimate partner violence (IPV) has prompted legislation in some states to make reporting by health professionals compulsory (Cole and Flannigan 1999).

For firearm injury surveillance in the US, although systems are being developed, systematic study of the extent to which there is correspondence between AED and police recording has yet to be done (Kellermann and Bartolomeos 1998). A study of violence-related injuries treated in a sample of 31 US AEDs in 1994, found that rates of injury inflicted by intimates (current or former spouse, boyfriend, or girlfriend) were four times higher than rates from the National Crime Victimisation Survey (Rand and Strom 1997). Since the purpose of this study was to estimate the overall burdens that violence imposes on AEDs, and not primarily to compare AED with criminal justice data, the reasons for lack of police recording were not investigated. It was assumed, however, that such major differences could be put down to method-ologic factors. Encouragingly for any future measurement of violence using AED records, however, there was close correspondence between overall rates of intentional injury when compared to rates from the 1994 National Hospital Ambulatory Medical Care Survey (ACDC 1994).

Successive editions of the International Victimisation Survey have demonstrated that substantial numbers of violent offences are not included in official crime statis-tics. They have also revealed that there are differences in rates of victimization between countries (Mayhew and Van Dijk 1997). For example, the 1996 survey showed that rates of victimization were highest in England and Wales, US, Sweden, and Finland, and lowest in the Netherlands, Austria, and Northern Ireland. In the eleven industrialized countries that took part in the survey, median reporting rate of violent offences was 39% (range 18–51%) (Mayhew and Van Dijk 1997).

Although it might be thought that it is predominantly assaults causing minor injury that are not reported, two UK studies have found that police recording could not be predicted on the basis of injury-severity scores and that many assaults causing severe injury are not reported (Shepherd 1997a; Shepherd and Lisles 1998).

Reasons to increase reporting

If AEDs and law enforcement worked together to enhance reporting of crimes, this could deter potential offenders, provide the police with information about violence that is not available from any other source, and help repair the wider damage done to victims and communities including, potentially, through the effects of restorative/reparative justice.

There is now strong evidence that the police and the criminal process have a deterrent effect. International comparisons of police and crime survey measures of violence have demonstrated negative correlations between the chances of conviction and levels of violence (Farrington and Langan 1992; Farrington et al. 1994; Langan and Farrington 1998). In 1981, the assault rate in England and Wales, according to victim surveys, was slightly higher than in the US, but by 1995 it was more than double (Langan and Farrington 1998). The same trend is evident for other categories of violence. For murder, in 1985, rates in the US were 8.7 times that of England and Wales, but by 1991 the excess risk had narrowed to 5.7 times. Over the same period, the proportion of assaults reported to the police in the UK did not change significantly, but improvements in recording rates for violence in the US (63% recorded in 1981 to 93% in 1995) were far greater than those noted in England and Wales (37% in 1981 to 46% in 1995).

At the same time, there were obvious but opposite changes in rates of conviction for assault in the two countries (Langan and Farrington 1998). Between 1981 and 1995, conviction rates rose steeply in the US from 0.16 to 0.44/1000 population, but fell markedly in England and Wales from 1.12 to 0.61/1000 population. A recent study of the effectiveness of urban closed-circuit television surveillance in Wales produced evidence consistent with this: only negative relationships were found between levels of community violence measured in AEDs and levels according to police data (Sivarajasingam and Shepherd 1999).

A recent authoritative review of research on criminal deterrence concluded that there had been negative correlations between likelihood of conviction and crime rates studied over 10 years in England, the US, and Sweden, and over 15 years in England and the US (Von Hirsch *et al.* 1999). This is consistent with previous research. Statistical associations between the *severity* of punishment and crime rates are much weaker than associations between *certainty* of punishment and crime rates, and generally have not reached statistical significance (Von Hirsch *et al.* 1999). Although attempts have been made to control for influences on crime rates other than deterrence (Reilly and Witt 1996), the methods used have not been reliable enough to draw reliable conclusions (Von Hirsch *et al.* 1999).

The principal source of quasi-experimental studies of deterrence is research on drink-driving (Nagin 1998; Paternoster 1987). It has been concluded that, 'There is considerable evidence that increasing the actual certainty of punishment for drunk driving in ways that also ensure adequate publicity of certainty of consequences can effect reductions in drunk driving' (Ross 1992).

Overall, the published evidence indicates that when would-be offenders perceive substantial risk of punishment, many are deterred from offending (Von Hirsch *et al.* 1999). This suggests that, based on a sound ethical framework, an important objective for primary and secondary injury prevention should be increasing the chances of punishment of violent offenders. This fits with the traditional public health strategy of targeting the agent of injury, in this case the offender or potential offender. Although treating violence as a public health issue is not new (Moore 1995; Shepherd and Farrington 1993), formal collaboration between health and criminal justice services to maximize the chances of arresting and convicting violent offenders as a means of injury prevention, has yet to be developed. An obvious application of this approach, given the low rates of recording by the police of offences that result in AED treatment, is for AEDs to facilitate and encourage increased rates of police reporting by, or on behalf of, the injured.

The second main reason to improve reporting is that the circumstances of a great deal of community violence are not known to the police. Although it is often assumed that the police know about where injuries are sustained and which weapons have been used, this is often not the case (Shepherd *et al.* 1989; Shepherd 1997b). Just because police are often in AEDs does not mean that they record and investigate all, or even the majority of offences. Information that can easily be obtained by AED personnel from victims (Goodwin and Shepherd 2000) is therefore often not available to the police and may be of substantial importance in targeting police resources to prevent violence or to arrest offenders. Where victims do not want to report, this can be provided by AEDs in aggregate, non-confidential form. For example, since in the UK only about one in nine assaults in licensed premises that result in AED treatment are recorded by the police (Shepherd *et al.* 1989), information from AEDs can identify the bars and night clubs that are the focus for violence. Similarly, AEDs can provide unique information about the locations of work-related, school, and drug-related violence.

In the UK, this AED perspective has even led to the identification and modification of a previously unrecognized weapon category, bar glassware; in fact the most frequently used weapon in UK violence (Shepherd 1998). Beer glasses in the UK are now manufactured almost exclusively of toughened glass. A recent randomized controlled trial shows that increasing the impact-resistance of bar glasses, reduces risk of injury (Warburton and Shepherd 2000). If it had not been for AED-derived information, this advance would not have been made.

It seems obvious that violence prevention should take account of risk of injury as well as offences reported to the police, but this does not seem to have been appreciated. Furthermore, a zero-tolerance policy demands that attention is paid to minor, as well as life-threatening, injury.

Third, increased reporting may not just be good for the community but good for patients since assaults are not usually isolated incidents in the lives of either victims or assailants. About half of assault victims treated in the AED have been assaulted before and most violent offences are committed by a small proportion of offenders (Blumstein et al. 1988; Shepherd 1990b). In a Philadelphia cohort study, it was found that 6% of males (18% of all offenders) accounted for 52% of all arrests of juveniles. This was even more noticeable for violent offences: 6% of 'chronic offenders' accounted for 69% of all aggravated assaults, 71% of homicides, 73% of forcible rapes, and 82% of robberies. In London, similar results have been obtained: about 6% of males (17% of all offenders) accounted for about 50% of all convictions (Farrington 1983). In Sweden, offending is even more concentrated (Farrington and Wikstrom 1993). These data help to explain the high risk of repeat victimization: in a recent study in Kansas City of domestic homicide, a substantial proportion of victims were found to have attended local AEDs for treatment of injuries sustained in domestic violence previously (Wadman and Muellman 1999).

A collaborative approach also helps to safeguard the social rights of patients, particularly their right to privacy and to prompt recognition and consideration of their wider circumstances, expectations, and needs (European Forum for Victim Services 1998). Since having somewhere safe to live is essential to physical and psychological well-being, re-housing on a permanent or temporary basis, and increasing levels of security through, for example, lock or window replacement, is important. Links between health and victim-support services help to safeguard the dignity and social rehabilitation of the injured, as well as providing help and advice with claims for compensation.

Obstacles to reporting

Several barriers to reporting have been identified: these may be categorized as attitudinal, logistic, ethical, and legal.

Attitudinal obstacles to reporting

A study of police–AED interaction carried out in five AEDs in Wales, UK, showed that barriers to police reporting were, in decreasing order of importance, perceived to be:

patient confidentiality, maintaining a neutral stance in relation to issues of blame, and protecting the patient (Shepherd and Lisles 1998). On the other hand, reasons for reporting, in decreasing order of importance were perceived to be: reducing risk to others, severe injury, use of a weapon, and vulnerability of the injured.

The scepticism with which the proposal that AED physicians in the UK should be more proactive in reporting community violence to the police was met, illustrates some of the attitudinal obstacles to the adoption of a more co-ordinated interagency approach to tackling violence (Shepherd *et al.* 1995). It was argued that violence prevention should not be medicalized, since this would let official crime-prevention agencies off the hook and divert some of the blame for violence to doctors. Advocacy for victims was attacked as 'unacceptable medical paternalism' (Shepherd *et al.* 1995). Trends towards partnership between public services to solve the problem of offending make these objections seem less appropriate now than previously (Graham *et al.* 1998). In contrast, in one study, half of AED doctors, nurses, clinical and managerial staff believed that they should have a role in victim protection and support, the detection of crime, and community crime prevention (Shepherd and Lisles 1998).

Fewer obstacles have been identified in relation to attitudes of the police. In Wales, the police generally understood the ethical constraints on AED staff but wanted more violence to be reported. However, some police officers found it hard to come to terms with the reality of so much unreported violence and of the extra work this might provide (Shepherd and Lisles 1998). The need to prevent violence and protect patients and staff in AEDs, for example, by ensuring that weapons are not brought into AEDs, may divert police attention away from undetected community violence. The way the police respond to a report can influence whether an offence is recorded as well: the injured may be categorized as offenders, evidence may not be deemed to be sufficient, the victim may be unwilling to make a formal complaint, or the incident may be dismissed as a 'family' affair (Clarkson *et al.* 1994).

Victims' attitudes are also important, since the burden for supporting the prosecution process falls predominantly on them at every stage (Clarkson *et al.* 1994; Cretney *et al.* 1994), including in the AED (Shepherd and Lisles 1998). The injured often do not go to the police because they cannot identify their assailant, because they are marginalized as a result of alcohol- or substance-misuse, because they are habituated to violence or they are unwilling to have their own conduct scrutinized, they are fearful of reprisals or have an ongoing relationship with their assailant (Clarkson *et al.* 1994). In this context, it is not surprising that even cases of serious gun-violence can go unreported.

However, many patients expect that, once their medical needs are addressed, AED staff will report offences on their behalf or at least rapidly summon police help to allow them to report (Shepherd and Lisles 1998). Victims and those who accompany them are not just concerned about physical injuries, but about the identification, arrest, and prosecution of the offender, prompt notification of the police and prompt collection of evidence. Particularly at this early stage, patients often want justice, and look to AED staff to help them achieve this (Shepherd and Lisles 1998).

Logistic obstacles to reporting

In the AED, logistic obstacles to reporting include lack of facilities for patients to report, lack of a software facility to record basic information about the circumstances of violence, the often exclusive health agenda of AEDs and lack of links/interface between AEDs and other community services, such as the police (Goodwin and Shepherd 2000; Shepherd and Lisles 1998). Immediate availability of a police officer, police politeness and pre-existing professional relationships with police officers influence whether AED staff report offences (Shepherd and Lisles 1998). The following case study illustrates these obstacles.

Case study

A dazed 20-year-old man with an obvious facial laceration and accompanied by his girlfriend reported to an AED receptionist having been assaulted in a bar. Although he was incapable of speech through his injuries, his girlfriend kept making comments about wanting police involvement, between trying to control her tears and physically supporting her boyfriend. She told the receptionist, 'The police don't know yet', and when an ambulance driver passed the reception area she asked desperately, 'Is that a policeman?'. The receptionist ignored all these comments. Later, when the man was lying on an AED trolley, the girlfriend asked the male nurse who was swabbing his face, 'Can you take photographs in here?', his reply was, 'No . . . you had better take them tomorrow when all the swelling comes out'. The girlfriend then immediately stated that after the attack in the pub, 'I asked them to ring the police . . . it was completely unprovoked'. Later, when the receptionist was asked by a research worker why she hadn't said anything about the police she said that, 'If she asked me, I would have told her . . . we can't do anything. They have to tell the police themselves'. When the research worker pointed out that people who had been attacked might not be aware of this, she agreed that, 'If he hadn't been assaulted before he wouldn't know the procedure'. Similarly, when the research worker asked the nurse why he had not responded more positively about taking photographs, he replied, 'We haven't got time to take photographs and anyway, I wouldn't want to go to court, it's bad enough meeting patients in Tesco's [a supermarket]'. At the time, this male nurse appeared to have plenty of time: he was eating a curry in the staff rest room. He stated that, in relation to supporting victims, 'We are taught not to be judgmental' (Shepherd and Lisles 1998).

In one study, the bureaucracy associated with reporting serious offences to the police led to informal police 'tip-offs' (Shepherd and Lisles 1998). Interestingly, in this study, individual clinicians had far more experience of contacting police officers than individual police officers had dealing with AED staff: relative inexperience of AED work may therefore be a logistic obstacle for the police. Neither group, however, knew about the other's formal guidance/protocols.

Conversations with AED receptionists were often perfunctory and limited to the recording of demographic information, cause of injury, and previous AED visits. A potential logistic problem is the often protracted nature of AED treatment, which in the Wales study involved waits of up to five hours for the patients surveyed, in waiting areas, treatment cubicles, and on trolleys. These waits nearly always reflected how busy AED doctors were, but they do provide clear opportunities and time for other staff, particularly receptionists and nurses, to institute discussion of reporting and victim-support issues (Shepherd and Lisles 1998).

Overall, victims of assault make up about 2–5% of all new AED attenders (Shepherd 1990b), a proportion that may make violence seem a relatively minor problem, particularly in countries where firearm injuries are comparatively rare. Late at night, this proportion is very much higher but at this time senior staff, who are in a position to develop violence-prevention strategies with the police, may not be present (Shepherd and Lisles 1998). Although links between AEDs and other medical services are well-established, active partnerships between AEDs and non-medical public services are relatively undeveloped.

Ethical barriers to reporting

The sequence of events exemplified in the case study from Wales was noted time and time again during observation of AED staff–patient interaction: the injured and those who accompanied them repeatedly presented AED staff with obvious cues to liaise with the police but, usually under the guise of 'confidentiality', these were not acted upon (Shepherd and Lisles 1998).

Respecting the confidential nature of the doctor–patient relationship is of course of major importance and, apart from exceptional circumstances, it should be for patients to decide whether offences are reported. However, patients should be advised, in their medical interests and in the medical interests of others, to report offences if there seems to be a risk of future harm. Importantly, the interests of patients and the wider community do not usually conflict (Shepherd et al. 1995). 'Conflict' may arise, however, when the victim is a potential suspect. In the UK, doctors are advised to report offences, without the patients' consent if necessary, where it appears that not doing so may hinder the detection, investigation, or prevention of a serious crime (Shepherd and Lisles 1998). 'Confidentiality' can be an obstacle to responsible, ethical reporting if it is used by health professionals as a reason not to consider the needs of patients, communities, and the public services that serve them. Failure to consider these needs when treating a victim could of course, lead to protection of offenders from prosecution.

Of importance, however, is the possibility that unauthorized disclosure, and a closer relationship between AEDs and the criminal justice system, might deter some people from seeking the medical help they need. Whether knowledge that information may be disclosed actually stops people seeking treatment is open to question (Crisp 1990).

Legal obstacles to reporting

Few countries have laws designed to ensure the reporting of violent offences by health professionals, though some US states have legislation to ensure that domestic violence (DV) is reported (Cole and Flannigan 1999). The reasons for this include the sometimes fatal consequences of repeat violence and the threat that DV poses to families and children. In the UK, reporting is left to the discretion of doctors. So far, however, on both sides of the Atlantic, there has been little or no requirement for AED staff to collect the information on which rational judgements about reporting can be made. In contrast to adult violence, in most countries, the investigation of child abuse has been the subject of legislation to ensure an appropriate multi-agency approach. Surprisingly, although legislative steps that involve unauthorized disclosure of information have been taken to protect society from communicable disease, these have rarely been taken and enforced to protect society from violence, even though violence has become a leading cause of death, disfigurement, and disability.

The lack of a legal framework to ensure that doctors make appropriate decisions about the reporting and investigation of adult violence may be an obstacle to protecting patients and communities. From an injury-risk perspective, the focus in the US on legislation concerning responses to DV seems narrow. Very importantly, however, although legislation should protect the interests of citizens and communities, some police responses to DV can do more harm to victims than good (Dunford *et al.* 1992; Pate and Hamilton 1992; Sherman 1997).

From an international standpoint, there are obvious potential abuses of closer collaboration between AEDs and the police in countries with poor human rights records. For example, in 1944 in France, attempts by occupying forces to oblige doctors to identify wounded members of the resistance prompted the President of the Ordre National des Medicines to remind all French doctors of their duty to preserve confidentiality. The text of his telegram still prefaces the *Guide d'exercise professionel* (Ordre National des Medicins 1988).

In the UK, advocacy for a multi-agency approach that breaks down barriers between services resulted in the Crime and Disorder Act of 1998 (Crime and Disorder Act 1998; Shepherd 1996). This Act formally identified health authorities as partners with whom Local Government and the police must work to audit and tackle crime.

Ideas about how obstacles can be overcome

Ideas about how these obstacles to reporting can be overcome are considered under the categories listed above. It is clear from past research that some attitudes need to be changed. Education and training of AED personnel is needed to provide understanding of the wider needs of patients and the community in relation to the causes of assault injury, violence prevention, the reporting of offences, deterrence, and the criminal justice process. Since the objective is ethical collaboration with the police, joint training seems important. An essential foundation of this training should be clear guidelines on circumstances in which reporting of offences, without the patients' consent if necessary, is justified.

AED reception personnel who record details of offences using suitably adapted software (see Table 11.1) also need training (see Case study). Since this group have been shown to be in the best position to record information about the circumstances of violence and whether the assault has been reported to the police, training is necessary to enable them to do more than simply record administrative details (Goodwin and Shepherd 2000). Minor changes to the organization of AED reception areas to facilitate the recording of what may be sensitive information may also be required. For example, patients and those who accompany them need to be able to have confidential, one-to-one conversations with receptionists away from lines or queues.

Table 11.1 Intervention strategies

Strategies to increase rates of police reporting/investigation:

◆ free direct phone lines from AED waiting areas to the police;

◆ incorporation of AED waiting areas into police patrols;

◆ asking all assault patients on AED registration whether they would like assistance to report;

◆ reporting by AED staff on behalf of patients if they wish;

◆ mandatory reporting of serious violence.

Strategies to target community policing more effectively:

◆ computerized collection of core data by admitting AED staff on the circumstances of community violence, particularly in the home, licensed premises, schools, and poor neighbourhoods;

◆ regular disclosure to the police of non-confidential aggregate information about assault time/weapons/assailants/location.

Strategies to measure community violence/police performance:

◆ core violence data set designed for AED use (Goodwin and Shepherd 2000);

◆ inclusion of AED aggregate data in community audits of violence;

◆ publication of local, state and national AED-derived information about community violence.

Practical ways in which reporting in the AED can be facilitated and encouraged have been identified (see Table 11.1).

Since police crime statistics are known to be unreliable measures of community violence, assault-injury rates are also potentially invaluable measures of local, state, and national police performance, and of the effectiveness of community violence prevention initiatives (Shepherd 2000). The UK Government have recently taken up the proposal that AED-derived data should be used for this purpose (Shepherd 1996; Simmons 2000). Further legislation in this area should be based on evidence of what works (see below) and should facilitate a co-ordinated approach to protect all adults and ensure access for victims to effective social and mental health interventions. It must also ensure that all serious violence is reported.

Directions for future research

Although the strategies outlined in this chapter are rational in terms of assault injury prevention, it is vital that AED–police partnerships based on sound ethical principles are evaluated to find out whether they are effective. This is true both for existing and new partnerships. In particular, evaluations are needed of the practical ideas set out in Table 11.1, of the use the police make of AED-derived reports of offences and non-confidential aggregate information about the circumstances of offences, and of joint interventions to target community violence. Evaluations should be focused, not just on injury outcomes, but also on process outcomes that local communities can adopt to ensure efficient and effective service co-ordination. In relation to the measurement of community violence and of police performance according to incidence and severity of assault injury, harmonization of police, criminal justice, and injury data-sets is required. The effectiveness of laws mandating the reporting of DV and, in the UK, of laws that include the health sector in community crime prevention, also needs to be assessed.

Conclusion

Health professionals who treat victims of assaults should not assume that the police know about all or most violence. In all countries where comparisons of police and crime survey data are possible this has been shown not to be the case, even for serious offences. Contacts with the AED are opportunities to improve reporting, deterrence, and violence prevention, as well as treatment and social care. Whilst safeguarding the rights of both offenders and victims to treatment without fear of inappropriate disclosure, this is a rational step towards safer and more just communities in which the fear of crime is kept to a minimum.

Note: This chapter is based on an article by the author which first appeared in the Annals of Emergency Medicine (2001).

References

Blumstein, A., Cohen, J., Roth, J.A., and Visher, C.A. (1988). *Criminal careers and career criminals.* National Academy Press, Washington DC.

Centres for Disease Control (1994). *National Hospital Ambulatory Medical Care Survey (NHAMCS).* Atlanta CDC.

Clarkson, C., Cretney, A., Davis, G., and Shepherd, J.P. (1994). Assaults: the relationship between seriousness, criminalisation and punishment. *Criminal Law Review,* Jan, 4–21.

Cole, T.B., and Flanigan, A. (1999). What can we do about violence? *JAMA,* **282**, 481–3.

Cretney, A., Davis, G., Clarkson, C., and Shepherd, J.P. (1994). Criminal assault: the failure of the offence against society model. *British Journal of Criminology,* **34**, 15–29.

Crime and Disorder Act 1998 (1998). *Clause five: authorities responsible for strategies.* Her Majesty's Stationery Office, London.

Crisp, R. (1990). Autonomy, welfare and the treatment of AIDS. In *AIDS: a moral issue* (ed. B. Almond), pp. 68–91. Macmillan, London.

Cummings, P., Grossman, D.C., Rivara, F.P., and Koepsell, D. (1997). State gun safe storage laws and childhood mortality due to firearms. *JAMA,* **278**, 1084–6.

Dunford, F.W., Huizinga, D., and Elliot, D. (1992). The role of arrest in domestic assault. The Omaha Police Experiment. *Criminology,* **28**, 183–206.

European Forum for Victim Services (1998). The social rights of victims of crime. *European Forum for Victim Services.* Brussels.

Farrington, D.P. (1983). Offending from 10 to 25 years of age. In *Prospective studies of crime and delinquency* (ed. K.T. Van Dusen and S.A. Mednick) Kluwer, Nijhoff, Boston.

Farrington, D.P., and Langan, P.A. (1992). Changes in crime and punishment in England and America. *Justice Quarterly,* **9**, 5–46.

Farrington, D.P., and Wikstrom, P-O.H. (1993). Criminal careers in London and Stockholm. In *Cross-national and longitudinal research on human development and criminal behaviour* (ed. E. Weitekamp and H-J. Kernen Hewer, Dordrecht, Netherlands.

Farrington, D.P., Langan, P.A., and Wikstrom, P.O. (1994). Changes in crime and punishment in America, England and Sweden between the 1980s and the 1990s. *Studies in Crime Prevention*, **3**, 104–31.

Goodwin, V., and Shepherd, J.P. (2000). Evaluation of a questionnaire to facilitate the contribution of Accident and Emergency departments to Crime and Disorder Act local crime audits. *Journal of Accident and Emergency Medicine*, **17**; 196–198.

Graham, J., Ekblom, P., Pease, K., Hope, T., Jordan, P., Moxon, O. *et al.* (1998). *Reducing offending: an assessment of research evidence on ways of dealing with offending behaviour.* Home Office Research Study 187. London.

Homel, R., Hauritz, M., Wortley, A., McIlwain, G., and Carvolth, R. (1997). Preventing alcohol-related crime through community action: the surfers' paradise. In *Policing for prevention* (ed. R. Homel). Crime Prevention Studies 7. Criminal Justice Press, Monsey, New York.

Joy, D., Probert, R., Bisson, J.I., and Shepherd, J.P. (2000). Post-traumatic stress reactions after injury. *Journal of Trauma* **48**; 490–4.

Kellerman, A.L., and Bartolomeos, K.K. (1998). Firearm injury surveillance at the local level: from data to action. *American Journal of Preventive Medicine*, **15**(3S), 109–12.

Langan, P.A., and Farrington, D.P. (1998). Crime and justice in the United States and in England and Wales 1981–96. (NCJ 169284). US Department of Justice, Washington.

Mayhew, P., and Van Dijk, J.J.M. (1997). *Criminal victimisation in eleven industrialised countries. Key findings from the 1996 International Crime Victims Survey.* WODC Ministry of Justice, Amsterdam.

Mirrlees-Black, C., Budd, T., and Partridge, S. (1998). *British crime survey: England and Wales 1998).* Home Office, London.

Moore, M.H. (1995). Public health and criminal justice approaches to prevention. In *Building a safer society* (ed.) D.P. Farrington and M. Tonry, pp. 237–62. University of Chicago Press, Chicago.

Nagin, D. (1998). Criminal deterrence research at the outset of the twenty-first century. *Crime and Justice: a Review of Research*, **23**, 51–91.

Ordre National des Medicins (1988). *Guide D'Exercise Professionel.* Conseil National des Medecine, Paris.

Paternoster, R. (1987). The deterrent effect of the perceived certainty of punishment. *Justice Quarterly* **4**, 173–217.

Pate, A.M., and Hamilton, E.E. (1992). Formal and informal deterrents to domestic violence: the Dade County spouse assault experiment. *American Social Review*, **57**, 691–8.

Rand, M.R., and Strom, K. (1997). *Violence-related injuries treated in Hospital Emergency Departments.* US Department of Justice, Washington.

Reilly, B., and Witt, R. (1996). Crime, deterence and unemployment in England and Wales: an empirical analysis. *Bulletin of Economic Research*, **48**, 137–59.

Rivara, F.P., Shepherd, J.P., and Farrington, D.P. (1993). Gun laws. *Lancet*, **342**, 809–10.

Ross, H.L. (1992). *Confronting drunk driving.* Yale University Press, New Haven, Connecticut.

Shepherd, J.P. (1990a) Fear of crime. *Lancet* **335**, 796–7.

Shepherd, J.P. (1990b) Violent crime: an Accident and Emergency department perspective. *British Journal of Criminology*, **30**; 289–305.

Shepherd, J.P. (1996). The casualty criminals. *The Times, London*, 16 July.

Shepherd, J.P. (1997a). Violence: the relation between seriousness of injury and outcome in the criminal justice system. *Journal of Accident and Emergency Medicine*, **14**; 204–8.

Shepherd, J.P. (1977b). Violent crime: using the NHS to unmask the scale of the problem. *Policing Today*, **3**; 20–22.

Shepherd, J.P. (1998). The circumstances and prevention of bar-glass injury. *Addiction*, **93**; 5–7.

Shepherd, J.P. (2000). Cause for hope on crime statistics. *The Times, London*, 31 January.

Shepherd, J.P., and Farrington, D.P. Assault as a public health problem. *Journal of the Royal Society of Medicine*, **86**; 89–9.

Shepherd, J.P., and Lisles, C. (1998). Towards multi-agency violence prevention and victim support: an investigation of police–Accident and Emergency service liaison. *British Journal of Criminology*, **38**; 351–70.

Shepherd, J.P., Morley, R., Adshead, G., Gillett, G., and Knight, M.A. (1995). Ethical debate: should doctors be more proactive as advocates for victims of violence? *British Medical Journal*, **311**, 1617–21.

Shepherd, J.P., Shapland, M., and Scully, C. (1989). Recording of violent offences by the police: an accident and emergency department perspective. *Medicine, Science and the Law*, **29**; 251–7.

Sherman, L.W. (1997). Family based crime prevention. In *Preventing crime: what works, what doesn't, what's promising* (ed. L.W. Sherman, D. Gottredson, *et al.* pp. 4–9. NCJ165366, National Criminal Justice Reference Service, Rockville, MD.

Simmons, S. (2000). *Review of crime statistics: a discussion document*. Home Office, London.

Sivarajasingam, V., and Shepherd, J.P. (1999). Effectiveness of urban centre CCTV to prevent violence. *Journal of Accident and Emergency Medicine*, **16**, 255–7.

Von Hirsch, A., Bottoms, A.E., Burney, E., and Wikstrom, P-O. (1999). *Criminal deterrence and sentence severity: an analysis of recent research*. Hart Publishing, Oxford.

Wadman, M.C., and Muelleman R.L. (1999). Domestic violence homicides: AED use before victimization. *American Journal of Emergency Medicine*, **17**, 689–691.

Warburton, A.L., and Shepherd, J.P. (2000). Effectiveness of toughened glassware in terms of reducing injury in bars: a randomised controlled trial. *Injury Prevention*, **6**, 36–40.

Wright, M., Wintemute, G.J., and Rivara, F.P. (1999). Effectiveness of denial of handgun purchase to persons believed to be at high risk for firearm violence. *American Journal of Public Health*, **89**, 88–90.

Where to find help

Association of University Teachers (AUT)

Egmont House
25–31 Tavistock Place
LONDON
WC1H 9UT

Tel: 0207 670 9700
www.aut.org.uk

Provides legal and contractual advice.
Legal and stress helplines.

British Association of Dental Nurses (BADN)

11 Pharos Street
FLEETWOOD
Lancashire
SY7 6BG

Tel: 01253 778631
www.badn.org.uk

Provides emotional support through local co-ordinators. Advises on sources of legal aid (e.g. Citizens' Advise Bureau). Legal helpline. Advice sheet on dealing with aggression, bullying, and violence.

British Association of Occupational Therapists

(BAOT)
106–114 Borough High Street
LONDON
SE1 1LP

Tel: 0207 357 6480
www.cot.co.uk

Publishes guidelines on dealing with violent behaviour. Membership benefits include personal injury insurance. Advises on contractual and legal problems.

British Association of Social Workers (BASW)

16 Kent Street
BIRMINGHAM
B5 6RD

Tel: 0121 622 3911
www.basw.co.uk

Membership benefits include personal injury and clothing insurance. Encourages staff care and 'buddy' support services. Provides representation of members in discussions and negotiations with employers. Publishes book: *Dealing with violence and stress in social services.*

British Dental Association (BDA)

64 Wimpole Street
LONDON
W1M 8AL

Tel: 0207 935 0875
www.bda-dentistry.org.uk

Advises on loss of earnings, statutory sick pay and contractual and legal problems. Advises on security. Refers members to Medical Defence organizations. Publishes advice sheet on violence at work.

British Dental Hygienists Association (BDHA)

64 Wimpole Street
LONDON
W1M 8AL

Tel: 01934 876 389

Advises on sources of legal assistance.

British Dietetic Association (BDA)

5th Floor, Elizabeth House
22 Suffolk Street Queensway
BIRMINGHAM
B1 1LS

Tel: 0121 616 4900
www.bda.uk.co

Provides counselling from its Industrial Relations Officers. Gives legal advice from BDA solicitors and provides representation.

British Medical Association (BMA)

British Medical Association House
Tavistock Square
LONDON
WC1H 9JP

Tel: 0207 387 4499
www.bma.org.uk

Refers members to Regional Industrial Liaison Officers. Gives assistance with contractual and legal problems. Refers enquirers to Medical Defence organizations.

British Orthoptic Society (BOS)

Tavistock House North
Tavistock Square
LONDON
WC1H 9HX

Tel: 0207 387 7992
www.bos.org

Provides representation in discussions and disputes with employers.

British Psychological Society (BPS)

St Andrews House
48 Princess Road East
LEICESTER
LE1 7DR

Tel: 0116 254 9568
www.bps.org.uk

Makes grants from welfare fund in some cases. Advises on sources of legal help. See also under MSF. Refers psychologists with a role in education to either the National Union of Teachers or the Association of Educational Psychologists.

British Union of Social Work Employees

(BUSWE)
BUSWE House
208 Middleton Road
Crumpsall
MANCHESTER
M8 4NA

Tel: 0161 720 7727
www.buswe.fsnet.co.uk

Provides legal advice and representation in discussions with employers. Communicates with police on behalf of members. Publishes policy statement *Dealing with violence at work*. Presses employers to support prosecution of assailants in all cases.

Chartered Society of Physiotherapy (CSP)

14 Bedford Row
LONDON
WC1R 4ED

Tel: 0207 242 1941
www.asp.org.uk

Gives free legal advice and assistance from CSP solicitors. Provides information and representation in relation to all aspects of safety at work and compensation claims. Publishes briefing packs: *Violence at work, Bullying at work* and *Lone working*.

Royal College of Speech and Language Therapists (RCSLT)
7 Bath Place
Rivington Street
LONDON
EC2A 3DR

Tel: 0207 613 3855
www.reslt.org

Refers enquirers to the union MSF. Publishes guidelines on violence. Emphasizes that employers are responsible for training, prosecution, and management of violence.

Employing authorities (self-governing trusts and health authorities)

Community Services

As for hospital services, but free personal alarms are provided for all staff in some Trusts. Portable telephones provided for staff in high-risk areas. Advice available from Security Officers. Training courses on handling aggression and self-defence, and staff counsellors are provided by some authorities.

Hospital Services

Provide Nursing/Junior Medical Staff Counsellors and Occupational Health/Personnel/Legal Departments. Advise on criminal/police procedures. Formal guidelines on safety/management of aggressive patients available in some Trust/Health Authorities. NHS Executive have developed concept of 'Zero Tolerance Zones'.

British Chiropractic Association (BCA)
Blagrave House
17 Blagrave Street
READING
RG1 1QB

Tel: 0208 9505950

Membership benefits include legal advice.

British Osteopathic Association (BOA)
Langham House East
Mill Street
LUTON
Beds
LU1 2NA

Tel: 01582 488455
www.osteopathy.org

Provides legal advice. Legal 'helpline' services purchased by BOA. Arranges informal support for colleagues.

Community Practitioners and Health Visitors Association (CPHVA)

40 Bermondsey Street
LONDON
SE1 1UD

Tel: 020 79397000

Ensures that incidents are recorded by employers and/or at premises where assaults took place. Arranges contact with local HVA representatives. Publishes guidelines on *Bullying at work, Violence at work* and *Working alone*. Membership benefits include personal injury insurance. Gives legal/contractual advice. Local representatives advise employers. Provides professional and employment advice in conjunction with parent union, MSF.

Health and Safety Executive (HSE)

Rose Court
2 Southwark Bridge
LONDON
SE1 9HS

Tel: 02077 176000
www.hse.gov.uk

Produces annual statistics on *Accident, injury and ill-health.* Employers are required under 'Reporting of Injuries, Diseases and Dangerous Occurrences' (RIDDOR) regulations to report incidents resulting in more than 3 days' incapacity. HSE or District Councils advise employers on injury prevention through area offices. Publishes *Violence and aggression to staff in health services. Evidence on assessment and management.* Area officers work with employers to ensure that appropriate staff training in prevention is being given and also that services for victims (e.g. counselling services) are available. Advises staff to contact local HSE inspector (based in regional office) or HSE Information Line (08701 545500).

Institute of Biomedical Science (IBMS)

12 Coldbath Square
LONDON
EC1R 5HL

Tel: 020 77130214
www.ibms.org

Refers enquirers to employing authorities. Runs 'legal helpline'.

Manufacturing, Science and Finance (MSF)

MSF Centre
32–37 Moreland Street
LONDON
EC1V 8HA

Tel: 0207 5053000
www.msf.org.uk

Publishes booklet *Working alone* for community staff. Publishes booklets on the topics of bullying, violence at work and stress-related issues.

Medical Defence Union (MDU)

230 Blackfriars Road
LONDON
SE1 8PJ

Tel: 0207 4866181
www.the-mdu.com

Membership open to broad spectrum of health-care workers. Advises on harassment and threatening behaviour by patients and their relatives, CICA claims, civil claims, criminal procedures. Publishes booklet *Confidentiality*.

Medical Protection Society (MPS)

33 Cavendish Square
LONDON
W1M 0PS

Tel: 0171 6370541
www.mps.org.uk

Membership open to broad spectrum of health-care workers. Advises on CICA claims, civil claims, criminal procedures. Helps members take out injunctions such as restraining orders on stalkers and in relation to harassment. Cases dealt with individually.

National Pharmaceutical Association (NPA)

38–42 St Peters Street
ST ALBANS
AL1 3NP

Tel: 01727 832161
www.npa.co.uk

Provides legal advice. Monthly supplement circulated to all members, which includes features on violence and threatened violence. Advises on CICA claims. Dedicated insurance arrangements for pharmacists in respect of premises, contents, and hold-ups.

National Union of Students (NUS)

461 Holloway Road
LONDON
N7 6LJ

Tel: 0207 272 8900
www.nus.org.uk

Refers victims to student union welfare officers at many schools, colleges, and universities. Welfare officers refer victims to counsellors (salaried posts: most are psychologists). Liaises with college authorities, such as Deans. Arranges legal aid certificates and liaises with solicitors regarding civil/criminal proceedings. Publishes booklets on alcohol problems, drug problems, racism problems at work, drug rape, and environmental safety.

Royal College of Midwives (RCM)

15 Mansfield Street
LONDON
W1M 0BE

Tel: 0207 3123535
www.rcm.org

Liaises with employing authorities about escorts and drivers for community midwives and about other safety aspects. Membership benefits include personal injury insurance.

Royal College of Nursing (RCN)

20 Cavendish Square
LONDON
W1M 0AB

Tel: 0207 409 3333
www.rcn.org.uk

Refers enquirers to regional offices. Has 24-hour information and advice line: RCN Direct (0845 7726100). Helps with CICA applications and police investigations. Individual counselling by RCN stewards (personal support). Offers and provides dedicated counselling service (0845 7697064). Publishes leaflets on the management of violence, aggression, bullying, and harassment.

Royal Pharmaceutical Society of Great Britain (RPSGB)

1 Lambeth High Street
LONDON
SE1 7JN

Tel: 0207 7359141
www.rpsgb.org.uk

Makes grants from benevolent fund in some cases. Runs 'Birdsgrove House' (Convalescent Home). RPSGB Regional Inspectors advise on security issues. Runs pharmacists Health Support Scheme to help pharmacists who experience problems that may affect fitness to practise. Has 'Listening friend' scheme offering free confidential advice to pharmacists suffering from stress.

Social Care Association (SAC)

Thornton House
Hook Road
SURBITON
KT6 5AN

Tel: 020 83971411
www.socialcareassoc.com

Carries out continuous negotiations with local authorities, charities and private residential home and schools, particularly in relation to staffing levels. Membership benefits include personal injury cover. Advises and represents members (mostly care staff in residential homes) concerning 'good practice', which includes dealing with violent/aggressive behaviour. Provides 'legal helpline' and emotional support from local officers.

Society of Chiropodists and Podiatrists (SCP)

1 Fellmonger's Path
Tower Bridge Road
LONDON
SE1

Tel: 0207 4863381
www.scpod.org

Negotiates enhanced salary levels for staff working in high-risk areas (e.g. in psychiatric units). Gives legal advice. Publishes *Minimum conditions of service*. Refers enquirers to the Department of Health Publication: *Violence to staff.*

Society of Radiographers

207 Providence Square
Mill Street
LONDON
SE1 2EW

Tel: 0207 7407200
www.sor.org

Provides legal advice.

Trades Union Congress (TUC)

Congress House
23–8 Great Russell Street
LONDON
WC1B 3LS

Tel: 0207 6364030
www.tuc.org.uk

Publishes booklet *violence to staff.* Publishes book *Hazards at work.* Co ordinates and initiates Trade Union policy on prevention, rehabilitation and compensation. Provides training for Safety Representatives of Trade Unions. Runs 'Know your Rights' information line. 0870 6004882.

Transport and General Workers Union (TGWU)

Transport House
128 Theobald's Road
Holborn
WC1X 8TN

Tel: 0207 6112500
www.@tgwu.org.uk

Provides legal support and representation. Negotiates with employers at national and local level. Helps with compensation claims.

UNISON

1 Mabledon Place
LONDON
WC1H 9AJ

Tel: 0207 3882366
www.unison.org.uk

Provides representation at tribunals. Assigns an officer to deal with each case. Publishes leaflets on *Harassment at work, Bullying, Domestic Violence, Employee Rights.* Gives legal advice. Provides advice on health issues through local representatives to ensure that members receive appropriate support from their employer including, where applicable access to the NHS injury benefit scheme. In appropriate cases, UNISON will also pursue legal action against the employer eg. in cases of negligence to secure compensation. UNISON will also help members secure social security benefits or criminal injuries compensation. UNISON also has a welfare service. For more information contact UNISON DIRECT on 0850 5979750. Seeks to ensure that violence is prevented.

Other useful addresses and telephone numbers

Citizens' Advice Bureau

see your local telephone directory

Criminal Injuries Compensation Authority (CICA)

Tay House
300 Bath Street
GLASGOW
G2 4JR

Tel: 0141 3312726

Law Centre Federation (referral to local centres)

Duchess House
18–19 Warren Street
LONDON
W1P 5DB

Tel: 0207 3878570

London Women's Aid

52–54 Featherstone Street
LONDON
E1Y 8RT

Tel: 0207 3922092

Northern Ireland Women's Aid

129 University Street
BELFAST
BT7 1HP

Tel: 01232 249041/249358

24 hour helpline: 01232 331818

Rights of Women (free legal advice)

52–54 Featherston Street
LONDON
EC1Y 8RT
Tel: 0207 2516577

Scottish Women's Aid

12 Torphicen Street
EDINBURGH
EH3 8JQ
Tel: 0131 2258011

Victim Support

Cranmer House
39 Brixton Road
LONDON
SW9 62Z
Tel: 0171 7359166

Welsh Women's Aid

4 Pound Place
ABERYSTWYTH
SY23 1LX
Tel: 01970 612748

Welsh Women's Aid

38–48 Crwys Road
CARDIFF
CF2 4NN
Tel: 01745 334767

Welsh Women's Aid

2nd Floor,
26 Wellington Road
RHYL
LL18 1BN
Tel: 01745 334767

Women's Aid Federation England

PO Box 4411
BRISTOL
BS99 7WS
National Helpline No: 0345 023468
Admin office: 01179 444411

Zero Tolerance Campaign

25 Rutland Street
EDINBURGH
EH1 2AE
Tel: 0131 2282500

Index